MUSIC AND MEDICINE:

INTEGRATIVE MODELS IN THE TREATMENT OF PAIN

Edited by

John F. Mondanaro

Gabriel A. Sara

Satchnote Press

The Louis Armstrong Center for Music & Medicine

Beth Israel Medical Center

New York, NY

Music and Medicine: Integrative Models in the Treatment of Pain

Satchnote Press
The Louis Armstrong Center for Music & Medicine
Phillips Ambulatory Care Center
10 Union Square East, Suite 2M 2060
New York, NY 10003
www.musicandmedicine.org

© 2013 by Satchnote Press. Printed and bound in the United States of America. All rights reserved. No part of this book may be reproduced or transmitted in any form by any means, electronic or mechanical, including photocopying, recording, or by information storage or retrieval system—except by a reviewer who may quote brief passages in a review to be printed in a magazine, newspaper, or on the Web without permission in writing from the publisher. For information, please contact Satchnote Press, The Louis Armstrong Center for Music & Medicine, Phillips Ambulatory Care Center, 10 Union Square East, Suite 2M 2060, New York, NY 10003.

Although the authors and publisher have made every effort to ensure the accuracy and completeness of information contained in this book, we assume no responsibility for errors, inaccuracies, omissions, or any inconsistency herein. Any slights of people, places or organizations are unintentional. Readers should use their own judgment or consult a holistic medical expert or their personal physicians for specific applications to their individual problems.

First printing 2013

Cover graphic design by John and Maurita Mondanaro

ISBN 978-0-615-72942-8
For purposes of confidentiality,
the names of patients and other details appearing throughout this book
are fictitious.
The Publisher of this book is not responsible for the
information, opinions, conclusions or views expressed
by its contributing authors.

ATTENTION CORPORATIONS, UNIVERSITIES, COLLEGES, AND PROFESSIONAL ORGANIZATIONS: Quantity discounts are available on bulk purchases of this book for educational, gift purposes, or as premiums for increasing magazine subscriptions or renewals. Special books or book excerpts may also be created to fit specific needs.

Related Titles Available from The Louis Armstrong Center for Music & Medicine

Music Therapy and Pediatric Pain
Edited by Joanne V. Loewy
Jeffrey Books
ISBN 978-0-9801355-0-3

Music Therapy in the NICU
Edited by Joanne V. Loewy
Satchnote Press
ISBN 978-0-9801355-1-0

Caring for the Caregiver: The Use of Music and Music Therapy in Grief and Trauma
Edited by Joanne V. Loewy & Andrea Frisch-Hara
American Music Therapy Association
ISBN 1-884914-07-1

Music Therapy at the End of Life
Edited by Cheryl Dileo & Joanne V. Loewy
Jeffrey Books
ISBN 0977027805

Music, the Breath and Health: Advances in Integrative Music Therapy
Edited by Ronit Azoulay and Joanne V. Loewy
Satchnote Press
ISBN 978-0-9801355-2-7

Music Therapy & Trauma: Bridging Theory and Clinical Practice
Edited by Kristen Stewart
Satchnote Press
ISBN 978-0-9801355-3-4

Available at www.musicandmedicine.org

ACKNOWLEDGEMENTS

The Editors offer gratitude and appreciation to each author whose unique contribution to the worldwide movement toward integrative treatment philosophy has inspired the fine chapters included here.

From John Mondanaro:

I thank my wife Maurita and son Adrian for their continued love, support, inspiration, patience and nurturance throughout the process of bringing this book into fruition. I also wish to dedicate this book to my late parents, Joseph and Phyllis Mondanaro for parenting me with unconditional love. My heartfelt appreciation goes to my co-editor and colleague, Gabriel Sara for his unending warmth, gentle candor and belief in the power of music to heal, soothe, bridge and commune. I would like to extend a very special thanks to my mentor and friend Joanne Loewy for her steadfast support of my most authentic self on the path of professional development, and in her tireless dedication to the music therapy profession through quality clinical care, outreach, research and education. Many thanks to Barbara Hesser, Susan Feiner, Peter Jampel, Alla Braverman and the many other fine professors at New York University for the education I received under their watch. I would like to express my gratitude to Erika Leeuwenburgh for her guidance and generosity of spirit. Finally, I wish to extend special appreciation to Tsz-Hei Fatima Chan for her valued guidance and assistance in the assembly of these most precious pages.

From Gabriel Sara:

I thank my wife Nada and children Albert, Aline and Paul for their continuous love and support, and for believing with me that we all have the mission to make a difference in the World. I thank my parents who during my upbringing surrounded me with love and the beauty of music. Special thanks and immense appreciation to my co-editor and friend John Mondanaro who is the driving motivation behind this book. His relentless efforts, his generosity, his dedication and compassion have been a true inspiration. I wish to dedicate this book to my dear friend Fuad Sawaya and his late wife Helen for being the source of "The Helen Sawaya Fund". Toward this endeavor, I am especially thankful for my dear friend and colleague, Dr. Louis Harrison who gave me his unconditional support to create a philanthropy program and also introduced me to the Louis Armstrong Center for Music and Medicine and the extraordinary team of music therapists who everyday create an environment of beauty for our patients. I offer additional heartfelt thanks to Dr. Michael Grossbard and the staff at 11G and 9A at

Roosevelt Hospital who welcomed and embraced the Helen Sawaya Fund. Finally, I am eternally grateful to our donors with whose generous support we are able to offer Music Therapy to our patients.

From The Louis & Lucille Armstrong Music Therapy Program and The Louis Armstrong Center for Music and Medicine:

We offer many thanks to the late Phoebe Jacobs and the Louis Armstrong Educational Foundation for making this a Wonderful World and continuing to support the Louis Armstrong Center for Music & Medicine at Beth Israel Medical Center. We also thank the late Richard Netter and the estate of John Slade, and to all who make our research and clinical work a reality. We are grateful that our work is supported by Dr. Gabriel Sara, Dr. Louis Harrison, Dr. Peter McCann, Dr. Edward Conway, REMO, the Heather on Earth Music Foundation, The Florence Tyson Foundation, and the Louis Armstrong Educational Foundation.

The staff at the Louis Armstrong Center for Music & Medicine have been understanding, attentive and devoted to the writing of this book: AIR/CAIR Coordinator Bernardo Canga, NICU Coordinator Angela Thompson, Radiation Oncology Coordinator Andrew Rossetti, AIP coordinator Wen Chang, Administrative Assistant Marie Grippo, Research Scholar Erik Baumann Cornejo and Medical Director Dr. Stephan Quentzel, whose profound understanding of the effects of music and medicine is appreciated. Our team has made this dream a reality. Thank you for your generous and thoughtful support.

Thank you to Fran Silverman, Vai Fa'agata and Dr. Martin Arron for your supervision and support, and to Carol Rubiano, Gloria Morton, Jim Mandler and Kathy McGovern-Kearns for your attention to our programs. Thank you to Dr. David Bernard and Dr. Harris Nagler for honoring our vision. We thank Dr. Russell Portenoy, Terry Altilio, Dr. Pauline Lesage, Dr. Serefe Eti, Dr. Katherine Leonard, Dr. Madeline Gittleman, and the Pain and Palliative Care Fellows for their inspiring collaboration toward integrating music therapy and pain care. We are grateful to our patients, interns, and Fellow's who have shared their clinical work and experiences, and in doing so have taught us so much.

FOREWORD

Joanne V. Loewy DA, LCAT, MT-BC

Pain is a difficult topic. Unpleasant to assess, tricky to treat, and often uncomfortable to evaluate, the experience of pain can evoke feelings of anxiety, fear, and hopelessness for patients, caregivers and practitioners alike. Evaluation of pain can be particularly frustrating when the etiology is unknown and/or all prescribed options have been maximized and still, horrific discomfort, with accompanying anger or sadness escalate to threaten the threshold of what a human being can endure.

It is hard to believe that it has been 16 years since the first text of our department, (then a small 'program') *'Music Therapy and Pediatric Pain'* was published. Pain was one of the first focuses of our team and this initial Pediatric book still remains as one of our best sellers in its current sixth reprint! It is assuring to me that the topic is still one of obvious critical interest to music therapists, and even perhaps of greater assurance is the growing interest of our colleagues in their wanting to know how music can address painful crises. Pain is an area that doctors, nurses, social workers, child life specialists and pastoral care staff have frequently sought out to learn about, with a desired interest in extending knowledge of music interventions and expressed efforts to expand treatment opportunities. We have steady requests from colleagues who want to observe how we use music therapy to treat pain; and other inquiries about suggested music therapy articles and texts to read on the subject. Indeed, there is an eagerness, to question, to learn, and to build strategies of how we might better treat pain.

Our team has grown a specialty in our efforts to better assess and provide best-practice applications of clinically applied live music to treat pain. We have addressed pain of all kinds in patients of varying ages and diagnoses-whether the episode is acute, chronic or procedural. We have studied the use of live music as a sedative, as an analgesic, and as a source of resilience to combat physical symptoms and their associated physiological effects. We have a protocol for implementing remedies inclusive of gonging and vibration to enhance blood flow. We initiate toning in an effort to integrate and balance one side of the body with the other, increasing a patient's capacity to rectify the cycle of expectancy that can frequently impair the ability to heal. Release-oriented techniques such as drumming are not uncommon options for the patient experiencing acute pain. We have built our foundation through the careful concurrent study of pain through actual patient care, weekly attendance at pain rounds, where we learn from our colleagues and patient-cases. We have upheld our knowledge of the guidelines set forth by the International Association for the Study of Pain (IASP). Understanding of the region of the body in pain, the actual system of dysfunction that is causing the pain, its duration, timing and patterns, as well as its intensity and source are as critical to assess as they are to treat. To further understand how pain is medically classified, as inflammatory, nociceptive, inflammatory; or pathological, or as a result of an irritation or dysfunctional has only helped our capability to treat it more astutely.

The current text is a mature expression of such understanding and growth in pain management, and is so clearly representative of the clinical diversity reflected in the cutting-edge music and pain work that the Editors have invited for inclusion in this wonderful book. How timely that two great master minds, John Mondanaro, and Gabriel Sara, music therapist and doctor have stepped into an integrative forum to weave together and edit this masterpiece. Each chapter is a jewel exemplifying a unique and diverse pain orientation or practice. The authors are representative of a variety of hospitals and universities situated within a broad array of departments, with each holding its own, distinct orientation.

The flavor of this book is fragrant and clearly reaps the knowledge, sensitivity and forward -thinking attitudes of its two brilliant and humble editors. I am aware of the frequent gatherings and deep thinking that went into the hours of editing and careful steering that John and Gabriel, the co-editors provided to each of the authors.

It is clear that the editors' hands are in the treatment of pain, and their direct, day-to-day care for human beings is apparent as evidenced by the passion they bring to this book. At the same time, within their writing and editing, they share their deep thinking and knowledge, with an evident and unique understanding of the pain experience. For this I am grateful. How fortunate we are to have this new and diverse text. I know it will be a strong addition to the music therapy and music medicine literature base for years to come.

Joanne Loewy, April 13, 2013

PREFACE

Gabriel A. Sara MD

On a cold November day, the early snowfall has delivered New York and its tenants into a sense of frenetic energy that infiltrates the windows and doors of the hospital. Disgruntled exchanges of greeting seem to melt away as I hear the gentle rolling of Bossa Nova drifting down the corridor from the Infusion Suite. Turning the corner into the space, the cold outside is all but forgotten as I see one of my regular patients playing the bongos with the music therapist. Music's power to transform and transport is again at work.

My contemplation of the preface I would write for this book became a journey of deep introspection as I reflected on the relationship I have had with music throughout my life. The innocence of my childhood, full of memories of singing with my parents during long car rides, laid the foundation for my experience as a medical intern serving in the Red Cross during the Lebanese War of the 1970s. Music seemed to anchor my military buddies and I into something real and unscathed by the war, even as our senses remained on hyper-alert through the barrage of constant civilian bombings of our homeland. It was here that my guitar provided auditory and psychological respite from the reality of war. In our shelter, surrounded by the sound of ricocheting bullets and echoing bombings, we existed in a perpetual state of not knowing whether we would survive, or of what we would find in the light of day. Sharing a human need for connection and affirmation of life's value and meaning, it was music that allowed us to persevere. In retrospect, I think that some of our comfort derived from creating music with harbored notions of generating our own version of Woodstock, and perhaps even flipping our fingers at the perpetrators of war, not unlike our American brothers 4000 miles away.

Since those years in Lebanon, I have honed my practice as a physician treating individuals journeying through the atrocity of cancer. Through my practice, I have been reminded time and time again that like the ravages of war, the diagnosis and treatment of cancer often strikes with the voraciousness of rape, forcing individuals onto a journey of sudden and unexpected reconciliation with life's meaning.

One such journey was that of my friends Helen and Fuad Sawaya. Helen's diagnosis of breast cancer was as close to home for me as the bombings and profound losses of friends, home, and culture I'd endured in Lebanon thirty-some years earlier. Helen traveled her road with dignity and a profound sense of what it meant to participate in life fully to the very end. It was Fuad's love for Helen that rendered the Helen Sawaya Fund, which in

Helen's memory endows many individuals living with cancer to inspirit their diagnosis and treatment with the same dignity with which Helen enlivened her own.

My work with Fuad to create this program led me to Dr. Joanne Loewy and the Louis Armstrong Center for Music and Medicine. Music therapy connecting body, mind, and spirit stands among various other offerings to patients including therapeutic art, healing touch, the unconditional love of animals through a pet therapy program, services focusing on beauty and cosmetic support, and opportunities for travel. On any given day, I can walk through the Infusion Suite and hear the transporting sounds of live music being rendered by a music therapist. Following my ears, I enjoy visible testament to the richness of the human connection and therapeutic relationship that ensues from the offering of music therapy. Be it Bossa Nova or the sounds of Motown, music again provides recluse from a seeming battlefield experienced by so many patients living with cancer.

When Clinical Director, John Mondanaro invited me to co-present with him on the importance of individualizing the medical treatment of pain through music therapy, at a symposium he was chairing for the Louis Armstrong Center for Music an Medicine, I was genuinely please to do so. My acceptance of his subsequent invitation to join in the editing of a forthcoming text, which you now hold in your hands, was equally gratifying.

The book stands as a testament to the Louis Armstrong Center's dedication to integration as a means to enriching patient care. Such conviction, depth of knowledge, and dedication is embedded in the working philosophy of the Louis Armstrong Center to which I bear daily witness.

It is an honor working with such esteemed individuals as the music therapists who have served our patients and families, and it was an additional privilege reading the written testament of the integrative work being done by so many others, from fellow physicians and psychologists to the host of music therapists represented on the following pages. Enjoy.

Gabriel Sara, April 14, 2013

TABLE OF CONTENTS

Foreword	Joanne V. Loewy DA, LCAT, MT–BC	vii
Preface	Gabriel A. Sara MD	ix
Introduction	John F. Mondanaro MA, LCAT, MT-BC, CCLS	1

Section I: Foundations — 9

Chapter 1:	Music Has Charms To Soothe A Savage Beast: An Integrative Medical-Psychiatric Perspective on Pain and Music *Stephan J. Quentzel MD, JD, MA*	11
Chapter 2:	Thirty-five Years Use of Anxiolytic Music (AAM) in Pain and Aversive Clinical Settings *Ralph Spingte MD*	29
Chapter 3:	Music Therapy for Pain Management *Suzanne B. Hanser EdD, MT-BC* *Susan E. Mandel PhD, MT-BC*	43
Chapter 4:	Ethical and Cultural Issues in Music Therapy for Pain Management *Cheryl Dileo PhD, MT-BC*	51
Chapter 5:	Measures of Pain Management and Patient Satisfaction as Core Factors in the Development of Medical Music Therapy Programming at Norton Healthcare *Jenny Branson BA, MT-BC*	59

Section II: Specific Treatment Approaches — 77

Chapter 6:	Music Therapy Improvisation and Reflection for Pain Relief with Hospitalized Adults *Paul Nolan MCAT, LPC, MT-BC*	79
Chapter 7:	Music Sedation and Pain *Joanne V. Loewy DA, LCAT, MT-BC*	95
Chapter 8:	Finding Relief from Pain through the Use of Music: A Gestalt Therapy Approach *Frank Bosco MA, MT-BC, LMT, RPP, SEP, LCAT*	115

Chapter 9:	Music Therapy Based Release Strategies for Acute and Chronic Pain: An Individualized Approach *John Mondanaro MA, LCAT, MT-BC, CCLS*	133
Chapter 10:	Analytical Music Therapy for Pain Management and Reinforcement of Self-Directed Neuroplasticity in Patients Recovering from Medical Trauma *Benedikte B. Scheiby MA, MMEd, DPMT, CMT, AMT, LCAT*	149
Chapter 11:	Backed into a Corner: The Use of Guided Imagery and Music in the Care of a Woman with Chronic Pain *Nancy A. Jackson PhD, MT-BC*	181
Chapter 12:	The Listening Room *Trisha Ready PhD*	193
Chapter 13:	Improvisational Singing: A Nordoff-Robbins Based Vocal Music Therapy Intervention in the Treatment of Pain *Melanie May Po Acosta, MA, LCAT, MT-BC, NRMT*	215
Chapter 14:	A Symphony of Life: Harvesting Emotions by Preserving Legacy and Honoring Pain *Brian H. Schreck MA, MT-BC*	237
Chapter 15:	Audio-Communication: An Integrative Approach to Pain Treatment with Music Therapy *Iris Valentin BM*	253
Chapter 16:	Environmental Music Therapy: Rationale for 'Multi-Individual' Music Psychotherapy in Modulation of the Pain Experience *Andrew Rossetti MMT, MT-BC* *Bernardo Canga MMT*	275

Section III: Specific Populations — 295

Chapter 17:	Pathophysiology of Pain and Stress: Music Therapy Implications for Perinatal, Perioperative, and Chronic Pain Patients *Fred J. Schwartz MD*	297

Table of Contents   xiii

Chapter 18:	Music Therapy for Pain and Stress in NICU Infants: A Developmental, Trauma-Informed and Family-Centered Approach *Angela Thompson MA, MT-BC*	309
Chapter 19:	"Hear My Song": Giving Voice to Adolescents with Sickle Cell Disease *Maya Charlton MA, MT-BC*	335
Chapter 20:	GIM: Deprivation and its Contribution to Pain in Eating Disorders *Annie Heiderscheit PhD, MT-BC, LMFT*	347
Chapter 21:	Music Therapy and HIV/AIDS Related Pain *John Mondanaro MA, LCAT, MT-BC, CCLS* *Christine Vaskas MS, MT-BC*	373
Chapter 22:	Music-Mediated Strategies for the Integrative Management of Pain in End of Life Care *Robert E. Krout EdD, MT-BC*	403

Section IV: Multicultural Perspectives   419

Chapter 23:	Culturally Informed Music Psychotherapy: Using Latin American Music and Repertoire in the Treatment of Pain and Anxiety Experienced by Individuals Receiving Chemotherapy *Jillian Hicks MA, MT-BC* *Erik Bauman Cornejo MMT* *Natalia Garrido MMT*	421
Chapter 24:	Confronting a Different Great Wall: Using Environmental Music Therapy to Provide Psychoemotional Support for Asian and Asian-American Patients in a Radiation Oncology Waiting Room *Thomas J. Biglin, Jr. MA, MT-BC* *Yi-Ying Lin MA, MT-BC*	451
Chapter 25:	Journeying through Cultures: Personal Explorations of Indian and Persian Music Traditions in Music Therapy Practice *Soniya K. Brar MA, MM, MT- BC* *Oksana Rosenblum MA*	473

Contributors	501
Index	513

INTRODUCTION

John F. Mondanaro MA, LCAT, MT-BC, CCLS

Pain and suffering have been inextricably connected and integral to the human experience since the beginning of recorded history. The early Greeks inspired their world with the myth of Pandora's box in which Pandora, unleashed pain and suffering among other afflictions upon the world from a box, when her curiosity prevailed.[1] Hope, remained in the box, signifying that no matter how dire the circumstances, she would be at mans' side. Almost 3000 years later, Oscar Wilde spoke of pain with the same reference to bleakness, "Behind Joy and Laughter there may be a temperament, coarse, hard, and callous. But behind Sorrow there is always Sorrow. Pain unlike pleasure, wears no mask".[2(p 99)] In neither reference is the experience of physical pain differentiated from emotional pain, leaving us to presume that the complexity of pain is like a tapestry woven of the many threads that make up the experience of being human.

Our reconciliation with pain as an expected component to the human experience has remained a venerable point of query across healthcare domains. Driven in recent decades by a heightening social awareness and acceptance of not only the universal immanence of pain, but of our entitlement to live without it, and the suffering it causes,[3] the existing paradigm of healthcare has continued to evolve. The acceptance and integration of nonpharmacologic therapies and modalities has gained momentum in the last thirty years with emphasis being placed on pain care that integrates pain control within a broader context focusing on the patient's overall quality of life [4].

This growing trend is visible even in the terminology used within hospital settings and clinics. Sixteen years ago, with the publication of our book, *Music Therapy and Pediatric Pain*, there was excitement that such therapies and practices referred to as alternative in the 1980s had been elevated to the status of complementary.[5] The days of acceptance of such therapies, but kept at a safe distance, had given way to treatment informed by an appreciation that these complimentary modalities could offer benefits alongside mainstream treatment. In this millennium, we have seen an even greater shift to a treatment philosophy defined as "integrative", in which nonpharmacologic therapies are being recommended as integrated aspects of interdisciplinary treatment planning. Specific to this book, the therapeutic benefits ascribed to many non-pharmacologic modalities and mind-body practices such as relaxation, imagery, meditation, release strategies, and cognitive skill training, are subsets of the scope of music therapy practice.

Music and Medicine: Integrative Models in the Treatment of Pain

Moving further into the spirit of true integrative, interdisciplinary care, music therapy with "its growing evidence base and widespread acceptance suggests that it too would be better classified as a conventional treatment with wide potential use".[4] Such enlightened thought seems to be heralding in an exciting paradigm of healthcare.

In the early part of 2011, Dr. Joanne Loewy announced to her team at the Louis & Lucille Armstrong Music Therapy Program, that with a gap of fifteen years since the First Symposium on Music Therapy and Pediatric Pain held at Beth Israel in 1997, the time was upon us to again provide such a colloquium that would give forum, and therefore testament to the growing body of work in the area of pain. That such a colloquium in 2012 would bring together a range of disciplines forging innovative practice and treatment approaches in pain medicine was clear to everyone. On January 30th and 31st, 2012, the symposium "Music and Medicine: Integrative Models in Pain Medicine", was hosted by the Louis Armstrong Center for Music and Medicine. True to our hopes and expectations, the gathering enticed rich participation of both presenters and attendees across a range of disciplines including doctors, nurses, social workers, psychologists, music therapists, contemplative and pastoral care workers, creative arts therapists, child life specialists, and educators.

Such was the context in which this book was planned and implemented into fruition. Even during the planning dialogues with my Director, colleague and friend Dr. Joanne Loewy, there was agreement that such an integrative book would benefit from the direct medical expertise of a physician whose philosophy was congruous with our own. My contemplation about with whom I would want to partner was brief, as I acted upon an already felt affinity for my esteemed colleague and friend Dr. Gabriel Sara. Dr. Sara's unhesitating "yes" was affirmation enough to proceed into what Joanne and I have laughingly referred to as giving birth to a baby. While I would never presume to know the experience of motherhood from conception to postpartum, I kind of think I may have more of a sense of it than ever before! Every juncture and aspect of bringing this book into fruition has been a personal experience of my own integration of body, mind, and spirit.

Love, a sense of beauty, and a mammoth dose of hyper vigilance, together became the driving force behind organizing such richly vast material into a book that could boast order and sensibility. The preservation of each contributing author's voice remained central to this process, as delivering a text as rich and diverse as the work itself was of cardinal intention. To this end, I have organized the chapters into four sections according to prevalent themes: Section I, "Foundations", Section II, "Specific Treatment Approaches", Section III, "Specific Populations", and finally Section IV, "Multicultural Perspectives". Each section has been organized

Introduction

sequentially as well so as to provide a foundation of understanding within each broad theme.

Section I: Foundations
The first section of the book establishes a foundation of understanding of music as an integrative treatment for pain.

In Chapter 1, Stephan J. Quentzel discusses pain medicine from an integrated medical-psychiatric perspective. Stephan's attention to medical and psychosocial assessment as precursory to effective and successful treatment and care management brings critical awareness not only to the value of therapeutic alliance but also to the necessity of patient conviction in optimizing treatment efficacy and outcomes.

In Chapter 2, Ralph Spingte delivers a review of research and literature spanning the use of music and music therapy as anxiolytic treatment of symptoms. The rich and comprehensive history provided, offers insight into how a dialogue thousands of years old has been reignited in such recent history, to the increased awareness and integration of music in medical care.

In Chapter 3, Suzanne B. Hanser and Susan E. Mandel lend clinical insight, up close and personal. Their descriptions of music therapy in the treatment of pain span a myriad of life circumstances, from chronic pain to acute surgical pain, and from childbirth to end of life. The authors' candor in this chapter exemplifies the nuance of human dynamics that raise therapeutic relationship to the pinnacle of consideration when discussing music therapy.

In Chapter 4, Cheryl Dileo introduces ethical and cultural considerations in the treatment of pain, bringing justified focus to the importance of patient autonomy and vulnerability as central themes in the work. The therapist's observance of beneficence and sensitivity is underscored as an ethical obligation to seek continued education toward best practice in music therapy, and clinical supervision toward continued self-awareness necessary to render competent and effective care.

In Chapter 5, Jenny Branson discusses the importance of pain scores and patient satisfaction in program building. Jenny's discussion of the chronological steps to building a program through continued outreach and education as to the efficacy of music therapy, reminds us that central to the use of music therapy in medical treatment, are the individual patients themselves.

Section II: Specific Treatment Approaches
Section II offers the reader entry into understanding the implementation of music and music therapy across a range of approaches and modalities.

Music and Medicine: Integrative Models in the Treatment of Pain

In Chapter 6, Paul Nolan discusses an approach to pain treatment that synthesizes verbal and nonverbal process through music improvisation and reflection respectively. His work again places the patient at the center of the care by bringing emphasis to the individual's existing strengths as opposed to deficits caused by the pain itself.

In Chapter 7, Joanne V. Loewy expounds upon her efficacious work with Music Sedation,[6] by highlighting its varied application in several case vignettes. Joanne's warmth and conviction to providing culturally competent care across a range of patient ages and diagnoses, sets a standard for effective integration of music therapy through the therapist's adherence to skilled assessment and interdisciplinary collaboration.

In Chapter 8, Frank Bosco describes his work with individuals experiencing pain through an approach informed by Gestalt Therapy. Here the individual learns to contextualize pain within the entire landscape of the self through the use of music and sound. Frank's individualized work addresses pain as an entity that can be better managed as an integrated experience, than as a compartmentalized one.

In Chapter 9, John F. Mondanaro illustrates the use of music therapy assisted strategies for the release of tension associated with acute and chronic pain. His work, informed from a Family-Centered perspective, again brings emphasis to individualized treatment, as presented in several clinical scenarios.

In Chapter 10, Benedikte B. Scheiby discusses the application of Analytical Music Therapy with individuals experiencing pain from medical trauma. Her rich presentation of an individual case introduces the idea of emotional healing and self-directed neuroplasticity through the use of improvisational songwriting within the safety of the therapeutic relationship.

In Chapter 11, Nancy A. Jackson provides a rich and moving profile of her work with a woman suffering from chronic pain. Nancy uses music, guided imagery, and the therapeutic relationship to empower this woman in her liberation from immobilizing thought processes toward the reclaiming of autonomy and quality of life.

In Chapter 12, Trisha Ready describes her work as a psychologist using recorded music, and the meaning of song as both an entry point and as an ongoing treatment modality with patients suffering from mental illness. Within "The Listening Room", Trisha looks at attunement with patients through their preferred song or music, and the therapeutic value of momentary recluse from their emotional pain, afforded by the experience of listening to a favorite song with a professional.

In Chapter 13, Melanie May Po Acosta shares her experience as a Nordoff Robbins trained therapist, using voice as a primary instrument in the therapy process. She deconstructs her vocal techniques and interventions

Introduction

with a pediatric patient experiencing pain, bringing into full scope for the reader, the therapeutic possibilities of connecting with the human voice.

In Chapter 14, Brian Schreck illustrates an approach to the individual's experience with illness and pain that is beautifully humanistic. His emphasis on the importance of honoring and sharing legacy further reinforces an understanding of the emotional catharsis that can occur within the safety and trust of a therapeutic relationship.

In Chapter 15, Iris Valentin defines "Audio-Communication", her integrative music therapy model initially created to address the pain and discomfort of those living with tinnitus. Over a period of twenty-five years while Iris lived and worked in Germany, she adapted the work to those living with cancer pain as well.

In Chapter 16, Andrew Rossetti and Bernardo Canga discuss the concept of Environmental Music Therapy in terms of its theoretical underpinnings, and its potential effects in modulating the perception of pain across medical milieus, particularly high stress areas like the ICUs and outpatient radiation and chemotherapy waiting areas.

Section III: Specific Populations

Section III offers the reader direct portal into the experience of pain within the context of specific diagnoses. As in Section II, music and music therapy approaches will be discussed but through the psychosocial lens of a given diagnosis.

In Chapter 17, Fred J. Schwartz looks at the relationship of emotional and physiologic responses to stress and pain, and their impact on physiologic pathology in the context of perinatal, perioperative, and chronic pain. Fred discusses and contrasts the clinical impact of music and music therapy with pharmacologic intervention on the autonomic nervous system's role in pain modulation, laying foundation for Chapter 18.

In Chapter 18, Angela Thompson moves us into the NICU, providing insight into the pain experience of neonates and caregivers from various theoretical perspectives. Her moving clinical vignettes offer unique perspective on the multidimensional role of the music therapist working in this fragile environment.

In Chapter 19, Maya Charlton identifies fragility of a different sort as she defines the psychosocial reality of adolescents living with Sickle Cell Disease. The extremes of physical and emotional responses to the pain of Sickle Cell crisis are given context and aesthetic meaning through songwriting and therapeutic relationship.

In Chapter 20, Annie Heiderscheidt takes us back into to GIM, but this time as a forum of support and process for individuals living with profound eating disorders. Deprivation as a contributing factor to pain is discussed in the context of a growing population of those living with Anorexia and Bulimia.

In Chapter 21, John F. Mondanaro and Christine Vaskas deliver a chapter that addresses the residual and continuous impact of HIV and AIDS over thirty years since the first documented case. Music therapy as a forum for both individual and group support is discussed in the context of a disease that carries emotional and social legacy into new generations of those infected by the disease.

In Chapter 22, Robert E. Krout describes his work with those at the end of life, again bringing emphasis to the importance of therapeutic relationship and integrative treatment. Music mediated strategies are introduced and explained by Robert, as he shares heart touching vignettes of his work with individuals and caregivers at this final phase of life.

Section IV: Multicultural Perspectives
This section to the book contributes to a growing trend in healthcare aimed at raising cultural diversity, sensitivity, and competence to primary consideration in defining initiatives foundational to healthcare.[7] The following chapters feature the work of newly emerging professionals in music therapy, and as such bring fresh insight to cultural understanding within music therapy practice. Each chapter offers musical and informational resources to the practicing clinician, and renders pragmatic considerations when working in culturally diverse settings.

In Chapter 23, Jillian Hicks, Erik Baumann Cornejo, and Natalia Garrido discuss the use of Latin American music and Spanish repertoire with patients receiving treatment within a chemotherapy infusion suite. The impact of such music on resilience and patient coping with physical and emotional pain encountered in this fragile environment is described in rich case scenarios.

In Chapter 24, Thomas J. Biglin Jr. and Yi-Ying Lin discuss their work providing Environmental Music Therapy in a radiation oncology waiting area serving a diverse population inclusive of Asian and Asian-American patients. Tom and Yi-Ying share personal process and clinical prowess honed from experiences integrating Asian repertoire with American music in an ever-changing milieu.

In Chapter 25, Soniya K. Brar and Oksana Rosenblum conclude the book by sharing with reverence, their affinity for Indian and Persian music traditions as potentially rich but minimally accessed musical resources in the treatment of pain. Both Soniya and Oksana reflect on personal connections to the respective music forms, as foundational to their explanations of each tradition's therapeutic potential.

Introduction

Conclusion

This book offers a testament to the integrative use of music and music therapy in the treatment of pain across a range of settings and diagnoses. From the use of entrainment[8-10] and music improvisation[11] to a myriad of other innovative approaches, each author's voice and philosophy is held in great esteem for its contribution to the important dialogue on best practice in pain treatment. Ever central to the dialogue, is the unique culture,[12] context, language,[13] and subjective experience of the individual patient.[14] As healthcare initiatives continue to evolve to the inclusion of music therapy and other non-pharmacologic services, the information presented here will hopefully serve to inspire others in contributing to the expanding body of literature supporting such growth.

References

1. Bulfinch T. *Bulfinch's Mythology.* Middelsex, England: The Hamlyn Publishing Group; 1964.
2. Keyes R, ed *The wit and wisdom of Oscar Wilde: A treasury of qotations, anectotes, and observations.* New York, NY: Gramercy Books; 1996.
3. Brennan F, Carr DB, Cousins M. Pain management: A fundamental human right. *Pain Medicine.* 2007;105(2):205-221. Accessed 4/2/2013.
4. Strada EA, Portenoy RK. Psychological rehabilitative and integrative therapies for cancer pain. *Uptodate.* 2010. http://www.uptodate.com/contents/psychological-rehabilitative-and-integrative--therapies-for-cancer-pain. Accessed March 31, 2013.
5. Loewy JV. Introduction. In: Loewy JV, ed. *Music therapy in pediatric pain.* Cherry Hill, NJ: Jeffrey Books; 1997:1-5.
6. Loewy J, Hallan C, Friedman E, Martinez C. Sleep/sedation in children undergoing EEG testing: A comparison of chloral hydrate and music therapy. *Journal of PeriAnesthesia Nursing.* 2005;20(5):323-331.
7. Carteret M. Dimensions of culture: Cross-cultural communications for healthcare professionals. *Cultural Aspects of pain management.* 2011. Accessed 4/1/2013.
8. Bradt J. The effects of music entrainment on posteperative pain perception in pediatric patients. *Music and Medicine.* 2010;2(2):150-157.

9. Bradt J. Music Entrainment for breathing regulation. In: Azoulay R, Loewy JV, eds. *Music, the breath and health: Advances in integrative therapy.* New York: Satchnote Press; 2009:11-19.
10. Dileo C, Bradt J. Entrainment, resonance, and pain suffering. In: Dileo C, ed. *Music therapy & medicine: Theoretical and clinical applications.* Silver Spring, MD: American Music Therapy Association; 1999:181-188.
11. Bruscia KE. A qualitative method of analyzing client improvisations. *Music Ttherapy Perspectives.* 2001;19(1):7-21.
12. Strada EA. *The helping professional's guide to end-of-life care: Practical tools for emotional, social, and spiritual support.* Oakland, CA: New Harbinger Publications, Inc.; 2013.
13. Altilio T. The power and potential of language. In: Altilio T, Otis-Green S, eds. *The Oxford Textbook of Palliative Social Work.* New York, NY: Oxford University Press; 2012:689-694.
14. Portenoy RK. *Contemporary Diagnosis and Management of Pain in Oncologic and AIDS Patients.* 3rd ed. Newtown, PA: Handbooks in Health Care Co.; 2001.

SECTION I

FOUNDATIONS

Music and Medicine: Integrative Models in the Treatment of Pain

CHAPTER 1

Music has Charms to Soothe a Savage Breast: An Integrative Medical-Psychiatric Perspective on Pain and Music

Stephan J. Quentzel MD, JD, MA

> *He has lain here for a terrible, motionless*
> *Decade, and talks through a system of winks*
> *And facial twitches. The nurse props a cigarette*
> *Between his lips, wipes his forehead. She thinks*
> *He wants to send the kid away, but decides*
> *To let him in – he's waited hours.*
> *Guitar case, jean jacket. A corduroy cap slides*
> *Down his forehead. Doesn't talk. He can't be more*
> *Than twenty. He straps on the harmonica holder,*
> *Tunes up, and begins his "Song to Woody,"*
> *Trying to sound three times his age, sandpaper*
> *Dustbowl growl, the song interminable, inept.*
> *Should he sing another? The eyes roll their half-hearted yes.*
> *The nurse grits her teeth, stubs out the cigarette.*
> David Wojahn
> (WOODY GUTHRIE VISITED BY
> BOB DYLAN: BROOKLYN STATE
> HOSPITAL, NEW YORK, 1961)

Introduction

Over the last several decades, there has been increasing attention to pain as a unique medical problem requiring focused and intentional clinical intervention. Because living with chronic pain often is so debilitating, any treatment that can add to relief is valuable. Music and music therapy are found to contribute to a comprehensive and integrative strategy for managing pain. First this chapter examines the physical and psychosocial aspects of the pain experience. Next the chapter outlines multiple features of current pain assessment and management. Establishing a foundational understanding of pain as a clinical entity informs the later discussion of the power of music as therapy to help manage medical and psychosocial aspects of pain. This chapter deliberately focuses on examining the psychosocial material to understanding and addressing pain because of great overlap between psychotherapeutic and music centered conceptualizations of, and treatments for, pain.

The Mechanics of Pain

Before a discussion of pain can be worthwhile, definitions of key words and concepts are needed. Some of the pain experience depends on how peripheral nerve cells register the painful stimuli on and in the body. Injury or dysfunction of the peripheral pain fibers can create pain messages or amplify existing ones, and, at times, can dampen pain impulses as well. At least as critical to defining the pain experience is how the brain translates the pain signal traveling from the body. For many reasons, people vary in how their brains interpret pain transmissions coming from the peripheral body. Various forms of pain management, including music therapy, focus in part on modulating the brain's processing of pain, regardless of the cause or intensity of the pain signal arising from the noxious stimulation of peripheral pain nerves.

Nociceptive pain[1] is normal pain, in which provocative stimuli drive rapid peripheral nerve signals along nociceptor sensory neurons to the spinal cord and the brain. It is here that pain is interpreted in proper character and proportion to the intensity and nature of the pain trigger. This is a key mechanism for human survival. At the first touch of pain, most people withdraw from the source of pain or otherwise recognize the pain source, thereby allowing themselves to avoid bodily injury from the pain-inducing stimulus.

Neuropathic pain[2,3] is a pathophysiological condition. The peripheral nerve is somehow damaged or dysregulated, thereby inducing a maladaptive chronic or exaggerated pain message to the brain, which registers the pain. Traumatic bodily injury and disease like diabetes are obvious examples of sources for peripheral nerve damage and sustained neuropathic pain.

Inflammatory pain is recognized increasingly as a unique but common type of pain. Inflammation driven by multiple potential causes can lead to tissue damage and the release of pain signals to the brain. Nociceptor sensory nerves can be functioning properly as they detect the inflammatory source for pain. In an adaptive fashion, they conduct the pain signal to the spinal cord and brain for self-preservation of the individual. Nevertheless, inflammatory activity and corresponding tissue damage can cause chronic pain that ultimately should be managed well if patients are to enjoy full global function.

Non-inflammatory/non-neuropathic pain comes from abnormal central nervous system processing that identifies pain despite the absence of any recognizable noxious trigger of, or damage to, the sensory nerve. Additionally, this type of pain occurs despite no detectable inflammatory problem with any tissue of the body. Brain dysfunction creates or amplifies feelings of pain, despite no classic cause for pain. This brain hypersensitivity, and the associated pain experience, can vary as other forces affect brain function and health. Fibromyalgia[4-6] is a common example of what often is referred to as a "hypersensitivity syndrome" of the brain, or a "central hypersensitivity syndrome."[7]

Due to problematic brain changes poorly understood, normal or low intensity pain signals are interpreted by the brain as being debilitating in nature in central sensitivity syndromes like fibromyalgia. Similarly, these problematic brain changes drive magnification of painful aspects of depressive symptoms or traumatic stress or other emotional illnesses. Hypersensitive creation of pain messages and hypersensitive magnification of existing pain signals offer one model for how pain syndromes and psychiatric ailments share pathophysiological origins and psychosomatic expressions.[8]

A painful stimulus generates a pain signal that travels down the peripheral nerve to the dorsal horn of the spine. There the pain message jumps to the central nervous system where the spinal cord (in part) and the brain (primarily) process the incoming pain signal in order to understand it and to produce a response. Ascending fibers transmit the pain impulse up the spinal cord to areas of the brain that also regulate mood and anxiety. In response to the pain recognition in the brain, descending pain pathways are excited to inhibit continuing incoming pain signals, thereby helping to modulate the pain experience.[9-11] Here the neurotransmitters serotonin and norepinephrine (noradrenaline), are, in part, released to carry the inhibitory message through the brain and down the spinal cord to ease the experience of pain.[12,13] These neurotransmitters also play key roles in the chemistry of depression, anxiety and cognition.

Because pain is processed in regions of the brain that also regulate mood and anxiety, and because pain transmission and mood and anxiety activity in the brain share common neurotransmitters, it is evident that pain and psychiatric problems provoke each other and co-exist when shared portions of the brain and/or shared neurotransmitter systems are somehow distorted.[14] In neuropathic pain and in central hypersensitivity syndromes, there are changes in peripheral and/or central neuronal structure and function, such that pain is felt or interpreted more and inhibited less.[15,16] Similar changes in central neuronal structure and function underlie psychopathological experiences. Enhancing serotonin and norepinephrine activity improves inhibitory signals to quell pain while simultaneously dampening brain interpretations of pain intensity. Similarly, such neurotransmitter activity also improves mood and anxiety. All of this goes to show again that pain and mental disorder are tied closely to one another.[17]

The interplay between mind and body, between the processes of psychiatric states and pain experiences, are profound. One concept to explain this link is based on a model of shared neurotransmitter dysregulation that creates or amplifies pain as well as depression/anxiety. It is evident, for example, that painful physical conditions are correlated highly with Major Depressive Disorder. In one study, 43% of depressives complain of physical pain as a component of the mood disorder, while only 16% of emotionally stable subjects experience varieties of somatic pain.[18]

Importantly, neurotransmitter models are far from the only theories to explain overlap and co-existence between pain and psychiatric problems. Take for instance Brain Derived Neurotrophic Factor (BDNF). It modulates the production, development and enriching of new and existing neurons well into human adulthood.[19] This influences regulation of mood and of pain perception.[20] Norepinephrine and serotonin levels seem to alter BDNF activity,[21] further exemplifying a cross-link between pain processing and psychiatric states.[22-24] BDNF promotes nerve cell neuroprotection, neuroplasticity and the networking of neurons,[25] which, in turn can promote brain cell health and enriched neuronal communication.[26] This then can translate to relief from depression. It additionally can result in effective quelling of pain signaling and of runaway central nervous system interpretation of pain.[26]

The interplay between the pain experience and the psychiatric experience is mediated, as just discussed, by neurotransmitter fluctuation and by BDNF function. It is affected, additionally, by the hypothalamic-pituitary-adrenal axis, the stress response and inflammatory activity.[27] A typical, temporary scare or physiological stressor stimulates firing of the brain's hypothalamus, which, in turn, ignites pituitary gland activation of adrenal gland release of stress hormones. The release of these hormones fuels, appropriately, the "fight or flight" response that is critical for survival in a threatening world. This is when the stressor is acute. But when the stress is unrelenting, as with prolonged pain, depression, anxiety, or difficult social or environmental conditions, the firing of the stress response continues until its feedback regulation is damaged. This results in perpetual stimulation of the stress hormones rather than the tactical use of brief "fight or flight" reactivity to address acute stressors or threats.[28] This plague of chronic stress and poorly regulated prolonged activation of the stress response defines much of what is at the core of many chronic diseases from which modern humanity suffers. Ongoing loss of the modulation of the stress response fuels chronic inflammation throughout the body. This results in enhanced pain and worsened depression and anxiety,[20] plus it functions as a risk factor for diabetes, obesity, atherosclerosis and heart disease, bowel diseases, neurological disorders, maybe even cancer.[29]

Additionally, pain, depression and physiological stress lower BDNF gene expression.[30] Reduced BDNF allows for diminished modulation of pain and depression, which in turn fuels a host of problems, including increased firing of a perpetual stress response, heightened systemic neuroendocrine dysregulation, more prolonged inflammation, elevated brain disease in the form of chronic pain and psychiatric illness, and enhanced multi-organ chronic disease. Psychiatric ailment and pain are inextricably linked the way mind and body are. Clinical intervention is necessary, through various means including the use of music as medicine, to restore adaptive homeostasis, or balance, to the neuroendocrine system, inflammatory regulation, and brain function.[31-33] Manipulating neurochemistry, through multiple approaches, including the use of music as medicine, can result in relief from pain and psychiatric blight.

Pain Management

The goal of pain management is to reduce, if not eliminate, pain, while freeing the patient to enjoy improved quality of life and global function.[34,35] Ultimately, it is uninhibited function across the major realms of life that matters most to real patients in the real world. The three cornerstones of pain management are precise pain assessment over time, patient education related to the pain experience, and a multifocal treatment plan for lowering, or, ideally, eliminating pain.

Pain Assessment

Pain can be measured and quantified over time through validated scales[36,37] like the Brief Pain Inventory[38] and the Visual Analog Scale,[39] to name but two. However, it is difficult and underproductive to measure pain outside the context of the individual experiencing the pain. Assessing the pain requires, in part, an indepth understanding of what the pain experience has been historically for a patient. Also, since the ultimate goal is to optimize function, measuring function across time is essential for pain management.[37,39-42] Reductions in pain itself do not necessarily correlate perfectly with improvements in function, so measuring both is important.

An interesting contributor to pain is the psychosocial meaning of the pain experience, both as a source for creating pain and as an outgrowth of living with pain. In other words, there can be psychosocial contributors to the pain experience occurring simultaneously with psychosocial consequences ensuing from the pain experience.[43] For example, depression and anxiety can make physical pain worse, while pain can feed development of depression and anxiety. This mind-body and mind-brain interplay that helps to define the pain experience offers a useful perspective on understanding and managing pain. Moreover, it provides a welcoming portal through which music can be applied to controlling pain.

Psychosocial Assessment

The psychosocial assessment of the pain experience is complex yet essential. As pain experts explain, the four subsets of the psychosocial assessment are psychological, social, role and "other."[43] These are discussed here.

Psychological Aspect of the Psychosocial Assessment
Psychological material relevant to understanding patients' pain experiences involves exploring the psychiatric symptoms and disorders that both fuel pain and are caused by living with pain. Equally important is to appreciate the psychological make-up of patients - their personality styles, traumas, coping mechanisms, vulnerabilities, interpersonal patterns, inner conflicts, substance abuse proclivities, cognitive status, and stress tolerance levels. These facets of human design are inextricably linked frequently with how pain develops and/or what results from living with pain. In addition, regardless of whether the psychosocial ailment or the physical pain comes first, the co-morbid existence of psychiatric/psychological problems and pain disorders is common. Part of this co-morbidity simply is the overlapping experience of living with pain and with psychiatric challenges. Beyond that, another aspect of this co-morbidity is explained by shared brain function for processing pain and for processing mood, anxiety, cognition and personality. Distortions in brain function can manifest in altered recognition of pain and, simultaneously, altered psychiatric condition.

So in developing a comprehensive assessment of pain, it is worthwhile to explore the psychological conditions that help to define the pain experience. Additionally, the assessment should examine the co-morbid existence between pain issues and psychiatric ailments, including facets of brain function that help to define both, as explained previously in this chapter. Finally, if the intent is to address both physical and emotional pains, and the interplay between the two, then clinical attention to both must be applied concurrently upon reaching the treatment phase of overall pain management.

Various psychological issues impact on how pain is experienced. In assessing this psychological contribution, it is beneficial to investigate with patients, their meaning for and interpretation of, pain. For example, does pain represent punishment, deserved or not? Is pain welcomed, as a perverse reward? Is there a history of physical or emotional trauma that leaves patients increasingly vulnerable to new trauma and pain? Are there physical or psychiatric co-morbidities that share in defining the pain experience of a person?

Importantly, are patients wed to the "sick role?" Has living as a person in pain, and has defining oneself as a person living in pain, become a central organizing principle in the daily life structure and self-definition of patients? Are there psychological rewards to being "sick," needy, dependent, helpless? Does being the "sick one" in the family or community create a role that the patient becomes reluctant to abandon? Does this schema then render the patient reluctant to get better, even if this all acts at an unconscious level? Are there conscious secondary gains, like monetary support, that incentivize patients to identify as "sick?"

Once patients are committed or unconsciously wed to the sick role, (no matter how mild their pain syndromes are), rarely will they get better, irrespective of treatment. On the other hand, patients with a sense of agency who are determined to work hard toward achieving pain relief and to find good health, inevitably will improve to a meaningful degree, even if their pain experiences are severe.

So we explore if the patient self-identifies as generally being ill with an occasional good day, or if he sees himself as being generally healthy but with a medical challenge? These are two very different psychological perspectives that are critical to understanding and treating the pain experience.

This mind-body, or mind-brain connection is not strictly a psychological phenomenon. It very much is a biochemical one as well. However, for purposes of categorizing and structuring the comprehensive work-up of pain, examination of the psychoneuroendocrinological overlap between experiencing pain and experiencing psychiatric hardship belongs in this exploration of the psychological aspects of the psychosocial assessment. But it could comprise its own focus of attention within the psychosocial assessment because this biochemical material itself is so critically important for pain management purposes.

Social Aspect of the Psychosocial Assessment
The social content relevant to understanding pain focuses on patients' interpersonal activity. Is support from family and friends available, or does input from such close connections actually undermine patient progress? Do supportive entities such as family members, clinicians and governmental programs help as intended or do they actually enable patients to remain in prolonged "sick roles" that do not correlate well with decreasing concrete

measures of pain? Is there intimacy in the life of pain patients? Are there social, medical, familial, financial and supportive resources available to help patients marshal their inner strengths to push against the debilitation driven by living with chronic pain?

Role Aspect of the Psychosocial Assessment
Life function, as highlighted by various roles that a pain patient can or cannot manage, is a useful measure for assessing pain since, ultimately, it is life function, not the pain level itself, that matters most. How does a patient lead a typical day? Can the patient work? If so, how much and at what? Can he parent? Does the patient have grounding structure day to day, or is he floating too much, wallowing in the pain experience? Can rewarding and positively distracting structure and routine be implemented for the patient? Can the patient be helped to identify passions and to utilize convincing reasons to jump out of bed in the morning, eager to engage the structured daily life awaiting?

"Other" Aspects of the Psychosocial Assessment
The psychosocial assessment of pain requires attention to a variety of issues not captured within the psychological, social and role aspects of that assessment.
 Personal history with pain, the travails of living with family members in chronic pain, and cultural expressions of pain all inform the overall assessment of a unique patient's current pain experience. One's pain history may mean that the individual patient is prepared more substantially to manage pain in the present moment. But equally likely, endurance and coping fail as a patient's involvement with pain lengthens over time. Adaptive success in handling pain in the past may empower similar success currently. On the other hand, maladaptive historical patterns may only worsen the ability to manage the pain now. In addition, from his family and culture, a patient may learn how to experience pain, to express it or not, to cope with it or not, and to integrate it well or not into his larger life narrative. So investigating a patient's historical, familial, and cultural lessons around pain, adds useful data to assessing thoroughly the pain experience of a patient. Again, comprehensive assessment dictates the nature of a broad and integrative treatment plan that maximizes the likelihood for success in treating the pain.
 Another source for understanding the pain experience of a patient and for personalizing a thorough treatment plan for the pain is to examine the spiritual, philosophical and religious particulars of a patient. This helps to identify potential inner strengths, conceptual principles, institutional supports, and individual allies for the patient involved in the long-term

management of pain. At the same time, such analysis may reveal vulnerabilities, limitations and themes of isolation and loneliness that threaten the optimal negotiation of a chronic pain journey.

Not only are historical, familial, cultural and spiritual factors relevant to understanding the potentials and the limitations of a patient tackling a chronic pain challenge, but also pertinent are financial, housing, insurance, legal and governmental limitations and strengths.

Finally, meaningful to the broad assessment of a patient's pain experience is study of his patterns of use and abuse with prescription medications and with illicit substances. Have patients demonstrated disciplined use of prescriptions for narcotics? Can the clinician predict how pending pain medications will be managed based on past use and abuse patterns with prescription and illicit agents? Have prescription medications been utilized by the patient for purposes other than those intended by the clinician who wrote the prescriptions? For example, is the patient redirecting opiates, knowingly or unconsciously, for legitimate psychiatric or sleep needs that are addressed more effectively with other interventions? Is the patient abusing prescribed pain medications or is it pseudo-addiction, whereby against doctor's orders, but with good intention to address unresolved or undertreated pain, the patient is using more opiate than prescribed?

Patient Education

The demands on a patient living with chronic pain are intense. A passive patient with chronic pain, expecting simply to receive treatment from outside sources like clinicians and supporters, has dramatically lower chances for full treatment success than does a pain patient who actively captains the treatment team and who takes disciplined responsibility for accumulating clinical progress. Patients who do not understand the process of pain and the nature of a comprehensive treatment plan for pain are destined to participate in their own care inadequately. So the patient needs to be taught about the origins of his pain, the pathophysiological underpinnings of it, the prognosis for where and how it will likely progress, and the lifestyle features that tend to exacerbate versus reduce pain and the hardship of the pain experience. Additionally, the patient should be educated about medication management and adherence, structured self-help, the toll that chronic pain and prolonged treatment can place on supportive family and friends, clinician expectations for degrees of success in relieving pain, and clinic rules and procedures around appointments, emergencies, complaints, medication mismanagement, and access to medication refills. A thorough pain assessment enhances the understanding of the unique patient so that broad patient education can be tailored to the needs and perspectives of that patient.

An active student is a better learner. It is the clinician's responsibility to find ways to reach, to motivate, to activate, and to engage the patient. If the education of the patient can approach a level of effectiveness that is optimal, then the patient can become driven to reject the sick role and to marshal his capacities to move beyond the pain experience, no matter how slow that process might be.

Treatment Plan

A medicinal intervention in the treatment of pain is considered a rousing success if it lowers the pain by half.[44] While that may be an impressive achievement given the limits of technology available in the clinical battle against pain, still, many real patients in the real world will require significantly more pain relief if they are to recapture full global function in life and an adequate quality of life. The addition of pain agents may reduce the residual pain,[13,45,26] but it is the rare case in which medication use alone brings full resolution of chronic pain. Additional integrative treatments of many kinds, including music therapy and music psychotherapy, are essential, often in combination to bring pain down far beyond what medication could do alone.

One area of adjunctive care is psychiatric attention when psychological or psychiatric conditions are precursors to the pain experience or are comorbid challenges alongside the pain experience. Psychopharmacology and natural psychoactive treatments may be useful. So may various types of psychotherapy, including music psychotherapy. Often proper psychotherapy is very useful even if there is no identifiable psychopathology. Just targeting the challenge of living with and managing chronic pain is a noteworthy goal for psychotherapy. Beyond that, psychotherapies may prove to be useful in addressing a host of psychological factors that are elicited in the comprehensive psychosocial assessment. Since there is high frequency for psychiatric problems to fuel the pain experience or to arise from the pain experience, a clinician typically can assume that in building a comprehensive treatment plan, he needs to include a thorough psychiatric/psychotherapeutic component.

Other frequently indicated sources of care for pain, to list a few, are music therapy, physical therapy, occupational therapy, rehabilitation medicine, acupuncture, chiropractic, body work, meditative practices, technological interventions for pain, mind-body approaches, biofeedback, orchestrated family support, and spiritual guidance. Finally, competent primary care is necessary to oversee all health matters because patients have medical needs far beyond just addressing their chronic pain.

Part of the comprehensive treatment plan for pain, and part of the benefits from intervention by many of the multiple sources for care listed just above, is stress management. With the physiology of chronic stress playing a significant role in fueling pain and numerous other significant psychiatric and medical conditions, and with chronic stress challenging the vast majority of pain patients, a plan to control the stress response often must be included in a broad pain treatment strategy.[47]

No treatment plan, no matter how thorough and well conceived, can be perfect nor static. As the pain experience evolves over time and in response to treatment, ongoing and dynamic reassessment of pain is essential.[39] Regular intervals between reassessments and the use of structured assessment tools over time all allow for proper therapeutic adjustments to meet the changing nature of the pain experience and related psychosocial material. In fact, with psychosocial factors playing such a substantial role in generating or amplifying pain, and with psychosocial problems arising so frequently from living with chronic pain, reapplication over time of the psychiatric/psychological/psychosocial evaluation is as appropriate as regular reassessment of the pain itself.

Music as Medicine for Pain
Music as medicine, music therapy, and music psychotherapy offer extensively utilized and well researched interventions for pain. The use of music in combination with multiple other forms of intervention makes sound sense based on theory and practice. Music therapy delivers clinical impact on various aspects of the pain experience.

Music psychotherapy offers broad clinical utility in the vein of most forms of psychotherapy. As a variation on psychotherapy, music therapy provides access into the inner life of the patient in pain and it offers the opportunity for the nurturing of a therapeutic relationship.[48] As well, it succeeds in supporting patient advancements in self-help and in developing a lifestyle geared toward dampening the pain experience. Music psychotherapy can be particularly useful around the issues of agency and avoiding the sick role, which are common and important when confronting long-term pain and its treatment. Music psychotherapy is a valuable modality for addressing patient autonomy, internalization of locus of control, and need for sustainable hope. Patients need to avoid loss of control to the pain and to the demoralization easily accrued under the ceaseless pressure of chronic pain.

Relationship and connectedness help buffer against the emotional onslaught of living with chronic pain. Music therapy works well to engage pain patients, to refocus them, and to make them feel connected to something bigger than the isolated self. Furthermore, it encourages them to find outlet for expression with an empathic partner, and it nurtures a therapeutic relationship that lies at the core of any and all successful clinical efforts.[48]

As a psychotherapeutic undertaking, music therapy serves as a potent tool for stress management.[49] From psychodynamic, cognitive and behavioral perspectives, music therapy provides multiple angles on aiding the pain patient to manage emotional and physiological stress productively. The therapeutic relationship itself relieves stress. In addition, music therapy nurtures outlets for thought, emotion and creativity, and it offers opportunity to find language through music to address stress and the consequences of stress. Music therapy affords the patient mindful and therapeutic refocusing. Furthermore, music therapy serves as a source for fun, playfulness, enjoyment, and passion, and it can serve as a path along which to transcend daily concerns and medical hardship. Overall, music therapy is a potent psychotherapeutic intervention for assisting pain patients to manage stress and, thereby, to ease the pain experience at emotional and behavioral levels.

Finally, music as medicine activates the regulation of breath and body rhythms, which counteracts the physiological stress response and dampens pain. In fact, as a biomedical intervention, music therapy activates numerous physiological processes recognized to add to the reduction of pain at biochemical levels. Clinical experience and research trials reveal that music used medicinally is a powerful instrument for modulating the psycho-neuroimmunoendocrine conditions of stress and pain.[50] It has a rich tradition as a means for reducing stress and anxiety before and after surgery,[51] thereby helping to control the associated pain experience. In addition, music therapy and music psychotherapy have established roles in treating depression and anxiety.[52] In managing emotional pain comes reduction of simultaneous physical pain.

Furthermore, music used as medicine influences a host of biochemical messengers broadly associated with pain. Various enzymes, peptides, proteins, hormones, neurotransmitters, neuromodulators, cytokines and inflammatory modulators all respond to music as medicine, and in doing so contribute to regulating the stress response and the biochemistry of pain.[53] Music activates dopaminergic centers in the brain that regulate pleasure-seeking and are, otherwise, stimulated by food, sex and drugs.[54] Music medicine stimulates particular sex hormones,[55,56] receptor proteins and stress hormones to enhance neurogenesis and improved learning.[57] Music, properly applied, moderates the stress response by regulating neurotrophins in the hypothalamus.[58] It also effects levels and activity of cortisol,[59] other stress hormones, tumor necrosis factor, adrenaline and norepinephrine, prolactin, interleukins[60] and plasminogen activator.[61,62] This all influences multiple pathways related to creating, amplifying and perceiving pain.[63] Music boosts levels and activity of endorphins,[64] oxytocin, growth hormone, T cells,[65] immunoglobulins and natural killer cells,[66] all helping to modulate pain through various biochemical avenues.[67,68]

In its totality, the physiological activity of music as medicine can result in improved emotions,[69] lowered stress response,[70] increased immune function,[71] reduced inflammation, enhanced BDNF production and impact,[58] stimulation of endogenous opiate effects[72] and activated parasympathetic drive to calm cardiovascular processes.[73] The outcome of all this constructive physiological activity is music's meaningful contribution to modulating the pain experience.[74] Ultimately, music therapy interferes with the production of pain signals,[75] with amplification of existing pain messages, with cerebral perception and interpretation of the character and intensity of pain, and with instinctual, behavioral, emotional and cognitive reactions to living the pain experience.

Music as psychotherapeutic and psychosocial medicine alongside music as biochemically active medicine has its clinically significant role in a comprehensive and integrative approach to managing pain. The music therapy model offers, as well, sensitive ongoing clinical engagement that allows for reassessing many of the variables in the pain experience over time as the pain is addressed.

Conclusion

The more we know about a health problem, the better we can target care. A thorough assessment of pain requires the proper physical exam[76] and diagnostic testing, but also elaborate investigation of associated psychosocial material. The results of the pain assessment are organized and understood within the context of our models explaining pain genesis – types of pain, physiology and biochemistry of pain, psychological/psychiatric causes of and consequences of pain, social contributors to the pain experience, life roles and life function as aspects of the pain experience, historical and familial and spiritual variables in the pain experience, and prescription medication and illicit substance use and abuse patterns relevant to the pain experience. The unique comprehensive assessment of the pain experience, including co-morbid diagnoses, then determines the corresponding integrative treatment plan.

This multifocal strategy to pain reduction addresses much more than mere analgesia. Attending to the full range of biological and psychosocial facets of the pain experience maximizes the likelihood of success in eliminating or minimizing the totality of pain elements. Because shared areas of the brain process both pain inputs and psychological/psychiatric material, the psychosocial and biological components of the pain experience are inextricably linked. So treating those psychosocial components, with a comprehensive strategy, is as critical as treating the physiological ones.

One tactic to modulate mind-body and mind-brain complexities is to apply music as medicine. Music therapy offers psychodynamic intervention as well as biochemical manipulation, lifestyle modification, and stress regulation, all toward managing the pain experience and its co-morbid co-conspirators. Finally, music therapy, as a longitudinal intervention, offers useful access for ongoing reassessment of the pain experience as it is addressed therapeutically over time.

Music has Charms to soothe a savage Beast...and a savage pain.

References

1. Woolf C. *Ann Intern Med.* 2004;140:441-451.
2. Portenoy RK, Kanner RM. Definition and Assessment of Pain. In: Portenoy RK, Kanner RM, Eds. *Pain Management: Theory and Practice*; 1998:4.
3. Galer BS, Dworkin RH. *A Clinical Guide to Neuropathic Pain*; 2000:8-9.
4. Wolfe F, et al. *Arthritis Rheum.* 1990;33(2):160-172.
5. Wolfe F. *Rheum Dis Clin North Am.* 1989;15:1-18.
6. Arnold LM, et al. *Arthritis and Rheumatism.* 2004;50(9):2974-2984.
7. Muhammad Y. The Concept of Central Sensitivity Syndromes. In *Fibromyalgia and Other Central Pain Syndromes*. Wallace DJ, Clauw DJ, Eds:29-44.
8. Bymaster FP, et al. *Current Pharm Des.* 2005;11(12):1475-1493.
9. Alpay M. Pain Patients. In Stern TA, et al. *Massachusetts General Hospital Handbook of General Hospital Psychiatry, 5th Ed.* 2004:314.
10. Fields H. *Nat Rev Neurosci.* 2004;5(7):565-575.
11. Fields H, et al. *Annu Rev Neurosci.* 1991;14:219-245.
12. McMahon SB, Koltzenburg M. In *Wall and Melzack's Textbook of Pain, 5th Ed.* Elsevier, 2006:125-142.
13. Bymaster FP, et al. *Neuropsychopharmacology.* 2001;25(6):871-880
14. Millan MJ. *Prog Neurobiol.* 2002;66(6):355-474.
15. Fields HL, Basbaum AI. Central Nervous Systems of Pain Modulation In Wall PD, Melzack R, Eds. *Textbook of Pain, 4th Ed.* Edinburgh: Churchill Livingstone; 1999:310.

16. Wall PD, Metzack R, Eds. *Textbook of Pain, 4th Ed.* London, UK: Churchill Livingstone; 1999:309-312.
17. Basbaum AI, et al. *Ann Neurol.* 1978;4(5):451-462.
18. Ohayon MM, Schatzberg AF. *Arch Gen Psychiatry.* 2003;60(1):39-47.
19. Duman RS, et al. *Arch Gen Psychiatry.* 1997;54(7):597-606.
20. Nestler EJ, et al. *Neuron.* 2002;34(1):13-25.
21. Gould E, et al. *Biol Psychiatry.* 2000;48(8):715-720.
22. Sheline YI, et al. *Proc Natl Acad Sci USA.* 1996;93(9):3908-3913.
23. Manji HK, et al. *Biol Psychiatry.* 2003;53(8):707-742.
24. Tsankova NM, et al. *Nat Neurosci.* 2006.
25. Lu B, et al. *Nat Rev Neurosci.* 2005;6(8):603-614.
26. Shimizu E, et al. *Biol Psychiatry.* 2003;54(1):70-75.
27. Heim C, Nemeroff CB. *Biol Psychiatry.* 2001;49:1023-1039.
28. Holtzheimer PE III, Nemeroff CB. *NeuroRx.* 2006;3:42-56.
29. Musselman DL, et al. *Arch Gen Psychiatry.* 1998;55(7):580-592.
30. Duric V, McCarson KE. *Neuroscience.* 2005;133(4):999-1006.
31. Mayberg HS, et al. *Biol Psychiatry.* 2000;48(8):830-843.
32. Brody, et al. *Biol Psychiatry.* 2001;50:171-178.
33. Duman RS. *Neuromolecular Med.* 2004;5(1):11-25.
34. Turk DC. *Clin J Pain.* 2000;16(4):279-280.
35. Belgrade MJ. *Postgrad Med.* 1999;106(6):127-140.
36. Brunton S. *J Fam Pract.* 2004:53(suppl 10):S3-S10.
37. Galer BS, et al. *Clin J Pain.* 2002;18:297-301.
38. Cleeland CS, et al. *Ann Acad Med.* 1994;23(2):129-38.
39. McCafery M, Pasero C, Eds. Pain: *Clinical Manual.* 2nd Ed. St.Louis, MO. Mosby, Inc; 1999:36-102.
40. APS. *Priciples of Analgesic Use in the Treatment of Acute Pain and Cancer Pain.* 5th ed. Glenview, IL: American Pain Society; 2003.
41. Ramelet AS, et al. *Aust Crit Care.* 2004;17:33-45.
42. Craig KD, et al. *Clin Perinatal.* 2002;29:445-457.
43. Portenoy RK, Kanner RM, Eds. *Pain Management: Theory and Practice.* Philadelphia, PA. FA Davis Co. 1996:248-276.
44. Argoff CE, et al. *Mayo Clin Proc.* 2006;8(suppl 4)S3-S11.
45. Bezchlibnyk-Butler KZ,et al. *Clinical Handbook of Psychotropic Drugs.* 2005:2-165.
46. Wang GK, et al. *Pain.* 2004;110(1-2):166-174.
47. Antoni MH, et al. Cognitive-Behavioral Stress Management Reverses Anxiety-Related Leukocyte Transcriptional Alterations. *Biol Psychiatry.* 2012;71(4):366-72.
48. Loewy & Schieby. *A Model of Integrative Medical Music Psychotherapy,* 2001.

49. Krout RE. Music Listening to Facilitate Relaxation and Promote Wellness: Integrated Aspects of Our Neurophysiological Responses to Music. Psychotherapy. 2007;34(2):134-141.
50. Abhishek G. The Effect of Music on the Production of Neurotransmitters, Hormones, Cytokines, and Peptides: A Review. *Music & Medicine*. 2012;4(1):40-43.
51. Migneault B, et al. The Effect of Music on the Neurohormonal Stress Response to Surgery Under General Anesthesia. *Anesth Analg*. 2004;98(2):527-532.
52. Erkkila J, et al. Individual Music Therapy for Depression: Randomised Controlled Trial, *Br J Psychiatry*. 2011;199(2):132-9.
53. Menon V, Levitin DJ. The Rewards of Music Listening: Response and Physiological Connectivity of the Mesolimbic System. *Neuroimage*. 2005;28(1):175-184.
54. Salimpoor VN, et al. Anatomically Distinct Dopamine Release During Anticipation and Experience of Peak Emotion to Music. *Nat Neurosci*. 2011;14(2):257-262.
55. Fukui H, Yamashita M. The Effects of Music and Visual Stress on Testosterone and Cortisol in Men and Women. *Neuro Endocrinol Lett*. 2003;24(3-4):173-180.
56. Hassler M, et al. Testosterone, Estradiol, ACTH and Musical, Spatial and Verbal Performance. *Int J Neurosci*. 1992;65(1-4):45-60.
57. Fukui H, Toyoshima K. Music Facilitates the Neurogenesis, Regeneration and Repair of Neurons. *Med Hypotheses*. 2008;71(5):765-769.
58. Angelucci F, et al. Music Exposure Differentially Alters the Levels of Brain-Derived Neurotrophic Factor and Nerve Growth Factor in the Mouse Hypothalamus. *Neurosci Lett*. 2007;429(2-3);152-155.
59. Khalfa S, et al. Effects of Relaxing Music on Salivary Cortisol Level After Psychological Stress. *Ann NY Acad Sci*. 2003;999:374-376.
60. Wachi M. et al. Recreational Music-Making Modulates Natural Killer Cell Activity, Cytokines, and Mood States in Corporate Employees. *Med Sci Monit*. 2007;13(2):CR57-CR70.
61. Mockel M, et al. Immediate Physiological Responses of Healthy Volunteers to Different Types of Music: Cardiovascular, Hormonal and Mental Changes. *Eur J Appl Physiol*. 1994;68(6):451-459.
62. Brownley KA, et al. Effects of Music on Physiological and Affective Responses to Graded Treadmill Exercise in Trained and Untrained Runners. *Int J Psychophysiol*. 1995;19(3):193-201.

63. Mockel M, et al. Stress Reduction Through Listening to Music: Effects on Stress Hormones, Hemodynamics and Mental State in Patients with Arterial Hypertension and in Healthy Persons. *Dtsch Med Wochenschr*. 1995;120(21):745-752.
64. Goldstein A. Thrills in Response to Music and Other Stimuli. *Physiol Psychol*. 1980;8(1):126-129.
65. Nunez, MJ, et al. Music, Immunity, and Cancer. *Life Sci*. 2002;71(9):1047-1057.
66. Hasegawa Y, et al. Music Therapy Induced Alterations in Natural Killer Cell Count and Function. *Nippon Ronen Igakkai Zasshi*. 2001;38(2):201-204.
67. VanderArk SD, Ely D. Biochemical and Galvanic Skin Responses to Music Stimuli by College Students in Biology and Music. *Percept Mot Skills*. 1992;74(3 pt 2):107-1090.
68. Conrad C, et al. Overture for Growth Hormone: Requiem for Interleuken-6? *Crit Care Med*. 2007;35(12):2709-2713.
69. Kreutz G, et al. Effects of Choir Singing or Listening on Secretory Immunoglobulin A, Cortisol, and Emotional State. *J Behav Med*. 2004;27(6):623-635.
70. Montello L. Music Therapy for Musicians: Reducing Stress and Enhancing Immunity. *Int J Arts Med*. 1995;4(2):14-20.
71. Bartlett D, et al. The Effects of Music Listening and Perceived Sensory Experiences on the Immune System as Measured by Interleuken 1 and Cortisol. *J Music Ther*. 1993;30(4):194-209.
72. Stefano GB, et al. Music Alters Constitutively Expressed Opiate and Cytokine Processes in Listeners. *Med Sci Monit*. 2004;10(6):18-27.
73. Okada K, et al. Effects of Music Therapy on Autonomic Nervous System Activity, Incidence of Heart Failure Events, and Plasma Cytokine and Catecholamine Levels in Elderly Patients with Cerebrovascular Disease and Dementia. *Int Heart J*. 2009;50(1):95-110.
74. Koch ME, et al. The Sedative and Analgesic Sparing Effect of Music. *Anesthesiology*. 1998;89(2):300-306.
75. Lepage C, et al. Music Decreases Sedative Requirements During Spinal Anesthesia. *Anesth Analg*. 2001;93(4):912-916.
76. APS. *Guideline for the Management of Cancer Pain in Adults and Children*. Glenview, Il: American Pain Society; 2005.

Music and Medicine: Integrative Models in the Treatment of Pain

CHAPTER 2

Thirty-five Years Use of Anxiolytic Music (AAM) in Pain and Aversive Clinical Settings

Ralph Spintge MD

*"Medicina sanat animam per corpus,
autem musica sanat corpus per animam."*
Giovanni Pico della Mirandola, (15th century)[*]

Introduction
Why Music?

Pain Medicine deals with two completely different entities of pain: acute and chronic. While chronic pain is seen as a biopsychosocial disease entity of its own, in acute pain an "emergency" triad of pain, acute distress and state anxiety does characterize the psychophysiological state of a patient. Furthermore, in all aversive clinical settings such as anaesthesia, surgery, obstetrics, intensive care, pain medicine, and other situations where a patient may endure invasive procedures, which themselves may cause procedural pain, unpleasant feelings, or may be perceived as dangerous, patients are also in what we may call a "state of negative emotional emergency".[1-6,21-23]

The so-called vicious circle of stress and pain may keep the patient in a state of anxiety, fear of pain and death, combined with impaired conscious perception, reduced self-esteem, anger, feeling of helplessness and disappointment.[1] The psychophysiological sequela include disturbances in central nervous (neurovegetative) regulation of cardiovascular and cardio respiratory systems with increased energy demand and oxygen consumption, inadaequate endocrinological control of metabolism with increased plasma levels of catecholamines, steroid hormones, endogenous opioids, lowered pain tolerance, general hyperaesthesia, ephaptic spreading of pain, accompained by vegetative disturbances such as nausea and vomiting, and motor dysfunction like tremor.[7-9] All lead to inadequate defence reactions, agression, reduced compliance, increased demand for sedatives, anesthetics

---

[*] Medicine heals the mind, soul, spirit by the body, but music heals the body by the mind, soul, and spirit.

and analgetics perioperatively, even to a prolonged postoperative rehabilitation phase.[1,10-20] Mainly two cognitive and emotional factors being responsible have been identified: lack of information and insufficient emotional support.[2,11,114]

Unfortunately, pharmacological interventions such as analgesics and sedatives often prove to be of limited value in alleviating stress response and resolving anxiety.[3,16,17,24] At the same time they may have undesired side effects and reduce a patient's ability to cooperate.[25-27]

Evaluation

Such clinical situations lead us to develop specific musical interventions called Medicofunctional Music, or more specifically, Anxioalgolytic Music (AAM). This means music designed and selected to reduce stress and pain. Over the last 35 years the concept of AAM has been refined using pre- and post-procedural patient questionnaires in about 160,000 patients, and evaluated in various clinical settings using state-of-the-art research protocols for traditional medical trials.[28,31] Each multimodal research protocol incorporates a selection out of psychological and physiological measurements such as self reports (open questionnaires, Thematic Apperception Test, e.g.[118]), observable behaviour and facial action coding system,[32] plasma levels of stress-hormones, EEG, PET, neurovegetative and cardiovascular responses, drug consumption, length of hospital stay and other economic parameters.[28,33,34] To date, AAM is widely applied in surgery and anaesthesia, dental care, pain medicine, palliative care, intensive care, obstetrics, pediatrics, geriatrics, ophthalmology and neurology.[2,5,22,24,28,33-43]

The effects of AAM we observed in clinical studies include: a decrease of heart rate and arterial blood pressure, harmonizing cardiac rhythm, increasing Heart Rate Variability, decrease of respiratory minute-volume and oxygen-consumptionl; a reduction of plasma levels of: catecholamines, ACTH, Cortisol, Prolactin, ß-Endorphin leading to a lower basal metabolic rate, and sleep induction; and marked reduction of vegetative symptoms such as nausea, sweating, and vertigo. Stimulation of neuroendocrine and neuroimmune receptors for catecholamines, endorphins, substance P, dopamine, interleukin-6 leading, result in a rise in IgA-saliva-levels, in T-cell counts, and in killer cells activity. Pain threshold and pain tolerance are increased, and relief of inflammatory pain is observable. Cognitve function is improved, for instance with less post-procedural confusion, and compliance is enhanced. Motor system performance is markedly improved through reduction of restlessness, muscle tonus and spasms. Economic benefits of these clinical improvements include both reduced drug consumption in premedication with Benzodiazepins (50% - 100%), and postoperative analgesics (opiod) demand. Also we found that hospital treatment period can be shortened, for instance on an average of 3 days in premature infants on ICU, and one day less in cataract surgery for high risk elderly patients. Additionally and notably, staff efficiency can be enhanced.

Evidence

Our first series of controlled studies today have been replicated and enlarged through a variety of clinical, randomized controlled trials in various clinical settings by researchers from quite a number of disciplines. These studies compare standard care during invasive and other aversive procedures to music alone, or, in addition to several other interfering variables, such as environmental sound. Clinical settings studied include:

Anaesthesia / induction room[44]
Anaesthesia / recovery room[45,46]
Anaesthesia / pediatric outpatient surgery[6,47,48]
Cardiac surgery[49,50]
Cardiology[51]
Dentistry[33,34]
Gastroenterology / endoscopy / abdominal surgery[52,53]
Gynecological surgery[54,55]
Intensive Care Unit, adults[56,57,58]
Intensive Care Unit, infants[59-69]
Obstetrical Caesarean Section[70]
Ophthalmic outpatient surgery[71,72]
Ophthalmic inpatient surgery[73]
Orthopedic surgery[74]
Pain Medicine[75,76]
Palliative Hospice Care[77-81]
Surgery, adults[82-85]
Surgery, infants[86]

Within these clinical areas, music is used either in competition with other means of analgesia or relaxation, such as analgesics and anaesthetics, or, complementing such other means. However, the question of whether there are direct beneficial effects during general anesthesia is still open.[85,87-89] The picture we get is becoming more complex, especially since brain imaging techniques were introduced. May we just mention one aspect, which is that some neurophysiological studies indicate that particularly effective parameters may be musical rhythm[90-94] as well as timbre.[95,96] Entrainment occurs, in which exogenous rhythms interact with bodily rhythms such as heart rate variability or cardiorespiratory variables, yet, further neurophysiological studies are necessary to finally identify the missing link between musical structure and biological function.[91,97,119] To this point for instance the significant issue of biorhythms is still widely embraced.

Music: Quality, Selection and Design

Quality standards have been established and published.[5,29,31,113,119] It is important to note that in order to secure reliability, validity, and reproducibility of concepts, methods and research results interfering variables, i.e. the musical stimuli themselves have to be defined in detail.

Situations with Acute Pain and Anxiety
As part of a clinical routine we applied and evaluated AAM now with about 160 000 pre- and post-procedural patient questionnaires. It became clear that in this situation, it has to be "popular" music of the patient's choice. In our population a selection of 10 different genres works with 95% of the patients. While frequency of genre chosen differed during the last 35 years, our patient controlled musical offer ranges from actual chart music such as Country Rock, Heavy Metal, Hip Hop, Techno, House etc, to western classical music from the Baroque and Romantic Period[5]. In certain genres a quarterly update of music selection is advisable, especially with younger patients due to this group's sensitivity and propensity for change. While technical and copyright considerations prevent listeners from choosing their favorite conductor or musician - about 30% do ask to do so.

Situations with Chronic Pain and Anxiety
Chronic pain patients often feel like they are living in a cage, thus they try to avoid any additional structure enforced from outside. Appropriate musical stimuli are completely different from those listed for acute pain situations. With chronic pain the music has to open new horizons, stimulate hopes and dreams, and enable a catharsis of heightened psychophysiological tonus, especially by avoiding stronger rhythmic structures. Our offered selection consists of New Age, Enya, natural sound scape, and Asian music for waiting situations (pre-/post-treatment for instance), plus specifically designed music programs for certain treatment itself. Their design may follow such clinical targets as Stress-Relaxation (Emotional Detonisation Training EDT), desired behavioural patterns through unpleasant treatments, as well as circadian biorhythm triggered activity levels of the 24 hours day, and sleep induction. Three very common target areas have been identified, which are routinely treated during every pain therapy session at our hospital: myofascial pain, distress, and sleep disorder. It is essential to transfer these programs as a tool for self-support into daily life of the patient. Such

programs comprise not only music alone, but also certain musically enhanced exercise programs, dream journeys, guided imagery, soundscapes of hiking through Australian bush at night, isometric muscle detonisation exercises guided verbally and non-verbally, and so forth. The patient himself must select his daily program out of such a variety of music and music-enhanced exercise programs to achieve pain control at home and at work. He/she should be enabled to meet individual needs in different situations over the course of the day (including the night) thus enhancing overall quality of life. Design, composition, notation, instrumentation, technical and artistic performance, all need to be of the highest quality. Artificial synthesizer music should be avoided. Our multidisciplinary production team consists of the highest quality experts, Music Therapists, physicians, composers from Germany and China, studio teams specialized on production of movie sound tracks, musicians from professional German symphony orchestras, and skilled sound technicians. The first programs established and published over a period of 20 years are still routinely used today. Further details are very complex and can be only roughly addressed here. A selection of programs is described and published elsewhere.[115-117]

The author wants to make very clear at this point, that not withstanding the obvious advantages of the above described receptive application of medicofunctional music, from our clinical experience of about 35 years, we are convinced that it is much more effective and beneficial to both patient and therapeutic team to include Music Therapists on a regular basis. Their expertise in diagnostic evaluation as well as active therapeutic sessions and exercises in many fields mentioned before is invaluable. This holds especially true in pain medicine and palliative care.

Conclusion

Medicofunctional music is now used in aversive clinical settings on a global scale.[37,39,98-105] While earlier studies focussed upon therapeutic benefits, current research also addresses clinical outcomes combined with economic benefits.[106-108] Music may contribute to cost containment with respect to medication, duration of hospital stay, effectiveness of staff utilization, and procedural times.[1,59,65,73,85,109]

Medicofunctional Music has established standards and definitions as in any other medical treatment. Medical standards and guidelines for research and application of music-based interventions are also necessary for informed discussions about evidence-based use of music in medicine in general,[28,29] which will immanently lead to a broad acceptance within the medical and scientific community.[112,119,120] Thus, an increasing number of practitioners and clinicians are incorporating medicofunctional music such as AAM into their practice, for both acute and chronic pain situations.[110-112]

References

1. Spintge R, Droh R. Die präoperative Angst [Preoperative Anxiety]. *Intensivmedizinische Praxis.* 1981; 4: 29 – 33.
2. Spintge R. Psychophysiologische Operations-Fitness mit und ohne anxiolytische Musik (Psychophysiological fitness for surgery with and without anxiolytic music). In: Droh R, and Spintge R, eds. *Angst, Schmerz, Musik in der Anaesthesie (Anxiety, pain, music in anesthesia).* Grenzach: Editiones Roche; 1983:77-88.
3. Badner N, Nielson W, Munk S. Preoperative anxiety: detection and contributing factors. *Canadian Journal of Anesthesia.* 1990; 37: 444-447.
4. Kain ZN, Mayes L, Cicchetti D. Measurement tool for pre-operative anxiety in children: the Yale Preoperative Anxiety Scale. *Child Neuropsychology.* 1995; 1: 203-210.
5. Spintge R. Musik in Anaesthesie und Schmerztherapie. (Music in Anaesthesia and Pain Therapy). *Anaesthesie Intensivtherapie Notfallmedizin Schmerztherapie AINS.* 2000; 35: 254-261.
6. Wang SM, Kulkarni L, Dolev J, Kain ZN. Music and preoperative anxiety: a randomized, controlled study. *Anesthesia Analgesia.* 2002; 94: 1489-1494.
7. Gellhorn E. Motion and Emotion. *Psychological Review.* 1964; 71: 457-472.
8. Spintge R, Droh R. Ergonomic Approach to Treatment of Patient's Perioperative Stress. *Canadian Anesthetist Society Journal.* 1991; 35(3): 104-106.
9. Keller V. Management of nausea and vomiting in children. *Journal of Pediatric Nursing.* 1995; 24(1): 280 – 286.
10. McGlinn JA. Music in the Operating Theatre. *The British Medical Journal.* 1931; 1(3654): 108.
11. Tolksdorf W. *Der präoperative Stress [preoperative stress].* Heidelberg – New York: Springer; 1985.
12. Norman JG, Fink GW. The effect of epidural anesthesia on the neuroendocrine response to major surgical stress: a randomized prospective trial. *American Journal of Surgery.* 1997; 63(1): 75 – 80.
13. Tolksdorf W. Preoperative stress. Research approach and methods of treatment. *Anaesthesiologie, Intensivmedizin, Notfallmedizin, Schmerztherapie AINS.* 1997; 32(3): 318 – 324.

14. Munafo MR. Perioperative anxiety and postoperative pain. *Psychology, Health and Medicine.* 1998; 3(4): 429 – 433.
15. Grossi EA, Zakow PK, Ribakove G, et al. Comparison of postoperative pain, stress response, and quality of life in port access vs. standard sternotomy coronary bypass patients. *European Journal of Cardio-Thoracic Surgery.* 1999; 16(2): 39 – 42.
16. Caumo W, Ferreira MBC. Perioperative anxiety: psychobiology and effects in postoperative recovery. *The Pain Clinic.* 2003; 15(2): 87 – 101.
17. Buyukkocak, U., Caglayan, O., Daphan, et al. Similar Effects of General and Spinal Anaesthesia on Perioeprative Stress Responses in Patients Undergoing Haemorrhoidectomy. *Mediators of Inflamation.* 2006; 1: 97257.
18. Shigeki M, Genyuki Y, Morio T. Postoperative pain and stress-related hormone responses to surgery in jaw deformities. *Japanese Journal of Oral and Maxillofacial Surgery.* 2006; 52(3): 162 – 166.
19. Stirling L. Reduction and management of perioperative anxiety. *British Journal of Nursing.* 2006; 15(7): 359 – 361.
20. Schön J, Gerlach K, Hüppe M. Einfluss negativer Stressverarbeitung auf postoperatives Schmerzerleben und –verhalten [Impact of negative stress upon postoperative pain experience and –behavior]. *Der Schmerz.* 2007; 21(2): 146 – 153.
21. Nolan P.Music therapy with bone marrow transplant patients: Reaching beyond the symptoms. In: Spintge R, Droh R, eds. *MusicMedicine.* St. Louis, MO: MMB Music; 1992: 209 – 212.
22. Nijkamp MD, Kenens CA, Dijker AJM, Ruiter RAC, Hiddema F, Nuijts RMA. Determinants of surgery related anxiety in cataract patients. *British Journal of Ophthalmology.* 2004; 88: 1310 – 1314.
23. Salimpoor VN, Benovoy M, Longo G, Cooperstock JR, Zatorre RJ. The rewarding aspects of music listening are related to degree of emotional arousal. *PloS One.* 2009; 16: 4(19), e7487.
24. Arts SE, Abu-Saad HH, Champion GD, et al. Age-related response to Lidocaine-Prilocaine (EMLA) Emulsion and effect of music distraction on the pain of intravenous cannulation. *Pediatrics.* 1994; 93: 797-801.
25. Fishman SM, Greenberg DB. Psychological Issues in the Treatment of Pain. In: Borsook D, LeBel AA, McPeck,BC, eds. *The Massachusetts General Hospital Handbook of Pain Management.* Boston; MA: Little Brown; 1996: 110.
26. Cunningham MF, Monson B, Bookbinder M. Introducing a music in the perioperative area. *AORN Journal.* 1997; 10: 67-69.

27. Sullivan M, Tanzer M, Stanish W, et al. Psychological determinants of problematic outcomes following Total Knee Arthroplasty. *PAIN.* 2009; 143. 23 – 129.
28. Spintge R, Droh R. *MusicMedicine.* Saint Louis, MO: MMB; 1992.
29. Robb SL. A Review of Music-based Intervention Reporting in Pediatrics. *Journal of Health Psychology.* 2009; 14 (4): 490-501.
30. Spintge R, Droh R. *The International Society for Music in Medicine ISMM – MusicMedicine, Music Therapy, Musicmedicine.* Book of Abstracts, Rancho Mirage; 1989.
31. Spintge R. Toward a research standard in MusicMedicine / Music Therapy: A proposal for a multimodal approach. In: Spintge R, Droh R, eds. *MusicMedicine.* Saint Louis, MO: MMB; 1992: 345 – 347.
32. Ekman P. Facial Expression of Emotion. In: Davidson RJ, Scherer KR, Goldsmith HH, eds. *Handbook of Affective Sciences.* New York: Oxford University Press; 2003: 415-131.
33. Hatano K, Oyama T, Kogure T, Ohkura I, Spintge R. Anxiolytic Effect of Music on Dental Treatment. Part 1: Subjective and Objective Evaluation. *Journal Japanese Society of Dental Anesthesiology.* 1983; 11(3): 332 – 337.
34. Hatano K, Oyama T, Tsukamoto A, Sakaki T, Spintge R. Anxiolytic Effect of Music on Dental Treatment. Part 2: Endocrine Evaluation. *Journal Japanese Society of Dental Anesthesiology.* 1983; 11(3): 338 – 345.
35. Fowler-Kerry S, Lander JR. Management of injection pain in children. *Pain.* 1987; 30: 169-175.
36. Spintge R, Droh R. *Music in Medicine.* Heidelberg-New York: Springer; 1987.
37. Maranto Ch. *Applications of Music in Medicine.* Washington D.C.: NAMT; 1991.
38. Steinke W. The use of music, relaxation and imagery in the management of postsurgical pain for scoliosis. In: Maranto Ch. *Applications of Music in Medicine.* Washington D.C.: NAMT; 1991: 141–162.
39. Pratt RR, Spintge R. *MusicMedicine* (vol. 2). Saint Louis, MO: MMB; 1996.
40. Bradt J. *The effect of Music Entrainment on postoperative pain perception in pediatric patients.* Dissertation submitted to the Temple University Graduate Board; 2001.
41. Arnon S, Shapsa A, Forman L, Regev R, Bauer S, Litmanovitz I. Live music is beneficial to preterm infants in neonatal intensive care unit environment. *Birth.* 2006; 32 (2): 131–136.

42. Leins AK. Heidelberger Musiktherapiemanual: Migräne bei Kindern [Heidelberg Music Therapy Manual: Migraine in Children]. Bochum: uni-edition; 2006.
43. Brice J, Barclay J. Music eases anxiety of children in cast room. *Journal of Pediatric Orthopedics.* 2007; 27: 831-833.
44. Oyama T, Sato Y, Kudo T, Spintge R, Droh R. Effect of anxiolytic music on endocrine function in surgical patients. In: Spintge R, Droh R, eds. *Music in Medicine.* Heidelberg - Berlin: Springer; 1987: 169–174.
45. Fredriksson AC, Hellström L, Nilsson U. Patient´s perception of music versus ordinary sound in a postanaesthesia care unit: a randomised crossover trial. *Intensive and Critical Care Nursing.* 2009; 13:
46. MacDonald RAR, Ashley EA, Davies MG, et al. The Anxiolytic and Pain Reducing Effects of Music on Post-operative Analgesia. In: Pratt R R, Grocke D, eds. *MusicMedicine 3.* Melbourne: University of Melbourne Press; 1999: 12-18.
47. Kain ZN, Wang SM, Mayes LC, Krivutza DM, Teague BA. Sensory stimuli and anxiety in children undergoing surgery: a randomized, controlled trial. *Anesthesia Analgesia.* 2001; 92(4): 897-903.
48. Kain ZN, Caldwell-Andrews AA, Krivutza DM, et al. Interactive Music Therapy as a Treatment for Preoperative Anxiety in Children: A Randomized Controlled Trial. *Anesthesia Analgesia.* 2004; 98: 1260-1266.
49. Nilsson U, Lindell L, Eriksson A, Kellerth T. The effect of music intervention in relation to gender during coronary angiographic procedures: a randomized clinical trial. *European Journal of Cardiovascular Nursing.* 2009; 1: 29.
50. Schwartz F. A Pilot Study of Patients in Postoperative Cardiac Surgery. *Music and Medicine.* 2009; 1(1): 70-74.
51. Micci N. The use of music therapy with pediatric patients undergoing cardiac catheterization. *The Arts in Psychotherapy.* 1984; 11: 261–266.
52. Ovayola N. Listening to Turkish Classical music during colonoscopy decreases patient´s anxiety, pain, dissatisfaction and the dose of sedative (Midazolam) and analgesic (Meperidine) drugs: A prospective and randomized controlled trial. *World Journal of Gastroenterology.* 2006; 14 (46): 7532-7536.
53. Chikamori F, Kuniyoshi N, Shibuya S, Takase Y. Perioperative music therapy with key-lighting keyboard system in elderly patients undergoing digestive tract surgery. *Hepato-gastroenterology.* 2004; 51 (59): 1384-1386.

54. Ikonomidou E, Rehnstrom A, Naesh N. Effect of music on vital signs and postoperative pain. *AORN Journal.* 2004; 80: 269–278.
55. Binns-Turner PG, Boyd GL, Pryor ER, Prickett C, Harrison L. Effects of Perioperative Music on Anxiety, Hemodynamics, and Pain in Women Undergoing Mastectomy. *Anesthesiology.* 2008; 109: A 1351.
56. Conrad C, Niess H, Jauch KW, Bruns CJ, Hartl W, Welker L. Overture for Growth Hormone: reqiem for Interleukin-6. *Critical Care Medicine.* 2007; 35(12): 2709–2713.
57. Gilad E. The Role of Music and Singing as a Stress-Reducing Modality in the Neonatal Intensive Care Unit Environment. *Music and Medicine.* 2010; 2(1): 18-22.
58. Nelson A, Hartl W, Jauch KW, et al. The impact of music on hypermetabolism in critical illness. *Current Opinion Clinical Nutrition Metabolic Care.* 2008; 11(6): 790-794.
59. Coleman JM, Pratt RR, Stoddard RA, Gerstman DR, Abel HH. The Effects of the Male and Female Singing and Speaking Voice on Selected Physiological and Behavioral Measures of Premature Infants in the Intensive Care Unit. *International Journal of Arts Medicine.* 1997; 5(2): 4–11.
60. Collins S, Kuck K. Music Therapy in the neonatal intensive care unit. Neonatal Network. 1991; 9(6): 23–26.
61. Golianu B, Krane E, Seybold J, Almgren C, Anand KJS. Non-pharmacological techniques for pain management in neonates on ICU: music clearly effective. *Seminars in Perinatology.* 2007; 31(5): 318-322.
62. Loewy JV. *Music therapy in the neonatal intensive care unit.* New York: BIMC by Satchnote Press; 2000.
63. Loewy J, Hallan C, Friedman E, Martinez C. Sleep/sedation in children undergoing EEG testing: A comparison of chloral hydrate and music therapy. *Journal of Perinatal Anesthesia Nursing.* 2005; 20(5): 323–332.
64. Lubetzky R, Mimouni FB, Dollberg S, Reifen R, Ashbel G, Mandel D. Effect of Mozart on energy expenditure in growing preterm infants. *Pediatrics.* 2009; 125(1): e24–28.
65. Schwartz F, Ritchie R, Sacks LL, Phillips CE. Music, stress reduction and medical cost savings in the neonatal care unit. In: Pratt RR, Grocke DE, eds. *MusicMedicine vol. 3.* Melbourne: University of Melbourne Press; 1998: 120–130.
66. Standley JM. *Music therapy with premature infants: Research and developmental interventions.* Silver Spring: American Music Therapy Association; 2003.

67. Standley JM, Moore R. Therapeutic effects of music and mother's voice on premature infants. *Pediatric Nursing*. 1995; 21(6): 509-574.
68. Stewart K. PATTERNS – A Model for Evaluating Trauma in NICU Music Therapy: Part2 – treatment Parameters. *Music and Medicine*. 2009; 1(2): 123-128.
69. Tramo MJ, Lense M, Van Ness C, Kagan J, Settle MD, Cronin JH. Effects of Music on Physiological and Behavioral Indices of Acute Pain and Stress in Premature Infants. *Music and Medicine*. 2011; 3(2): 72-83.
70. Laopaiboon M, Lumbiganon P, Martis R, Vatanasapt P, Somjaivong B Music during caesarean section under regional anaesthesia for improving maternal and infant outcomes. *Cochrane Database Systemic Review*. 2009; 15, (2): CD006914.
71. Allen K, Golden LH, Izzo JL. Normalization of Hypertensive Responses During Ambulatory Surgical Stress by Perioperative Music. *Psychosomatic Medicine*. 2001; 63: 487-492.
72. Fernell J. Listening to music during ambulatory ophthalmic surgery reduced blood pressure, heart rate, and perceived stress. *Evidence Based Nursing*. 2002; 1 (5): 16-26.
73. Reilly MP. *Music, a cognitive behavioural intervention for anxiety and acute pain control in the elderly cataract patient*. San Antonio: Dissertation Faculty of the University of Texas Graduate School of Biomedical Sciences; 1999.
74. McCaffrey RG. The Effect of Music on Cognition of Older Adults Undergoing Hip and Knee Surgery. *Music and Medicine*. 2009; 1 (1): 22-28.
75. Siedlecki SL. Racial variation in response to music in a sample of african-american and caucasian chronic pain patients. *Journal of Pain Management in Nursing*. 2009; 10 (1): 14-21.
76. Silvestrini N, Piguet V, Zentner MR. Music and Auditory Distraction Reduce Pain - Emotional or Attentional Effects? *Music and Medicine*. 2011; 3(4): 264-270.
77. Canga B, Hahm CL, Lucido D, Grossbard ML, Loewy JV. Environmental Music therapy - A Pilot Study on the Effects of Music Therapy in a chemotherapy Infusion Suite. *Music and Medicine*. 2012; 4(4): 221-230.
78. Clements-Cortes A. Portraits of Music Therapy in Facilitating Relationship Completion at the End of Life. *Music and Medicine*. 2011; 3(1): 31-39.

79. Dun B. All in Good Times: A Music Therapists Reflection of Providing a Music Therapy Program in a Pediatric Cancer Center Over 20 Years. *Music and Medicine.* 2011; 3(1): 15-19.
80. Krout RE. The effects of single-session music therapy interventions on the observed and self-reported levels of pain control, physical comfort, and relaxation of hospice patients. *American Journal of Hospice and Palliative Medicine.* 2001; 18 (6): 383-390.
81. Magill L, O'Callaghan C. Music therapy and Supportive Cancer Care. *Special Issue, Music and Medicine.* 2011; 3(1).
82. DeMarco J, Alexander JL, Nehrenz G, Gallagher L. The Benefit of Music for the REduction of Stress and Anxiety in Patients Undergoing Elective Cosmetic Surgery. Music and Medicine. 2012; 4(1): 44-48.
83. Good M, Stanton-Hicks M, Grass JA, Anderson GC, Choi C, Schoolmeesters LJ, Salman A. Relief of postoperative pain with jaw relaxation, music, and their combination. PAIN. 1999; 81: 163-172.
84. Leard R. Randomized clinical trial examining the effect of music therapy in stress response to day surgery. *British Journal of Surgery.* 2007; 94 (8): 943-947.
85. Nilsson U, Unosson M, Rawal N. Stress reduction and analgesia in patients exposed to calming music postoperatively: a randomized controlled trial. *European Journal of Anaesthesiology.* 2005; 22 (2): 96-102.
86. Bradt J. The Effects of Music Entrainment on Postoperative Pain Perception in Pediatric Patients. *Music and Medicine.* 2010; 2(3): 150-157.
87. Gross MAF, Nager W, Schalk F, Piepenbrock SA, Münte TF, Münte S. Unbewußte Wahrnehmung bei Patienten im Operationssaal unter Allgemeinanaesthesie[Unconscious awareness in patients with general anaesthesia]. *Anaesthesiologie Intensivmedizin Notfallmedizin Schmerztherapie AINS.* 2003; 11(43): 755.
88. Nilsson U, Rawal N, Unosson M. A comparison of intraoperative or postoperative exposure to music – a controlled trial of the effects on postoperative pain. *Anaesthesia.* 2003; 58(7): 699-703.
89. Kölsch S, Heinke W, Sammler D, Olthoff D. Auditory processing during deep propofol sedation and recovery from unconsciousness. *Clinical Neurophysiology.* 2006; 117(8): 1750-1759.
90. Rider MS. Entrainment mechanisms are involved in pain reduction, muscle relaxation, and music-mediated imagery. *Journal of Music Therapy.* 1985; 22: 183-192.
91. Koepchen HP, Droh R, Spintge R, Abel HH, Kluessendorf D, Koralewski E. Physiological rhythmicity and music in medicine. In:

Spintge R, Droh R eds. *MusicMedicine vol1*. Saint Louis: MMB; 1992: 39–70.
92. Thaut MH. *Rhythm, music, and the brain*. New York, N.Y.: Routhledge; 2005.
93. Avanzini G, Lopez L, Koelsch S, Majno M. *The Neurosciences and Music vol 2. From Perception to Performance*. New York, NY: Annals of the New York Academy of Sciences. 2005: 1060.
94. Bernardi L, Porta C, Balsamo R, Bernardi NF, Sleight P. Dynamic interactions between musical, cardiovascular, and cerebral rhythms in humans. Circulation. 2009; 22.
95. Cook ND. The Sound Symbolism of Major and Minor Harmonies. Music Perception. 2007; 24 (3): 315–319.
96. Cook ND, Hayashi T. Die Biologie des Wohlklangs (The Biology of Harmonics). *Spektrum der Wissenschaft*. 2009; 3: 64 – 70.
97. Gomez P, Danuser B. Relationships between musical structure and psychophysiological measures of emotion. *Emotion*. 2007; 7/2: 377-387.
98. Standley JM. Music Research in Medical/Dental Treatment: Meta-Analysis and Clinical Applications. *Journal of Music Therapy*. 1986; 23: 56-122.
99. Thompson JF, Kam PC Music in the operating theatre. *British Journal of Surgery*. 1995; 82: 1586-1587.
100. Standley JM. A meta-analysis of the efficacy of music therapy for premature infants. *Journal of Pediatric Nursing*. 2002; 17: 107-113.
101. Dileo C. *A meta-analysis of the literature in medical music therapy and MusicMedicine with an agenda for future research*. Volume of Abstracts VIII. International Symposium for Music in Medicine of the International Society of Music in Medicine. Hamburg: ISMM; 2003: 100-101.
102. Pelletier C. The effect of music on decreasing arousal due to stress: A meta-analysis. *Journal of Music Therapy*. 2004; 41: 192-214.
103. Hilliard RE. Music therapy in hospice and paliative care. A review of the empirical data. *Evidence-Based Complementary and Alternative Medicine*. 2005; 2: 173-178.
104. Cepeda MS, Carr DB, Lau J, Alvarez H. Music for pain relief. *The Cochrane Database Systematic Reviews*. 2006; 2.
105. Bradt J, Dileo Ch. Music for people with coronary heart disease. *Cochrane Database of Systematic Reviews*. 2007; 3: CD006577.
106. Goodman O, Sims E. *State of the Field Report: Arts in Healthcare*. State of the Field Committee. Washington, DC: Society for the Arts in Healthcare; 2009.

107. Romo R, Gilford L. A Cost-Benefit Analysis of Music Therapy in a Home Hospice. *Nursing Econoimics*. 2007; 25(6): 353-358.
108. Walworth D. Procedural-support music therapy in the healthcare setting: A cost-effectiveness analysis. *Journal of Pediatric Nursing*. 2005; 20(4): 276 – 284.
109. DeLoach D. Procedural-support Music Therapy in the Healthcare Setting: A cost-Effectiveness Analysis. *Journal of Pediatric Nursing*. 2005; 20 (4): 276-284.
110. Pölkki T, Vehviläinen-Julkunen K, Pietilä AM. Nonpharmacological methods in relieving children's postoperative pain: A survey on hospital nurses in Finland. *Journal of Advanced Nursing*. 2001; 34(4): 483–492.
111. Mathur A, Duda L, Kamat DM. Knowledge and Use of Music Therapy Among Pediatric Practitioners in Michigan. *Clinical Pediatrics*. 2008; 4 (2): 15-159.
112. MacDonald RAR, Kreutz G, Mitchell L. *Music, Health, and Wellbeing*. Oxford: Oxford University Press; 2012.
113. Spintge R, Loewy JV. At a Crossroads: Big Questions - Little Knowledge in Achievements, With Issues of Translation. *Music and Medicine*. 2011; 3/4: 209-211.
114. Trevena LJ, Davey HM, Barratt A, Butow P, Caldwell P. A systematic review on communicating with patients about evidence. *Journal Evaluation Clinical Practice*. 2006; 12: 13-23.
115. Spintge R. *Selbsthilfe bei Verspannungsschmerz [Help Yourself in Myofascial Pain]*. A Handbook and Audio Program. Hamburg: Universal Music - Polymedia; 1998.
116. Spintge R. *Selbsthilfe zur Stressbewältigung [Help Yourself against Stress]*. A Handbook and Audio Program. Hamburg: Universal Music -Polymedia; 1998.
117. Spintge R. *Selbsthilfe bei Schlafförderung [Help Yourself to Sleep]*. A Handbook and Audio Program. Hamburg: Universal Music - Polymedia; 1999.
118. Westen D. Clinical Assessment of Object Relations Using the TAT. *Journal of Personality Assessment*. 1991; 56(1): 56-74.
119. Spintge R. MusicMedicine: Applications, Standards, and Definitions. In: Pratt R R, Grocke D. eds. *MusicMedicine vol 3*. Melbourne: University of Melbourne Press; 1999: 3-11.
120. Spintge R. Musik im Gesundheitswesen [Music in Healthcare]. Schwäbisch Gmünd - Skt.Augustin: Asgard GEK Edition; 2007.

CHAPTER 3

Music Therapy for Pain Management[*]

Suzanne B. Hanser EdD, MT-BC
Susan E. Mandel PhD, MT-BC

*"I have been looking for a tool
to use as an antidote for pain and tension.
Music is a wonderful choice.
It makes me feel more secure and optimistic.
I truly believe it will help me."*
Barbara, 55 years old

Music for pain? Surely such a benign modality could not be much of a panacea. But perhaps we take music for granted. After all, it is everywhere—from grocery stores to elevators—and these days we can hear almost anything we like on radio, iPods, mp3s, YouTube, and the latest digital media. Most of us are fully aware of the impact of music on mood and emotion, but can music help us feel better?[2] Actually, research has demonstrated that music can reduce opioid requirements, and that postoperative pain may be lessened.[1] In a Cochrane Review conducted by Cepeda et al, investigators examined the effect of music on acute, chronic, or cancer pain intensity; pain relief; and analgesic requirements.[1] Of the 51 studies evaluated, four studies reported that subjects exposed to music had a 70% higher likelihood of having pain relief than unexposed subjects (95% CI: 1.21 to 2.37). In three studies evaluating opioid requirements 2 hours after surgery, subjects exposed to music required 1.0 mg (18.4%) less morphine (95% CI: -2.0 to -0.2) than unexposed subjects. Additionally, in five studies assessing analgesic requirements 24 hours post-surgery, the music group required 5.7 mg (15.4%) less morphine than the unexposed group (95% CI: -8.8 to -2.6) (1).

---

[*] This article first appeared in *Practical Pain Management*, and is reprinted with permission from Music Therapy in Pain Management. *Pract Pain Manage*. 2012, Volume 12, Issue 5, pgs. 16-20. © 2012 Vertical Health Media, LCC.

In addition, music therapists have designed clinical protocols that are effective in helping people manage different forms of pain. Part of the music therapist's job is to help people find the music that is significant to them so the patient can use this music in a specific, functional way to help cope with stress and pain. Music therapists teach people to fully listen to that music and also to listen to the effect that the music has on many aspects of their whole selves. These non-traditional therapists show people how to create music and engage the brain actively so the perception of pain is overcome by multiple sources on multiple levels. Some interventional techniques that may be used by music therapists in pain management include singing, playing instruments, rhythmic-based activities, improvisation, composing/ songwriting, and listening to music.[2]

A person is more than a sum of individual parts. Thoughts, emotions, and sensations are interconnected parts of the human condition, and one's entire self is affected when in pain. Whether chronic or acute, pain is exacerbated by stress and anxiety. Thus, the most effective pain management strategies are holistic, taking into account the body, mind, and spirit. Music is a unique component of holistic pain management because the influence of music is felt on physical, mental, emotional, and spiritual levels (Table 1). Music therapists are privileged to work with the power of music to transform the perception of pain and the experience of suffering. In this review, we highlight five different patient cases where music therapy was effectively used to help manage signs and symptoms associated with various pain-related illnesses and procedures.

Table 1. Positive Characteristics of Music Therapy*
- Acts upon the brain's limbic system—specifically the nucleus accumbens, which is part of the brain's "pleasure center"—and has generalized/widespread effects
- Helps activate self-repair mechanisms throughout the body and brain, promoting healing and mental health
- Can be used to supplant or reduce the use of pharmaceuticals, reducing the cost of medical care
- Can be easily incorporated into multimodal pain management programs due to few side effects *based on Reference 3

Cancer Treatment

Anxiety has been shown to frequently exacerbate the perception of pain. Reducing this emotion prior to any pain-inducing procedures improves patients' quality of life.[3] In a study conducted by Bradt et al comparing the effects of music therapy plus standard care versus the effects of standard care alone, results suggested that music interventions may have a beneficial effect on anxiety in patients with cancer.[4] Investigators reported an average anxiety reduction of 11.20 units (P=0.009) on the State-Trait Anxiety Inventory Scale and -0.61 standardized units (P=0.0007) on other anxiety scales.[4]

When 55-year-old Barbara was diagnosed with metastatic breast cancer, she sought treatment to deal with a constellation of fear, anxiety, depression, and physical pain. In music therapy, she found a coping tool to help. Barbara wrote in her pain journal: "I had to go up for a blood test, which was particularly distressing to me. I had been having repeated problems with the test and had been overly emotional about having it again. I was in tears as the nurse tried over and over to get my vein. She asked me to take a deep breath, but I knew that wouldn't help. Without even thinking, my brain must have automatically felt that music would help me. I found myself singing to myself in my head ... The music sounded so loud and powerful that I could not focus on the blood test and the singing at the same time. The music won, the test was over, and I was *thrilled* to realize that I had found a tool to help me with these procedures. I have tried it on a few other occasions, and it has been successful for me, even with other songs."[5]

Barbara's strong sensory engagement while singing, and the concomitant positive affect and emotion, contributed to her ability to block the sensation of pain.

Spine Surgery

Barbara is not alone. Here are words from Susan's journal that describe her experience of listening to music through spine surgery:

"Through 30 years of undergoing spine surgeries and medical procedures, I have experienced the power of music to comfort, to distract, to accompany, and to allow my feelings. Prior to my most recent operation, I prepared playlists on my mp3 player. The topics ranged from Broadway to spiritual music, from light opera to music-assisted relaxation and imagery. In the days preceding the surgery, I listened to relaxing music to ease my anxiety. On the morning before surgery, my mother died. I needed my music more than ever before.

Immediately after donning the hospital gown on the morning of surgery, I put on my headset and let the music play. Listening to 'Defying Gravity' from *Wicked* allowed me to escape the surgical waiting area and travel to the fantastical world of *Wicked* where a person can fly above the pain. 'The Prayer,' sung by Josh Groban and Charlotte Church, led me to a place—oceanside—where I felt safe. As the anesthesiologist inserted the intravenous needle, I was guided by music-assisted imagery and did not feel the prick. My deep state of relaxation removed any resistance that might have impeded the procedure.

As I was wheeled into the operating room, I felt my mother's spirit present with me and eased into a gentle sleep, listening to familiar sounds of Daniel Kobialka's soothing music based on classical themes. The music remained with me throughout the 4-hour procedure, and my first awareness upon waking in the recovery room was the sweet sound of music. I felt calm, comforted, and present. I knew the surgery was complete before I could speak. I recognized the sounds of John Barry's music from movie soundtracks, which I had pre- selected to help me rouse in the recovery room. The music was less sedative than the music to which I listened before and during the surgery.

Although a pain pump had been inserted, I was reluctant to push the button to release the medication into my bloodstream. For me, opioids are a two-edged sword. Though they may relieve the sharp edge of pain, they adversely impact my gastrointestinal system and I find that discomfort far more difficult to bear. Surgical pain is reflective of healing, so I listened to music and allowed myself to remain in a calm, protected zone. My mind was filled with thoughts of gratitude, relief, and hope. I knew that the worst of my ordeal was behind me. After a 5-day stay in the hospital, I returned home to my own bed and eased into a sound sleep with my headset and music right beside me—waiting to be listened to.

A few weeks after my mother's funeral, I hesitantly sang my first notes. My spirit soared as I sang: '*Wake up, bestir yourself, it's time that you disinter yourself. You've got a spot to fill, a pot to fill. And what a gift package of shower, sun, and love, you'll be met above everywhere with*'.[6] [Lyrics are from the musical, 'On a Clear Day You Can See Forever.'] That gift package is also filled with music."

When Susan closed her eyes and concentrated on her music, she immediately discovered pleasant memories and positive associations. The music evoked beautiful imagery that offered the sense of calm and peace that she sought at a time of extreme distress. Anticipatory anxiety prior to surgery was dispelled when relaxing music flooded her brain with positive affect, hopeful thoughts, and sensory stimulation involving all her senses. Susan then had a conditioned relaxation response to the musical selections that accompanied her during surgery. All she had to do was turn on the music to evoke a state of mind exuding beauty and peacefulness.

According to Bernatzky et al, the fear and dread of pain caused by an impending surgical procedure pro-mote suffering. Negative emotions, such as anxiety prior to surgery and pain after surgery, can be successfully alleviated through the use of music therapy.[3]

Waking from anesthesia can be disorienting and traumatic, but Susan was spared an introduction to consciousness through the mechanical sounds of medical equipment in the recovery room, and she was treated to familiar music that could immediately soothe. Singing during the weeks following surgery brought another dimension to Susan's recovery. Her positive psychological attitude was supported by listening to, and singing her favorite songs. The physical requirements of singing necessitated taking deep, healing breaths, while the process of singing songs with strong, positive messages comforted her through the days of pain and loss.

Cardiac Illness

George underwent coronary artery bypass graft surgery. He learned to manage his pain and stress by listening to a recording that blended the music therapist's spoken voice with music that George identified as relaxing.

"By the end of the time, you feel very, very calm and just very relaxed. [Music therapy] relaxes [the] physical body [and] slows down thinking, too. Getting a chance to just stay in one spot and listen to something that's slower and wants you to relax, tries to help you relax, makes a big difference."[7]

Many people living with cardiac illness cope with ongoing pain, stress, and anxiety about the future. A randomized controlled trial involving 68 individuals enrolled in a cardiac rehabilitation program found that music therapy improved regulation of blood pressure, decreased stress and anxiety, and improved selected quality of life measures. Music therapy interventions included playing and listening to live music as well as learning techniques to evoke the relaxation response.[8] These techniques involved strategies that could be practiced at home. Compliance with these methods was high, and participants learned that they could take control of their blood pressure using a benign and enjoyable activity.

Childbirth

Meredith was in labor with her first child. As a participant in a research experiment that investigated the impact of music listening on pain-related outcomes, Meredith prepared her playlist of favorite songs, meaningful melodies, and music that was associated with good times in her life.[9] The music therapist then categorized these pieces into slow, medium, and fast tempi, and asked Meredith to simulate the experience of having a 60-second contraction while breathing to her specially selected music. Beginning with the slow music, Meredith rehearsed listening while she closed her eyes and imagined a beautiful, healthy baby. Next, she practiced a gradually faster pace of breathing, while hearing music of a slightly faster tempo. Here she focused her attention on making different sounds, like "hoo" and "hee," as she emphasized her exhalation along with the rhythmic cue provided by the music. Finally, she listened to the fastest, most energetic music with strong beats and an easy rhythm to follow. She breathed directly with the music, as she prepared for the transition stage of labor, the most arduous time immediately before the birth of the baby.

As part of the experimental protocol, Meredith listened to her music for the duration of 10 contractions, and then discontinued the music for the next 5 contractions, followed by 10 contractions with more music, then 5 without music, and so on, throughout labor. The music therapist observed pain-related behaviors during these contractions, consisting of vocalizations of pain, requests for medication, and obvious signs of tension in body parts (eg, clenched jaw or fist, flexed feet, or raised shoulders). These pain-related behaviors were documented, and an average number was calculated so that they could be compared across conditions of music versus no music. Meredith and the six other research participants in this experiment emitted fewer pain-related responses during the periods of music listening than when no music was playing (range of 3 to 30 fewer pain responses with a mean of 12).[9] This study was, thus, instrumental in demonstrating the impact of music as a focus of attention during episodes of acute pain, and identifying the potential of music as an "auditory focal point" akin to the "visual focal point" recommended as an efficacious methodology for managing the contractions of childbirth.

End of Life

At the other end of the life cycle, Jay was dying of brain cancer. In what was to be his final hours of life, the music therapist visited his bedside with the hope of providing some comfort to Jay and members of his family who were standing vigil through his ordeal. The music therapist began playing a Native American flute, while breathing along with Jay's shallow gasps and irregular breathing rhythm. She alternated between long, flowing phrases and short, punctuated breaths that matched Jay's. Slowly, she stretched the musical notes and lines into extended melodies. Jay's oncologist, who was witnessing this scene, noted an elongation in the pattern of Jay's breathing, and a relaxation of his muscles.

Whether or not the sounds of the flute were responsible for Jay's response, family members reacted to the mood inspired by the flute, and expressed their gratitude for the peaceful atmosphere that accompanied Jay's passing. This "entrainment" of breathing, rhythm, and tempo was another tool in the music therapist's repertoire to gently guide Jay and his surrounding family to a more relaxed way of breathing and of being.

Conclusion

In these examples, music, whether heard passively or along with guided imagery, had an impact not only on the senses, but also on perception, and the perception of pain, in particular. Music, sung or performed, was able to serve as a source of concentration for people experiencing various types of pain. The key for most was identifying music that resonated with their needs, like Barbara's powerful song, Susan's meaningful musical selections, George's relaxing music and imagery, and the pieces that guided Meredith's and Jay's breathing. These cases were meant to inspire the use of music listening, singing, and other musical activities to help manage the signs and symptoms associated with pain[10] and it is the hope of the authors that this simple, cost-effective medium will be helpful to individuals who are coping with different sorts of discomfort and pain. In the case of music, there are few side effects and there is much creative potential to heal.

References

1. Cepeda MS, Carr DB, Lau J, Alvarez H. Music for pain relief. *Cochrane Database Syst Rev.* 2006(2):CD004843.
2. World Federation of Music Therapy. FAQ music therapy. http://www.wfmt.info/WFMT/FAQ_Music Therapy.html. Accessed April 30, 2012.
3. Bernatzky G, Presch M, Anderson M, Panksepp J. Emotional-Foundations of music as a non-pharmacological pain management tool in modern medicine. *Neurosci Biobehav Rev.* 2011;35(9):1989-1999.
4. Bradt J, Dileo C, Grocke D, Magill L. Music inter- ventions for improving psychological and physical outcomes in cancer patients. *Cochrane Database Syst Rev.* 2011(8):CD006911.
5. Hanser SB. Music therapy to enhance coping in terminally ill adult cancer patients. In: Dileo C, Loewy JV, eds. *Music Therapy at the End of Life.* Cherry Hill, NJ: Jeffrey Books; 2005:33-42.
6. Lerner A, Lane B. Hurry! It's lovely up here. In: Walters R, editor. *The Singer's Musical Theatre Anthology Volume 5: Mezzo-Soprano.* Milwaukee, WI: Hal Leonard; 2008:188-193.
7. Mandel SE, Hanser SB, Ryan LJ. Effects of music- assisted relaxation and imagery on health-related outcomes in cardiac rehabilitation. *Music Ther Perspect.* 2010;28(1):11-21.

8. Mandel SE, Hanser SB, Secic M, Davis BA. Effects of music therapy on health-related outcomes in cardiac rehabilitation: a randomized controlled trial. *J Music Ther.* 2007;44(3):176-197.
9. Hanser SB, Larson SC, O'Connell AS. The Effect of Music on Relaxation of Expectant Mothers During Labor. *J Music Ther.* 1983;22(2):50-58.
10. Hanser SB, Mandel SE. *Manage Your Stress and Pain Through Music.* Boston, MA: Berklee Press; 2010.

CHAPTER 4

Ethical and Cultural Issues in Music Therapy for Pain Management

Cheryl Dileo PhD, MT-BC

*"May I never see in the patient anything
but a fellow creature in pain[1]"*
Oath of Maimonides

Although there are ethical issues common to a range of music therapy practices, there are ethical concerns specific to the use of music therapy for pain management. The purpose of this chapter is to present several ethical challenges that occur when using music therapy to treat persons in pain. Although it is not possible to present a comprehensive coverage of this topic within the limits of one chapter, ethical concerns are presented according to the standard ethical principles of autonomy, beneficence, and nonmaleficence. The impact of culture is emphasized within each of these principles.

In essence, persons who are in pain have a self-evident right to be free from unnecessary pain and suffering. At the same time, those providing treatment for the patient in pain have ethical obligations to avoid causing pain to the patient (more than what is necessary for diagnoses or treatment), and to use every means, based on available knowledge and resources, to alleviate pain to the greatest extent possible. These obligations should be executed only according to the wishes of the patient who provides informed consent.[2(p517)]

Autonomy

In practice, acting autonomously "requires independence from undue or controlling influence and cognitive capacity to make rational decisions."[3(p148)] Although a patient's autonomy is a primary concern for music therapists and other healthcare professionals, there are a number of factors that may inadvertently minimize the freedom of the pain patient to exercise self-determination.

Autonomy is a culture-bound phenomenon. The emphasis placed on autonomy in the United States is consistent with its dominant individualist culture[4]; this emphasis is seen in healthcare in the requisite practice of informed consent, the concept of advanced directives[5] and the Patient Self-Determination Act.[6] However, not all cultures value autonomy in a way similar to the dominant culture. For example, the choice of the patient to relinquish decision-making and allow a family member to make his or her healthcare decisions may still represent an autonomous act. In a similar manner, a patient's trusting of the knowledge of his or her physician to make the healthcare decision may also represent self-determination. To force a patient to act otherwise may be a violation of his or her autonomy.[7]

Intense and/or unrelenting pain may compromise or impair a patient's ability to provide true informed consent for treatment and to adequately ascertain a treatment's risks and benefits. The consumption of high doses of pain medication may interfere with the patient's judgment. At the same time, taking narcotic drugs may increase the patient's exercise of true autonomy if withholding consent for a particular treatment might jeopardize his supply of analgesics. Conversely, the patient also may be readily coerced to provide informed consent to treatment that is inconsistent with his or her will if this consent will ensure access to needed pain medication.[3]

In addition to optimizing patients' autonomy to decide if they will engage in music therapy treatment, it is also essential to allow patients to decide how they prefer to cope with their pain both within and outside of the music therapy session.[8]

There are numerous ways in which individuals cope with (i.e., are predisposed to react to) acute and/or chronic pain; these ways of coping may be culturally determined. Coping styles may be categorized as active or passive with regard to the pain, may involve approaching or avoiding the pain, or may be problem-focused or emotion focused. Not all coping styles have positive outcomes for the patient; some may exacerbate the pain experience. Thus, the music therapist is challenged to offer music therapy strategies that are consistent with the patient's coping preferences and that also help the patient to achieve positive outcomes, i.e., reduce the pain.[8]

Beneficence and Nonmaleficence

"Beneficence or 'doing good' for others stems from the Hippocratic Oath and implies the responsibility to actively help others according to what is in their best interest and welfare.[4(p7)]" Beneficence implies doing good over and above avoiding harm.[3] Nonmaleficence implies "the responsibility to avoid at all costs intentional or unintentional harm or injury through either a specific action or neglect."[4(p7)]

Failing to do good or causing harm may result from a number of factors. It is clear that music therapists cannot always provide pain relief to all of their patients. However, providing a music therapy intervention that does not have the potential to help the patient may be considered unethical.[3]

An important issue for music therapists in "doing good" for their patients is competence in the music therapy treatment they provide. There are a number of music therapy techniques used in pain management, and these strategies can be categorized into various levels of a hierarchy corresponding to: 1) the therapeutic goal or intent, 2) how specific or comprehensive the technique may be, 3) the coping preferences of the patient, 4) the position of the patient in relationship to the pain, and 5) the skill and training required of the therapist.[8]

For example, for the category at the bottom and most basic level of the hierarchy, "Distraction/Refocusing," the intent of interventions is to engage either actively or passively the patient's attention in a music activity, thereby diverting his attention away from the pain and reducing the amount of pain he experiences. A range of active and passive music therapy strategies may be used at this level, and entry-level training may be sufficient to ensure the competence of the therapist.[8]

At the top of the hierarchy, the intent of interventions in the "transformational," category is to support the patient in a music experience that involves an interaction with or entrance into the pain.[8] Specialized, advanced training is required for the therapist to be competent at this level of practice, for example in using the Bonny Method of Guided Imagery and Music[9] or the process of music therapy entrainment.[10] A list of advanced competencies for music therapy interventions in pain management have been suggested by Dileo and Loewy.[11]

Perhaps the most common form of "failing to do good or causing harm" in pain management is the undertreatment or inadequate treatment of pain, known as oligoanalgesia.[12] This problem has been noted in pediatric pain patients and caused by caregivers' inadequate understanding of the pediatric pain experience as well as their fears of inhibiting respiration and contributing to addiction.[13-15] Oligoanalgesia is associated with a range of negative and potentially devastating consequences for this population.

Pain, Culture and Oligoanalgesia

The problem of oligoanalgesia is common to other populations of pain patients besides pediatrics and is compounded by issues of race, culture, gender, age, and socioeconomic status.[12,14]

"Pain is a culturally defined physiological and psychological experience." Calister,[16(p207)] According to the Biocultural Model of Pain[17,18] neurophysiological mechanisms of pain perception are similar among all persons, regardless of ethnic background. However, social/cultural learning influences psychological and physical factors and may affect how pain is perceived and modulated. Thus, the way an individual reacts to, expresses and copes with pain is highly influenced by culture.[19,20]

There are a number of cultural factors that influence an individual's experience and expression of pain. The meaning of pain, as culturally determined, may contribute to how much pain can be tolerated. Also, cultures vary according to the language available for the expression and description of pain. In some languages, there are many terms for pain; in other languages, there are fewer words available to classify pain. Thus, the reporting and description of an individual's pain may be limited or enhanced by the words available.[19]

Religion and/or spirituality also play a key role in determining the meaning a person ascribes to pain, as well as how one copes.[8] In addition, these beliefs may inhibit a person's willingness to discuss pain or seek appropriate treatment.[21]

Although cultural factors influence individuals' perception and expression of pain, a patient's culture is also associated with differential treatment of their pain. There are major disparities in pain treatment based on race, ethnicity, socioeconomic status, gender and age for all types of pain in all settings.[5,22,23] Many examples of this phenomenon exist in the literature. For example, there are differences in the provision of pain medication based on ethnicity.[23] There is evidence also of untimely and inadequate treatment of pain for elderly individuals[24] and also for older and minority persons with cancer.[25] Moreover, minority individuals may have less adequate pain assessments than those in the majority culture, and the pain issues of women and elderly patients may be treated less aggressively than those of male and younger patients.[22,26,27]

Patient factors may also contribute to disparities in pain management among ethnic and racial groups. For example, in these groups there may be a lesser degree of treatment compliance as well as a delay in seeking treatment,[22,28] potentially due to a mistrust of white medical staff, a negative history with the healthcare system and/or inadequate health literacy.[22,29]

Countertransference Issues among Therapists Working with Persons in Pain

Perhaps the most disturbing factors in the inadequate or undertreatment of pain are differences in perceptions of patients' pain among medical staff, attributed to stereotypes, lack of empathy, stigma, blatant discrimination or poor cross-cultural communication skills.[22,29,30] Also, the cultures of members of the medical staff may contribute to this equation. For example, nurses of different cultures were found to vary in a substantive manner in their perceptions of patients' pain.[31]

Chronic pain patients, especially those on long-term opioid treatment, are often at risk for stigmatization by medical staff and the public in general. As these patients may also have concomitant substance abuse and behavioral issues, they may be viewed as "burdens" on the system and subject to receiving inadequate care.[21] It has been suggested that there may be misconceptions or lack of information among medical professionals regarding opioid tolerance and addiction, opioid side effects, and pain vs. disease severity in opioid treatment.[32,33]

The music therapist's ability or inability to empathize with pain in a way that is beneficial to the patient and safe for the therapist is a major ethical issue in pain treatment. Training and supervision are crucial in ensuring that the therapist is able to empathize in a way that is meaningful but without loss of the therapist's boundaries. Awareness of boundaries is of particular importance for the therapist who uses advanced music therapy approaches, such as music therapy entrainment.[10]

The therapist's awareness of his or her own coping style regarding pain and the ability to be open to other coping styles requested by the patient is critical so that the therapist does not impose his or her own beliefs about managing pain onto the patient.

Conclusions and Recommendations

Music therapy for pain management has unique areas of ethical concern, in addition to the potential ethical issues common to all types of music therapy practices. Upholding the core ethical principles of autonomy, beneficence and maleficence requires the therapist to be aware of his or her competence according to the level of music therapy intervention used and to seek additional training and supervision for implementation of interventions beyond the therapist's knowledge and skill level. The therapist must exercise caution with the use of new or untested music therapy approaches so as not to risk causing additional pain for the patient.

Therapists must also be particularly sensitive to issues that may diminish the patient's autonomy in consenting to treatment, including extreme vulnerability, coercive factors and also preferences for coping with the pain. The therapist should have the competence to adapt music therapy to the patient's preferred ways of coping with pain to achieve a positive outcome.

Patients' cultural factors (age, ethnicity, race, etc.) may predispose them to increased vulnerability and inadequate or undertreatment of their pain. Thus, music therapy assessment should take into account cultural issues that may impact on clients' expression of pain, including their religion, spirituality, meaning of the pain, and specific language for the pain. Music therapists must commit to ongoing education and supervision regarding the cultural factors that may compromise appropriate treatment for the patient, exercise sensitive self-awareness of potential cultural biases and stereotypes, understand how their own cultural backgrounds influence their perceptions of their patients' pain, and understand how their own pain history and reactions to pain may affect their ability to provide empathic and non-imposing treatment.

Music therapists must strive to remove barriers to the establishment of trusting relationships with their patients in pain and work diligently in understanding as accurately as possible their patients' reports of pain. Moreover, as members of the treatment team, music therapists should continually advocate for appropriate and adequate treatment for all of their patients. To do less than this is to cause additional suffering, loss of dignity, discrimination, and alienation of the most vulnerable among us.

References

1. Maimonides M. Oath of Maimonides. Translated by Harr Friedenwald. (1917).*Bull Johns Hopkins Hosp 28*: 260-261.
2. Edwards RB. Pain and the ethics of pain management. *Soc Sci Mrd.* 1984; IX(6):515, 523.
3. Taylor ML. Ethical issues for psychologists in pain management. *Pain Med.* 2001;2(2): 147-154.
4. Dileo C. *Ethical thinking in music therapy*. Cherry Hill, NJ: Jeffrey Books; 2000.
5. Werth JL Jr.,Blevins D, Toussaint KL,Durham MR. The influence of cultural diversity on end-of-life care and decisions. *Am Behav Sci.* 2002; 46(2): 204-219.
6. Omnibus Budget Reconciliation Act of 1990, Pub.L.No.101-508, §§ 4206 and 4751, 104 Stat.1388, 1388-115, and 1388-204 (classified respectively at 42 U.S.C. 1395cc(f) and 1396a(w)(1994)).
7. Ersek M, Kagawa-Singer M, Barnes D, Blackhall L,Koenig BA. Multicultural considerations in the use of advance directives. *Oncol Nurs Forum.* 1998;25: 1683-1690.
8. Dileo C. Cultures of pain: A meta-perspective on decision-making in music therapy. Paper presented at the Integrative Models of Pain Conference, Beth Israel Medicine Center, January, 2012.
9. Bruscia K, Grocke DE. *Guided imagery and music: the Bonny Method and beyond.* Gilsum, NH: Barcelona Publishers; 2002.
10. Dileo C. Reflections on medical music therapy: Biopsychoscial perspectives of the treatment process. In: Loewy JV, ed. *Music Therapy in Pediatric Pain*. Cherry Hill, NJ: Jeffrey Books; 1997: 125-144.

11. Dileo C, Loewy J. Advanced music therapy training in end-of-life care. In: Dileo C, Loewy JV, eds. *Music Therapy at the End of Life*. Cherry hill, NJ: Jeffrey Books; 2005:259-274.
12. Popenhagen MP. Undertreatment of pain and fears of addiction in pediatric chronic pain patients: How do we stop the problem? *JSPN.*2006;11(1):61-67.
13. Walco G, Cassidy R, Schechter N. Pain, hurt and harm: The ethics of pain control in infants and children. In: Loewy JV, ed. *Music Therapy in Pediatric Pain*. Cherry Hill, NJ: Jeffrey Books; 1997: 23-32.
14. Rupp T, Delaney KA . Inadequate analgesia in emergency medicine. *Ann Emerg Med.*2004; 43(4): 494–503.
15. Wolfe J, Grier HE, Klar N. et al. Symptoms and suffering at the end of life in children with cancer. *N Engl J Med*. 2000;342:326–333.
16. Calister LC. Cultural influences on pain perceptions and behaviors. *Home Health Care Manage Pract*. 2003;15(3):207-211.
17. Bates MS. Ethnicity and pain: A biocultural model. *Soc. Sci. Med.* 1987; 24,(1):47-50.
18. Bates MS. Chronic pain: theories and research and treatment approaches. In: Bates MS, ed. Biocultural Dimensions of Chronic Pain: Implications for Treatment of Multi-Ethnic Populations. Albany, NY: Suny Press; 1996:7-22.
19. Al-Atiyyat NMH. Cultural diversity and cancer pain. *J Hosp Palliat Nurs*. 2009;11(3): 154-164.
20. Zborowski M. Cultural components in response to pain. *J Soc Issues*. 1952;8:16-30.
21. McGee SJ, Kaylor BD, Emmott H, Christopher MJ. Defining Chronic Pain Ethics. *Pain Med.* 2011; 12: 1376–1384.
22. Green C, Todd KN, Lebovits A, Francis M.Disparities in Pain: Ethical Issues. *Pain Med.* 2006; 7 (6): 530-533.
23. Todd KH, Samaroo N, Hoffman, J.R. Ethnicity as a risk factor for inadequate emergency department analgesia. *JAMA*. 1993; 269: 1537-1539.
24. Jones JS, Johnson K, McNinch M. Age as a risk factor for inadequate emergency department analgesia. *Am J Emerg Med*. 1996;14: 157-160.
25. Bernabei, R., Gambassi, G., Lapane, K., Landi, F., Gatsonis, C., Dunlop, R., et al. (1998). Management of pain in elderly patients with cancer. *JAMA*. 1998; 279: 1877-1882.
26. Bonham VL. Race, ethnicity, and pain treatment: Striving to understand the causes and solutions to the disparities in pain treatment. *J Law Med Ethics*. 2001;29:52–68.

27. Green CR, Anderson KO, Baker TA, et al. The unequal burden of pain: Confronting racial and ethnic disparities in pain. *Pain Med.* 2003;4: 277–94.
28. Blanchard J, Lurie N. R-E-S-P-E-C-T: Patient reports of disrespect in the health care setting and its impact on care. *J Fam Pract* 2004; 53(9): 721–30.
29. Betancourt JR, Green AR, Carrillo JE, Ananeh-Firempong O 2nd. Defining cultural competence: A practical framework for addressing racial/ethnic disparities in health and health care. *Public Health Rep.* 2003;118(4):293–302.
30. Lasch KE. Culture and Pain. *Pain.* 2002; 10(5): no page numbers.
31. Davitz LJ, Sameshima Y, Davitz J. Suffering As Viewed in Six Different Cultures. *Am J Nurs.* 1976;76:1296-1297.
32. Cousins MJ, Brennan F, Carr DB. Pain relief: a universal human right. *Pain.* 2004; 112: 1–4.
33. Bennett D, Carr D. Opiophobia as a barrier to the treatment of pain. *J Pain Palliat Care Pharmacother.* 2002;16:105–9.

CHAPTER 5

Measures of Pain Management and Patient Satisfaction as Core Factors in the Development of Medical Music Therapy Programming at Norton Healthcare

Jenny Branson BA, MT-BC

*"The problems of the world cannot possibly be solved by skeptics or cynics whose horizons are limited by the obvious realities.
We need men who can dream of things that never were."*
John Keats

Introduction

Grumbling at performance improvement reports for an upcoming meeting, I was frustrated to hear the library door swing open-again. Thinking to myself that "music therapy is the easy part of the job," I turned to welcome this most recent interruption. It was one of our dietitians, stopping in with a referral. "Jenny, I know it's late, but Jan is back, and I know she wants to see you today if you can make it up to the unit. She doesn't look too bad, but she's really upset about another admission."

Worried about my long-time patient, I thanked Phyllis for letting me know. "I hate to hear that she's back in here; she's had such a rough spring already! Yes, I can stay over and spend some time with her. Do you know the reason for this admission?" I took down the room number and gathered instruments and recorded music to take with me. I've had the privilege to work with Jan over the past six years. In her sixties, she has taught me volumes about working with patients with chronic pulmonary disease and motivated me to stay current with latest research in music therapy group intervention for persons with chronic illness, stress management, music therapy in the intensive care unit, and counseling in music therapy techniques.[1-5] Heading upstairs, I hoped I was prepared for whatever lay behind that door.

Individual Casework as a Context for Care

I first met Jan in 2006, during her hospitalization and diagnosis with chronic obstructive pulmonary disease (COPD). I was paged to the intensive care unit, where she was struggling with claustrophobia, air hunger, and intense fear of intubation for ventilator support. A respiratory therapist paged me to the unit, hoping for an intervention that would help decrease Jan's anxiety without depressing her breathing. Through a nonverbal, "yes/no" interview with Jan and a more extensive interview with her close friend, I was able to determine her music preferences and history with music. Most importantly, I was able to find ways to help her cope with her fears while she struggled with the bipap machine.[6]

This first visit lasted more than two hours, as her family and treatment team helped me create a more calm and supportive environment that would help decrease her anxiety and facilitate more regular breathing. Throughout this session, I utilized the iso principle, techniques from neurologic music therapy, and music-assisted relaxation techniques to match the music to Jan's emotional state, entrain her breathing, focus her attention away from her anxiety, provide musical structure to the noisy ICU environment, and gradually de-escalate her stress response.[1-5]

I returned later in the day to see how she was coping, and to provide education to Jan and her treatment team about the use of recorded music and diaphragmatic breathing techniques to help her rest during the nighttime when no music therapy services were available. I provided Jan with recordings of her preferred instrumental relaxation music, and we discussed the possibility that she may later associate music that she finds relaxing with a very stressful experience.

These techniques were used in individual music therapy treatment with Jan throughout several hospitalizations. Later in the same year, Norton Audubon Hospital opened an outpatient pulmonary rehabilitation center, and music therapy was integrated into the standard of care for this department. Since then, I have had ongoing opportunities to work with Jan in both individual and group settings. Walking up the stairs, I tried to anticipate what we might be working on in this session.

When I got upstairs, Jan was tearful. Trying to remain calm and quiet in the shared room, she reported that she just needed a friendly presence. Today, as on some other days, the music would be "too much." Jan knew that many difficult emotions lay just under the surface, but she felt that she did not have the energy to engage in that work today. Instead, she asked me to update her on recent developments in our department. She knew that I had recently traveled to give a presentation, and that we had been working on a survey of medical music therapists across the country. I got fresh coffee for both of us, and shared the updates regarding one of our recent projects.

Founding Philosophy

In 2010, I met with a potential donor who was executing an estate gift that had strict parameters regarding the types of services or projects the gift could support. Some of the parameters were that the fund must support some type of music activity in the community, involve musicians from the Louisville Orchestra, and provide education to students or members of the community. Working with the Norton Hospitals Foundation, I created a proposal for the donor. His response to our request was valid: "what sets you apart from other music therapy programs?" In response, we pursued a national survey of medical music therapy programs.

We learned that we are a comparatively large and productive department. Surveys were sent to 381 music therapists listed by the Certification Board of Music Therapists (CBMT) as working in a medical or hospital setting; questions were in regards to work during the 2010 calendar year. We received responses from 106 (28%), and 91 of those qualified for inclusion in our study. Compared to the average number reported, our program provided a more broad scope of services than many other programs. Respondents reported an average of 976 individual music therapy interventions were provided in 2010, and 512 persons received music therapy intervention in a group setting. In comparison, the Norton Audubon Hospital music therapy staff reported 2,197 individual interventions and 689 persons attending group music therapy intervention.

We learned that our department is unique in its staffing and reporting structure. We are one of only five departments that reported having a designated clerical staff member. My position is similar to other music therapy positions in the number of hours I work (32 hours per week) and my job description. We have our own cost center and report directly to hospital administration. The majority of respondents (45%) report to the child life department, while 55% report to a variety of departments that include rehabilitation, expressive therapies, palliative care, pastoral care, and arts in healthcare.

Norton Audubon Hospital music therapists, working exclusively with adults, are in the minority in the demographic we serve. More than 65% of respondents work with children at least some of the time, while only 11% work exclusively with adults. Most respondents work just over 32 hours per week, with 70% of their working hours dedicated to patient care. Participants reported that 17% of their time is spent in administrative tasks, 6% in staff development, 4% in research, 2% in community education, and 2% on other duties. As music therapy matrix coordinator, I dedicate 40% of working hours to patient care, 20% to interface with system music therapists, and 20% to interface with the community and the Children's Hospitals Foundation.

"Wow! You have come a long way since we met!" said a visibly calmer Jan. "I remember when you were the only therapist here."

We reflected for a while on all of the changes in our department as well as on potential directions for music therapy services in pulmonary rehab. Jan voiced her hope that more patients would enroll in outpatient rehab and that we could have enough group members for another choir. As we were brainstorming ideas for recruitment to the choir, her pulmonologist stopped in for afternoon rounds. I departed, making plans to follow up with her on the next day. As I walked out of the room, the physical therapist paged me to another unit for co-treatment with a patient who had experienced an acute stroke.[8] Walking up the stairs, I thought about the evolution of our department, which is the first medical music therapy program in our area.

Beginnings

Established in 2002, the Robert Lerman Memorial Music Library and Music Therapy Department at Norton Audubon Hospital is the product of the combined vision and effort of a broad range of people. Led by Joanie Lerman and Chaplain Keitha Brasler, a steering committee of community members collaborated with Norton Audubon Hospital, the University of Louisville, members of the music and music therapy community, and the Norton Healthcare Foundation to create the space, resources, vision, and mission that would bring medical music therapy, a visiting artist program, and a listening library to the patients, families, and staff served by Norton Audubon Hospital. What began as a vision for a beautiful space, listening library, and performance program is now a music therapy program that employs eight music therapists, a music librarian, a team of library volunteers, and a roster of volunteer musicians who provide a range of services throughout a five-hospital system. Each hospital operated by Norton Healthcare provides some medical music therapy intervention, whether hospital-wide or specific to certain units or diagnoses. Each facility also provides recorded music and music listening equipment for use at the bedside and during diagnostic or surgical procedures. Norton Healthcare music therapy departments coordinate visiting artist programs in the public spaces of the facilities, and are building a strong partnership with The Kentucky Center Arts in Healing Program, which provides monthly arts experiences to outpatients and staff in the facility.

Driving this patient-centered, sustainable program are a dynamic network, the efficient utilization of existing resources, the application and generalization of current research and best practice in music therapy, and consistent monitoring of the effects of music therapy in patient outcomes. Consistent and evolving collaboration with other clinicians, volunteers, and members of the community have created the extensive network that supports, inspires, and motivates music therapy at Norton Audubon Hospital. Existing resources include advocates, clinical processes and protocols in other departments, physical space and supplies, and experienced music therapy staff.

Some key strategies have been in place since the department was established, while others have evolved with the changing needs and objectives of the department or Norton Audubon Hospital. Objectives for education, outreach, and interdisciplinary collaboration rely heavily on effective networking, maintaining an understanding of the processes for other services in the facility, and staying informed regarding the growth and improvement focus areas for the hospital. A working knowledge of the current literature regarding medical music therapy, arts in medicine, and the use of music by other allied health care providers remains a top objective to effective communication and collaboration. The efficient utilization of existing resources helps maintain and sustain growing programs.

Launched in 2001, the vision for the department was created through the shared effort and vision of Joanie Lerman and Keitha Brasler. Joanie, the widow of Dr. Robert Lerman, sought to provide the hospital with a visiting artist program as a memorial to her late husband. The Lerman family had received care from the music therapy department at Memorial Sloane Kettering; the experience made such an impression on the family that they sought to establish something similar at the hospital where Joanie and Dr. Lerman had worked. At the same time that Joanie Lerman was collaborating with the volunteer services coordinator, Connie Billharz, to create a visiting artist program, Keitha Brasler began to envision a listening library that would be available to patients, families, and staff as a respite from the noise and stress of the clinical environment. Connie Billharz connected Keitha Brasler with Joanie Lerman, and their vision was well-received by hospital administrators, who were willing to donate a space within the hospital for a music library. Norton Audubon Hospital administration requested formation of a steering committee to coordinate the efforts and multiple layers of project management that would be involved in the development of this project. The committee included hospital administrators, hospital engineering staff, infection control staff, an architect, Keitha Brasler, Joanie Lerman, Connie Billharz, and volunteers from throughout the community. Their collective knowledge, resources, and energy equipped the team to create the vision and design that would ultimately create a sustainable, patient-centered department, unique in its scope and impact.

Music and Medicine: Integrative Models in the Treatment of Pain

During this incubation and growth period, Keitha Brasler contacted Dr. Joy Berger, a music therapist and chaplain who attended her church. Dr. Berger provided the steering committee with vital information regarding music therapy and emphasized the importance of having a music therapist in the hospital. She advised the committee that the most vital component to a successful program would be a music therapist to oversee the listening library, recruit and coordinate the visiting artists, provide music therapy intervention, and educate hospital staff regarding the role of music and music therapy in the hospital setting. Dr. Berger facilitated connections among the committee, Dr. Deforia Lane, and Dr. Barbara Wheeler. Dr. Lane was Director of Music Therapy at University Hospitals of Cleveland, Seidman Cancer Center and Rainbow Babies & Children's Hospital. Dr. Wheeler was the head of the University of Louisville undergraduate music therapy program. Dr. Lane, actively directing a dynamic medical music therapy program, fielded program development and process questions for the committee, and reinforced the importance of the connection with the University of Louisville. Dr. Wheeler, in the process of building the new music therapy training program, was actively seeking partners in the community to educate the community about music therapy, facilitate student training opportunities, and conduct demonstration and research projects to further the profession. One key development as a result of this collaboration was the creation of a dynamic partnership between Norton Healthcare and the University of Louisville music therapy program. This partnership addresses several objectives: student education, staff education, patient care, collection and presentation of patient outcome metrics, opportunities for future collaboration, and an expert music therapy resource for the growing department.

Beginning in 2002, Dr. Wheeler worked approximately four hours per week to provide music therapy intervention, student supervision, and staff education. Demonstration projects, conducted for ten weeks each in the summers of 2002-2004 provided hands-on music therapy education and experience for music therapy students while delivering quality group and individual music therapy intervention to patients throughout the hospital. Designed and supervised by Dr. Wheeler, each project focused on different units in the hospital and various patient outcomes, including perceived pain, anxiety, stress, depression, and relaxation just before and following the music therapy intervention. While not research projects, these demonstration projects provided the facility with important opportunities to learn about medical music therapy and its potential impact on patient care.

By early 2004, Dr. Wheeler had collected and presented sufficient data to help the committee provide a strong case for a larger and more consistent music therapy program at Norton Audubon Hospital. Expanded grant funding was requested from the Norton Hospitals Foundation, the now-annual fundraising concert was planned, and a proposal was written to provide a basic job description and objectives for a contract music therapist to work twenty hours per week throughout the facility for one year. Objectives for this first year included provision of more focused staff education regarding medical music therapy and patient outcomes; music therapy intervention in critical care, cardiac care, and skilled nursing units; supervision of music therapy students; interface with donors and the hospital foundation; quarterly reports to administration regarding the impact of the program on patient outcomes related to pain and coping; and pursuit of third party reimbursement for medical music therapy services.

Growth

In June 2004, I was hired as an independent contractor to provide music therapy services 20 hours per week throughout Norton Audubon Hospital. On my first day, I walked into a beautiful office equipped with a brand-new personal computer and a summer intern collecting data for a university-supervised demonstration project. There were no forms, business cards, or processes in place – for anything. No one outside of administration knew that a music therapist had been hired, or how or why to request a consult. It was exciting and terrifying. Drawing from clinical experience, business experience, coursework, and current research in music therapy, I set out to establish a presence and a process for music therapy in the facility. With the independent contractor model, providers typically reported to management outside of Norton Healthcare, who would coordinate and negotiate contracts and services with the corporation. As the owner of the private music therapy practice contracted with Norton Healthcare, I initially had no formal reporting structure or supervisor within or without the facility. I was oriented alongside Norton Healthcare employees and held to the same clinical and ethical standards, but had no connections with management. Besides oversight, supervisors provide guidance, support, and advocacy for their teams. Without a guide and advocate to help me navigate the who, how, and why of corporate healthcare, I faced a maze of protocols and reporting lines.

As staff chaplain, Keitha Brasler had strong connections to a wide variety of care providers, leaders, and innovative thinkers throughout Norton Healthcare and the community. As a strong and informed advocate for music therapy, as well as an informed and connected employee, she agreed to serve as my first supervisor and mentor. Her guidance and relationships have proven invaluable to networking, navigating administrative politics, and making connections with the committees and leadership that support, inform, and collaborate with music therapy initiatives. Her expertise in communication, advocacy, and basic management helped me build a strong foundation as a clinician and collaborator. By connecting first with the staff and leaders who were known supporters of this new program, we were able to demonstrate the efficacy of music therapy intervention and the potential for interdepartmental collaboration, and to use a "top-down" approach for educating other allied health care providers in building an understanding for the role of music therapy in every unit of the hospital. Observation and word of mouth provided effective and efficient opportunities for advocacy, as leaders and staff had the opportunity to observe and request music therapy intervention and collaboration, as well as to hear quarterly presentations regarding the impact of music therapy on coping, pain scores, satisfaction, and other patient care metrics.

Keitha facilitated introduction to various persons throughout the hospital, and I was invited to join nursing and leadership committees assigned to address key quality metrics. These committees worked to improve or develop processes to improve patient outcomes related to pain, palliative care, joint replacement, COPD, stroke, and acute care for elders. I have worked with each team to review, adapt, and apply current, evidence-based research from a variety of disciplines to develop music therapy protocols for various initiatives in the facility. By including music therapy as the standard of care for these new initiatives, the teams can collect data and demonstrate the efficacy of music therapy intervention. By identifying the priorities for the facility, hospital leaders provide me with direction for specific objectives and data reports to support program development. The metrics collected and presented evolve to meet the needs of the facility and the system. The original data sets are still in use, with additional data collected each year as the program expands into more and varied service lines. This longitudinal data allows the program to examine several trends, including collaboration, reasons for referral, patient outcomes, demand for music therapy intervention, and department productivity. Current metrics include number of:

- patients referred
- attempts made to assess/treat patients
- individual interventions provided
- members in group intervention
- patients not seen due to time/availability
- patients that refuse intervention
- music library services provided
- music in surgery services provided
- arts visits in public spaces

- hours music therapy services are available
- patient satisfaction scores for patients receiving music therapy services.

These metrics are presented to administration quarterly, with specific information highlighted for the purpose of corporate performance improvement. As reports of referrals and the efficacy of interdisciplinary collaboration increase, the budget for the music therapy department increases.

The addition of a second music therapist in 2006 significantly increased the visibility and availability of services. Kerry Willis was hired to assist with a perioperative music pilot study requested by the anesthesia department. The study, informed by research in anesthesia, nursing, and music therapy[9-11] was launched in October 2006, and was planned to last through the end of the year. Due to unforeseen complications with retrieving project data from a new electronic medical records system, the information needed to address the research question became unavailable. Three months into the study, the project was suspended. Despite the end of the research project, nurses in the recovery room reported an observed decrease in anxiety and nausea for patients receiving music in surgery. They began to request that music therapy and recorded music services be made available for all patients undergoing surgical intervention. Perioperative music therapy and the use of recorded music in surgery were made available to all patients, additional iPods were purchased, and Kerry Willis was reassigned to provide music therapy intervention throughout the facility. This proved to be a pivotal moment for the program, in terms of growth and the integration of music therapy as a standard of care.

With the increase in the availability of services and increased staff awareness of the efficacy of music therapy, we experienced significant growth in the number of referrals we received throughout the building. The music therapy department reported a 63% increase in individual music therapy intervention between June 2004 and June 2007 (J. Branson, MT-BC, unpublished data, 2007). By documenting and reporting this information to administration, we were able to present a solid rationale for the creation of both a full-time and a part-time music therapy position, increasing the availability of music therapy services from 32 to 52 hours per week. This move by the hospital demonstrated support for the program, and also highlighted for us the need for a formally recognized supervisor.

Keitha Brasler had proven a strong and effective leader, and was willing to continue in her supervision, but her position as a staff chaplain did not have the administrative status or access to a cost center with the budget needed to help the program continue in its growth. This newly established department needed a supervisor who would advocate for the program, guide growth, provide reliable evaluation of the program, and help build a sustainable budget for the department. Various clinical departments were considered: rehabilitation, nursing administration, service excellence, quality. The director of quality, Shirley Schilling, stepped forward to claim music therapy as part of her team. A member of administration, Shirley Schilling was part of the team that helped bring the music therapy pilot project to Norton Audubon Hospital. Given that her focus was quality, evidence-based practice, and that she had advocated for the program since its inception, it seemed like a good fit. My full-time position, the summer internship program, and the new part-time position were established in the cost center for Quality and Risk Management. This provided the department with an energetic supervisor committed to growth, quality, and best practice initiatives in the hospital.

With no precedent for a music therapy position or intervention formalized in the system, every aspect of these new job descriptions and department processes had to be created and vetted to meet both current and anticipated needs of the department and facility. The interface between music therapy and other departments in the hospital was broad, and the new documents required input from a wide variety of clinicians, educators, and administrators. Shirley Schilling coordinated these efforts, and the job descriptions and policies created in 2007 are still in use for all five music therapy departments.

Kosair Children's Hospital, a freestanding, full-service pediatric facility owned by Norton Healthcare, launched its music therapy program in 2006. Under the supervision of Service Excellence, this part-time position provides music therapy in the NICU and in the adolescent psychiatric inpatient unit. Many of the policies and protocols for referral, interdisciplinary collaboration, documentation, continuing education, visibility, and fundraising that were built at Norton Audubon Hospital were duplicated or adapted for use at Kosair Children's Hospital. The Service Excellence director provides administrative supervision to this music therapist.

Similar collaboration and adaptation took place as other departments and facilities began to build their own music therapy programs. In 2006, the Norton Cancer Institute began to provide music therapy intervention to oncology patients and their families at three Norton facilities: Norton Hospital in downtown Louisville, Norton Suburban Hospital on the east end of the city, and Norton Audubon Hospital. Music therapy services expanded to include pediatric oncology services at Kosair Children"s Hospital in 2009, with supervision provided by the Director of Support Services.

Program Development

Throughout program growth, the partnership with the University of Louisville has remained an important objective. The Norton Healthcare music therapy department supervises students in all levels of music therapy training including observation, practicum, data collection, summer internship, and university affiliated internship experiences. This partnership provides a broad and rich experience for the students as well as the staff.

To further the partnership with the University of Louisville, a shared position was created in 2007. With funding and supervision shared between the University of Louisville, the Norton Hospitals Foundation, and Norton Audubon Hospital, this position created an opportunity for an adjunct music therapy professor to focus on student education, clinical supervision, and medical music therapy research at Norton Audubon Hospital. A three-year contract outlined the objectives, which included teaching coursework, supervising practicum hours, grant writing to support medical music therapy research, and publication of the research. This shared position provided additional opportunities for student clinical experience that had been unavailable due to time constraints and staffing needs at the hospital, as well as opportunities for outreach in the community. Supervision of the position was shared between Norton Audubon Hospital and the University of Louisville.

By the time Norton Brownsboro Hospital opened in 2009, music therapy services were considered a standard component of care throughout Norton Healthcare. Project managers and administrators planning the design of the facility included music therapy from the outset of the project. This part-time position provides services throughout the adult acute-care facility and is supervised by the Director of Rehabilitation. As the music therapy departments expanded, the objectives on my annual evaluation expanded. I continued to address the original patient care, education, and student supervision objectives. I also began to assist new departments and supervisors in planning and development, interface with the Norton Hospitals and Children's Hospital Foundations for fundraising and grant writing, and write protocols for care and continuing education for the music therapists, and organize visiting artists. In 2010, my job title and status were changed from "staff music therapist" to "music therapy matrix coordinator" to reflect the changes in my role.

Funding
Like many creative arts therapies programs, the Norton Healthcare music therapy program has received funding and support from a variety of sources, while consistently working towards sustainable growth. Initial funds and

resources were provided by a combination of donations from steering committee members, proceeds from fundraising concerts, a grant from the Norton Hospitals Foundation, donation of space from Norton Audubon Hospital, extensive volunteer support in the library, and an agreement that the hospital would assume responsibility for the program, contingent upon outlined objectives. This initial arrangement, in use from 2002-2004, provided a solid start for the project by allowing the construction of the music library and office space, purchase of listening materials and musical instruments, and grant funding to pay for a music therapist to supervise student clinical training and demonstration projects. The program was initially designed to be partially sustained through third-party reimbursement of medical music therapy services. Additional funding was projected through grants for research and outreach projects, donations, and the hospital operating budget.

Early in this first year of the program, it was determined that third-party billing would not be an option. Due to the per diem reimbursement model used in the acute care setting and the resources potentially required for insurance coding and appeals, it was determined that it would be much more cost effective to simply pay the music therapist to provide evidence-based intervention without charging patients or departments. From 2004-2007, funding for music therapy services was provided exclusively by a designated Norton Hospitals Foundation fund. This fund was supported by donations, employee support through the Norton Healthcare Combined Giving Campaign, and fundraising events held in the community. In 2007, with increasing demand for services and data to support the efficacy of music therapy intervention in the hospital, Norton Audubon Hospital began to assume partial responsibility for the music therapy budget. Over time, the hospital assumed increasing responsibility for the service, and in 2012, the department was assigned a separate cost center and was fully integrated into the hospital's operating budget.

The music therapy departments at other Norton Healthcare facilities have been funded in a variety of ways, but are now in the various facilities' operating budgets, with occasional support from grants and fundraising events. Each position or department collects and reports data to support and direct program growth. These reports have proven effective; in May 2012, 100% of the operating costs for each of the ten music therapy positions was included in hospital operating budgets. Each of the five facilities has plans to expand music therapy services in 2013. Music therapy department operating costs include music therapist salaries, anticipated equipment purchase and maintenance, office supplies, music library equipment, stipends for continuing education, textbook and journal purchases, and marketing needs. Operating budgets for the departments provide the essentials, but facility growth and innovations in evidence-based music therapy intervention often create needs beyond the established annual budget. Music library volunteers, visiting artists, project grants, and collaboration with the University of Louisville help bridge the occasional budget gap.

Resourcing
Access to volunteers, a library of resource binders, and collaboration with hospital educators are essential to sustain day-to-day operations, continued growth, as well as special projects. Volunteers share their time and talents in a variety of ways: providing performances in public spaces; carrying out clerical tasks; hosting visitors in the music library space; delivering, disinfecting, and filing music listening equipment; and brainstorming fundraising and publicity events. The growth of the various departments provided a catalyst for development of resource binders that outline consistent processes within each music therapy department and throughout the hospital system. Protocols for communication, progress towards measurable objectives, and a shared vision and growth plan are essential to ensure collaborative work towards common goals, and to enable that work to continue through inevitable changes in staffing and programming needs. Hospital staff education requires ongoing effort. A variety of approaches are used to educate staff regarding the integration of music therapy services and the importance of interdisciplinary collaboration for improved patient outcomes and experience.

Visibility
At Norton Audubon Hospital, visibility and presence may or may not be subtle. Music therapists usually wear business casual gear with the Norton Healthcare Music Therapy logo embroidered on the front pocket. This dressed-down, practical attire clearly communicates to patients and staff that each music therapist is a member of the care team, and that while clinical, music therapy is a less physically invasive intervention that does not require scrubs. The team strives to provide visibility on every unit, every day. Music therapists and interns check in with nurses and other allied health care providers in the halls and at the nursing stations for further music therapy or music library needs on each unit. Often, the physical presence and visible reminder is more effective than a 'music therapy and pain' flier in the break room or a cue on a patient pain assessment flow chart. Four times each day, seven days per week, nursing leadership and representatives from each

department gather for "bed huddle." Monday through Friday, a music therapist attends the 9:30 A.M. bed huddle to share announcements and brainstorm special patient needs.

The presence of the music therapist prompts departments to make referrals and our consistent presence encourages nursing leaders to think more holistically during their early morning rapid rounds and bring those referrals with them to the bed huddle.

Each Norton Healthcare facility publishes a weekly e-newsletter that is required reading for all clinical staff. These newsletters provide need-to-know information and are required reading for all nursing staff. They also provide for delivery of music therapy information, such as the addition of a service, dates for visiting artist performances, or data regarding patient outcomes. To maintain visibility and remind staff to make referrals, we maintain a rotation of monthly topics and related music therapy objectives for inclusion in the newsletters. The entries typically relate to a national awareness initiative for a demographic served by that hospital, and will include a few bullet points regarding potential music therapy objectives for that population (e.g., heart health in February, breast cancer in October, etc).

Outreach and Education
Continuing education is required for allied health care providers. By offering and providing continuing education credits for the various departments throughout the system, the music therapy department has found an efficient way to address multiple objectives. Continuing education presentations are tailored to specific questions, to suit the programming needs of the audience. Well-planned, one-hour "lunch and learn" presentations can provide as much impact and ignite as much curiosity as a four-hour workshop. Often, clinicians attending the presentations generate more questions, request further collaboration, or develop ideas for pilot projects in departments or facilities currently without music therapy services.

Our music therapy staff provides outreach presentations to several allied health care programs in the area that have incorporated medical music therapy information into the syllabi, and schedule an experiential lecture for their students each semester.

Informal networking is another important factor in the success of the program. Music therapists are encouraged to take breaks and meals with other clinical staff in a variety of areas throughout the facility. Non-clinical interactions can provide opportunities to build rapport on a variety of levels, and help to personalize the relationships between departments. The pursuit of continuing education alongside other allied health care professionals reinforces that music therapists have clinical standards and expectations to meet, and also allows for informal discussions regarding various aspects of music therapy and programming. Connections made over lunch or during training can carry over into additional clinical, as well as non-clinical networking.

Music therapy staff members are often contacted as resources or references for other music and arts services in the community. Internally, music therapy team members are recognized for their contributions, and the team makes an effort to recognize others. Through both established, corporate channels - as well as more personal efforts - each member of the music therapy department is encouraged to "manage up" by recognizing other employees for their contributions to better care and for professional or personal achievement. Handwritten notes to individuals and their supervisors are an effective way to say "thank you," and to maintain a connection with other departments.

Externally, the music therapy department at Norton Audubon Hospital has received local, regional, and national recognition in the form of nominations, awards, and invitations to contribute to symposia, conferences, and publications. Some of the awards include AMTA 2005 Music Therapy Advocacy Award recognizing Keitha Brasler and Joanie Lerman; 2005 Sodexho Spirit of Excellence Award for Service; 2006 Anthem Blue Cross Blue Shield Quality Award; 2012 Nomination for Medistar Seven Counties Healthcare Advocacy Award; and multiple Norton Healthcare Better Care Awards. Presentations have been made at conferences of the American Music Therapy Association, Southeastern Region of the American Music Therapy Association, and the Great Lakes Region of the American Music Therapy Association; the Louisville Cardiopulmonary Summit; and the Louis Armstrong Center for Music and Medicine's 2012 symposium, *Music and Medicine: Integrative Models in Pain Medicine.*

Networking outside of the walls of the facility is vital to the growth and sustainability of this program. Since its opening, the music therapy department has worked to build mutually beneficial relationships with a wide variety of partners in the community. Partnership with the Kentucky Center Arts in Healing program provides juried artists with a regular stipend as they provide monthly arts experiences to patients and staff. Through partnership with the Parkinson's Support Center of Kentuckiana, the music therapy department receives funding to provide a free, weekly outpatient music therapy group to persons with Parkinson's Disease.[12] Twice a year, Arts at Audubon hosts the 202nd Army Reserve Band Woodwind Quintet, who are grateful to have a scheduled, indoor space for required community outreach performances. Collaboration with the University of Louisville music therapy department provides clinical training and research opportunities for both entities. Local musicians volunteer in a variety of roles to give back to the community, complete community service, and hone performing skills in a low-stress environment.

Patient Satisfaction
Healthcare facilities rely heavily on patient satisfaction scores and core measures of specific clinical data for continued quality in care, as well as for third party reimbursement for specific diagnoses. Important patient satisfaction measures for healthcare facilities often include patients' perceptions of pain management, the extent to which patient feel their emotional needs are addressed, the perceived noise level near patient care areas, and patients' overall assessment of their experience.

In 2011, administration asked us to determine whether music therapy or music library services have a demonstrable, positive impact on patients' Press Ganey satisfaction scores regarding pain, emotional needs, noise, overall satisfaction, and likelihood of recommending the facility. Press Ganey surveys were sent only to patients who were discharged directly home. Patients who may have had multiple admissions received a maximum of one survey every 90 days. A total of 3,062 surveys were returned; of these, 160 were from patients who had received music therapy and/or music library services. Patients who received any service from our department rated their satisfaction with the noise level, overall experience, and likelihood of recommending the facility higher than patients that did not receive music therapy or music library services. While music therapy patients did not rate their satisfaction with pain or emotional needs higher than patients that did not receive music therapy, the differences between the ratings for noise, overall experience, and likelihood of recommending the facility were significant enough that the overall mean score for music therapy patients was higher than for patients that did not receive music therapy. These findings were comparable to those reported by Yinger and Standley in 2011.[13]

We will continue to track and report this information to administration quarterly; this information will help guide program development. The survey questions and distribution guidelines changed for 2012 to ensure that more patients will receive the survey. This change will yield a larger sample size and additional opportunities to examine trends in the data.

Conclusion

These patient satisfaction reports are sprawled on my desk as I return to document my visit with Jan and my co-treatment with physical therapy. Working quickly, I add this data to the presentation for the Performance Improvement committee later in the day.

The phone rings; it's Jan. "I know you already came up today, but I wondered if you had time to stop by again later."

"Sure, Jan. It won't be until about 5 o'clock. Will that work?"

"Of course, honey. Just come when you can. I'm not going anywhere."

With the sun low on the trees, I sank into a chair while Jan finished a breathing treatment. The respiratory therapist in the room knows both of us, and took her time, hoping to hear the music she anticipates we'll make. Handing over the nebulizer, Jan turned to me.

"You know, it really bothers me that more people don't know about pulmonary rehab or music therapy. It really *does* help, if folks would just try it."

Nodding in agreement, I asked what changes she'd like to see. "I'd really like to be able to teach people about some of the wonderful things available."

References

1. Ademek, M.S.; Codding, P.A.; Darrow, A.A.; Gervin, A.P.; Gfeller, K.E. *Effectiveness of music therapy procedures: documentation of research and clinical practice.* Silver Spring, MD: AMTA; 2000.
2. Miller, S. The sound of music: respiratory therapy coupledwith music therapy benefits health, well-being. *Adv for Resp Care Prac.* 2005; 18(6); 10-12, 18.
3. Wong, E.H. Clinical guide to music therapy in adult physical rehabilitation settings. Silver Spring, MD: AMTA; 2004.
4. Bizek,K. S.,Fontaine,D. K. 2009. The patient"s experience with critical illness. In Morton,P. G., Fontaine,D. K. (Eds.) *Critical Care Nursing: A holistic approach.* Wolters Kluwer Health/Lippincott Williams & Wilkins: Philadelphia. 12-26.
5. Johnson, S.L. Therapist"s guide to clinical intervention: the 1-2-3"s of treatment planning. San Diego, CA: Academic Press; 2003.
6. Bilevel positive airway pressureThaut, M.H. Training manual for neurologic music therapy. Colorado State University: Center for Biomedical Research in Music; 1999.
7. Standley, J., et al. Medical music therapy: a model program for clinical practice, education, training, and research. Silver Spring, MD: AMTA; 2005
8. Koch, M. E.; Kain, Z.N.; Ayoub, C.; Rosenbaum, S.H. The sedative and analgesic sparing effect of music. *Anesthesiology.* 1998; 89 (2), 300-306.

9. Clark, P.A., Drain, M., Malone, M.P. Addressing patients" emotional and spiritual needs. *Jt Comm J Qual Patient Saf.* 2003; Dec; 29(12): 659-670.
10. Mitchell, L. A.; MacDonald, R. A. R. An experimental investigation of the effects of preferred and relaxing music listening on pain perception. *J Music Ther*, XLIII (4), 2006, 295-316.
11. Pachetti, C., et al. Active Music Therapy in Parkinson's Disease: An Integrative Method for Motor and Emotional Rehabilitation. *Psychosom Med.* 2000 (62) 386–393.
12. Yinger, O.S.; Standley, J. The effects of medical music therapy on patient satisfaction: as measured by the Press Ganey inpatient survey. *Music Therapy Perspectives.* 2011; 29(2)149-156.

SECTION II

SPECIFIC TREATMENT APPROACHES

Music and Medicine: Integrative Models in the Treatment of Pain

CHAPTER 6

Music Therapy Improvisation and Reflection for Pain Relief with Hospitalized Adults

Paul Nolan MCAT, LPC, MT-BC

"Music...it's very structure transforms feelings into an objectified form that can be reflected upon."
Gilbert Rose

Introduction

This chapter describes the rationale and description of an individual music therapy protocol to address a hospitalized patient's pain experience. The treatment protocol is intended for a single music therapy session or for short- term care. The intention of the protocol is to elicit positive emotions for neurological gaiting of pain signals through music therapy improvisation and verbal reflection.

When music therapists work with hospitalized adults we usually do not know how many sessions we can anticipate. Hospital schedules, patient fatigue, patient visitors, our own schedule with other patients, and the typical suddenness of discharge or transfer to another facility often limits treatment planning beyond the single session. I became concerned that our graduate students or I may not be able to be as effective as possible with the limited time for our therapeutic relationships to develop within the general hospital setting. I imagined that it could be possible to develop a single session protocol that could include just one or two treatment goals that addressed the patient's chief complaint, yet have the work continue with a prescriptive component so the patient could possibly replicate at least part of the therapeutic effect after the termination of music therapy.

The most frequent treatment issues that we face in the general adult hospital setting that can be addressed within a short period of time are pain issues, most often persistent pain, and anxiety, or depressed mood. In my work, I have noticed that when any of these issues are effectively reduced for the patient, that the other issue(s) are in turn affected. Apparently, other music therapists and those medical personnel who use music interventions have observed this combination of effects as well. Music therapists,[1] reported in their Cochrane Review on music interventions for improving psychological and physical outcomes in cancer patients that "...music interventions may have beneficial effects on anxiety, pain, mood, and quality of life in people with cancer." I've learned that whenever goals to address pain, anxiety and/or depressed mood were met in any way, a common factor in all cases was a decrease in negative affect and usually an increase of positive emotions. Both of these changes in affective states are associated with changes in pain. Anxiety increases pain, positive emotions decrease pain.[2] Finucane, et al reported in their study of basic emotions among healthy, chronic pain, depressed and Post Traumatic Stress Disorder (PTSD) subjects that chronic pain subjects experience more negative emotions (anger, sadness and fear) than healthy subjects.[3] It seemed likely that hospitalized oncology patients with persistent pain may also experience more negative emotions than healthy individuals. If these patients can experience positive emotions through music therapy then we may be able to find a way, or a protocol, that can help in altering their pain experience.

This chapter will suggest a method for a positive change in the pain experience that focuses on creativity as a primary forum in which to facilitate openness to such change. Music therapy improvisation and reflection to activate positive emotions; a known means to reduce the pain experience are central to this method. The music is intentionally structured to facilitate a psychological movement by the dyad toward positive emotions through an experience of beauty or transcendence. The induction of positive emotions through the musical experience and the revisiting, with amplification, of the music-facilitated emotional experience through a phenomenological-oriented reflection interview, seems to activate one or more of the known neurological mechanisms through which pain is reduced. This method came into fruition as a result of its effective implementation in short-term music therapy treatment where it appeared to be effective in helping patients positively alter their pain experience. It is suggested that patients can use adaptations of this method prescriptively when they are alone.

To Use a Music Therapy Protocol or Not?

There is lack of music therapy literature identifying treatment approaches that are specific to any given disorder within the myriad of health care issues being addressed. A systematic understanding of how music therapists select methods for conducting therapy across receptive and expressive approaches, as well as the musical instruments they use in relation to treatment goals, is still in development for most populations. Music therapists report various approaches, methods and instrument use even within similar populations. It seems to me that music therapists choose methods that use music in ways that they tend to personally enjoy. Also, the medium of music, such as improvisation, song writing, or group singing, tend to be selected based upon the therapists areas in which they have the greatest personal interest or musical mastery. Music therapists who are primarily vocalists seem to choose singing as their most often used instrument. Those who are pianists seem to prefer the piano as their primary approach to music therapy. Songwriters like clinical song writing and those who enjoy composing music and improvising tend to rationalize those uses of music primarily across a wide range of clinical populations. Therapists with an interest and experience in technology use electronic means in therapy. There are probably good reasons for these selections. Therapists can create music environments that are the most aesthetic when they choose to work with musical elements that are specific to their talents and skill.

There is however logic in trying to use evidence based practices by embracing what the literature reports to be effective for specific clinical populations and goals. Therapists can then develop music therapy interventions that use both approaches: 1) therapist comfort in instrument selection; and 2) method development based upon evidence. With this said, there are few, if any, evidence based practice guidelines in music therapy that specify a medium for specific populations and goals.

In creating a protocol within music therapy, especially for hospitalized adults, one needs to consider the ongoing discussion about whether music therapy is more of an art than a science. Although these discussions are important within the field, they also postpone the development of protocols that employ clinical methods that can foster known therapeutic responses that are directed toward the alleviation of the patient's experience of pain. This next section will describe some of this quandary and provide a rationale for the combination of methods, or protocol, suggested in this chapter.

Rationale for a Music Therapy Protocol with Pain Patients

As an art, music therapists and patient(s), know how and when music therapy is working implicitly, without explanation. As a science, it is less clear. Due to the incredibly robust brain responses to music, the mechanism, not to mention the effects, cannot lead us to an explanation, nor give specific predictions of the therapeutic effects. Very little seems to be known about what contributes to the outcomes of music therapy.[4] For example, it is unclear as to what within the music therapy experience is the therapeutic mechanism of action. Is it the passive reception of music or creating music? Is it the group cohesion between members or people having creative and positive experiences together in the music, or the special therapeutic relationship to the music therapist? Or is it any of the numerous other therapeutic possibilities? Little is known about which ingredients or processes specifically contribute to the outcomes of music therapy.

How do music therapists know which methods to use for specific therapeutic goals? From the collective experiences and documentation across the field of music therapy there are research and clinical reports that document the often, consistent effects of the use of music and music therapy to positively alter the pain experience, although most of these are not based upon randomized controlled trials. Reports from an analysis by Cepeda, et al of studies from a broad range of disciplines that employ receptive methods state "Listening to music reduces pain intensity levels and opioid requirements, but the magnitude of these benefits is small and, therefore, its clinical importance unclear…".[5]

The protocol used within this chapter relies upon the co-creating of music through a structured music therapy improvisation approach. This approach attempts to elicit positive emotions through the invocation of known responses to music, described here as realms. These music response realms are then explored via a structured interview. The interview is designed as a type of phenomenological inquiry meant to both learn about the patient's realm activations, as well as to facilitate a reflective expression which again activates positive emotions through the patient's deepened awareness of physical, emotional, cognitive, interpersonal and spiritual responses to the music improvisations. The reflection helps to bring awareness to the self-generated positive emotions in response to music. Such emotional responses may be able to be harnessed by the patient as needed when singing, playing rhythms along with recorded music or even audiating (internally generated music).

Realms of the Response to Music

Within this theoretical knowledge we have ways of knowing and limiting some of the possibilities of the "what" works, as in a positive change in the pain experience, referring to methods, approaches, and ways of working with patients. To get closer to the "how" there are places where we can begin. Responses to music take place within and between five realms: physiological, cognitive, emotional, interpersonal, and spiritual. Each of these realms of responses contains related sub realms, which often overlap with every other realm. Each realm also functions independently depending upon the individual and the immediate musical event. Although it is not the purpose of this chapter to demonstrate all of the research studies associated with these realms, the following are operational descriptions on the realms.

Cognitive Realm: includes all: 1) thoughts about the music making experience itself, related to music cognition, that begins with listening, comprehending, and recognizing familiar musical processes; 2) creating rhythms and melodic motifs that fit together with the tempo, harmonic structures and style of the therapist; 3) adding variations to the rhythm, melody, accents, phrasing timbre, form of the music, as well as; 4) simply exploring a melodic or percussive instrument within the context of the on-going style or idiom of the music. Also any memories about anything related to music can be thought of as cognitive, even though these remembrances may also fit into other realms as well. Everyday creativity, as a form of cognition, comes into play during music therapy improvisation and can result in self-efficacy and controllability, which can reduce pain.[2]

Emotional Realm: the emergence of feelings or moods in response to the listening to, or playing, music. This can include emotional responses to extramusical associations as well as emotional responses to the interpersonal dyad musical encounter.

Physiological Realm: Our physiological responses to music begin in the ear in the form of sound wave pressure. Eventually, the musical process involves many brain regions, depending upon the music listening, or playing task. Physiological responses to music are related to chemical processes, including the expression of neurotransmitters and hormones that create responses in all of the realms, such as activating the basic emotions via the limbic system. Additional brain/mind interplay can manifest as physical behavioral responses to unconscious and conscious music-elicited imagery processes. Any awareness of the body during the music event can be considered to be a musical response.

Interpersonal Realm: Virtually every activity within the musical experience can be linked to a memory trace of another person. Memory traces of music teachers, family members, friends, music performers, or even introjected components of people from our remote past and early object relations may consciously or unconsciously play a role in our overall listening or playing music experience.

Spiritual Realm: includes any experience that connects the person with something ineffably felt as inside or outside of him or herself, sometimes described as "a presence bigger that my self." This phenomenon may be linked with a deity but not necessarily. Sometimes an unconscious process that manifests as unexplainable crying during music listening is associated with a spiritual experience. Beck[6] adds the following characteristics to a spiritual experience: 1) insight and understanding; a sense of context and perspective; 2) awareness of the interconnectedness of things, of unity within diversity, and of patterns within the whole; 3) optimism; 4) acceptance of the inevitable; 5) gratitude, gladness, humility; 6) love (the characteristic par excellence of the spiritual person).

Other responses that may become apparent from body movements, postures, facial expressions, and verbal reports can include those that can be categorized as aesthetic. These responses can be difficult to discern from affective and emotional responses. An aesthetic response may be associated with the spiritual realm because both are types of peak experience.[7] It typically incorporates more than one, and perhaps all five realms of responses to music.

Within my medical music therapy experience I have heard many patients, who in their report of having an experience of beauty during music therapy, use very similar language as those who describe a spiritual experience within music therapy. For the purposes of this chapter the experience of beauty is included within the spiritual realm of responses.

Pain Perspective

Persistent pain is a very complex phenomenon. The perspective used in this chapter focuses upon emotions and their relation to pain, however Lumley et al recognize other contributing factors that are important in the understanding of persistent pain. These include genetic factors, environmental factors, behavior, placebo effects, and cognitions.[2] Psychopathology and personality traits also factor into the person's experience of pain. Within our psychiatric/medical care unit, the patient's pain experience, was in many cases further complicated by external factors such as a pending personal injury law suit, and other types of litigation.

Method: General Premise

A general premise in this chapter is that the occurrence of positive emotions within music therapy is a result of variable interactions between multiple realms. These positive emotions are an initiating stage of the neurological processes that are associated with the gating of pain. Positive emotions within the pain experience may be driven by a stronger activation of one realm over another. However since all of the realms can be associated with both music and pain reduction, it is likely that activation of any realm within a creative, interpersonal music therapy improvisation, and subsequent reflection, can initiate one or more of the known physiological mechanisms responsible for positive changes in the pain experience.

Pain reduction can be understood through various neurochemical and neuro suppression mechanisms. The term "affective analgesia," from the review of pain and emotion by Lumley, et el, is associated with the release of opioids from positive emotional experiences. Their review also cites that "...activation of the brain reward circuitry contributes to the positive emotional state created by pleasant music, which reduces pain through mechanisms that may involve inhibition in the amygdala.[2] Attention shifts, also known as distraction, seem to additionally play a role in pain reduction, however, the effects of emotions on pain are partially independent from the effects of attention.

Finally, gaiting (the closing of pain signal transmission) occurs when descending analgesic fibers synapse on short spinal interneurons. The interneurons synapse on the ascending pain fiber and secrete enkephalins (opiods) into the synapses to block the pain message from sending the signal to the brain.[8]

Method
Part one of a protocol is the use of music therapy improvisation designed to decrease negative emotions, such as anxiety and fear, as well as to increase positive emotions. The improvisation is intended to increase the awareness of positive emotions by helping the patient move toward an experience of beauty within music making. An experience of beauty is assumed to be associated with positive emotions and is considered within this protocol to be a transcendent experience.

Protocol Stages
Referral for music therapy can occur through communication from the physician, nurse or from the music therapist. The music therapy assessment begins with an initial introduction and conversation about the patient's stay in the hospital. The therapist may inquire about the patient's pain experience, although following the initial assessment the therapist does not ask about pain in order to maintain a state of positive emotions. The therapist can use the Mini Mental Status Exam for an indication about the patient's mental state. The therapist inquires about the role of music in the patient's life. This is followed by an explanation and demonstration of the uses of the instruments. The therapist explains that for many people musical experiences can disrupt the pain experience. The music engagement begins as soon as the patient is ready to play. The music therapist's approach is based upon the following understandings:

1) Engage the patient in an aesthetic experience so that higher needs are being addressed instead of the pain experience.
2) Improvisation is a creative, interpersonal, and cooperative expressive music experience. In this method, the therapist attempts to use music to move toward an experience of beauty, by using well-chosen musical elements and expressions. With patient's who may desire more concrete ways to focus attention on movement toward an experience of beauty within the music making, the therapist can use paper and colored markers to write words to construct a compo-

site image that describe what it is like to experience beauty. Words such as "flowing," "calm," "tranquil," and "uplifting" have been suggested by patients.

3) Mutual responsiveness to expressions of musical gestures associated with positive emotions can access interpersonal factors that modulate negative emotions and elicit empathy, which in turn increases positive emotions.[2]

4) Accessing everyday creativity within improvisation (referential or non-referential) adds to adaptability, increased self efficacy, and encourages patients to become aware of his or her own problem solving abilities. I have observed that patients experience joy as they discover a melody or a rhythm that they regard as a perfect fit with the therapist's music. They also become aware either during the music or during the listening of the recorded improvisation(s) that their creations enhance the overall music quality.

Following each improvisation the therapist assesses if the patient is capable of verbal expression about the effects of his or her experience in the music. If the patient shows signs that a conversation is possible he initiates an interview based upon the author's model of reflection. This model is based upon verbal therapy methods that focus upon the process of accessing and reflecting upon the patient's own emotions. Reflection can enhance adaptation and reduces the tendency for pain catastrophizing, which is the tendency "…to ruminate upon pain sensations and feel helpless about pain…".[2] If possible, the therapist attempts to limit direct verbal references to the pain experience and instead responds to, and encourages, the patient's description of any positive emotions that have emerged from the music making. If the patient desires to instead ruminate on pain descriptions, then the therapist encourages the patient toward another music making experience based upon the patient's preference. The therapist may also create another composite image upon which the improvisation is structured. Either way, the therapist attempts to gently shift the patient's focus away from the sensation of pain and toward emotional expressions in the music.

Thomsen et al reported that positive emotional stimuli, in this case the music, enhances conscious reporting, which is observable in the way that patients expressively use verbal and physical gestures.[9] If a post-music conversation can continue toward reflection of the music experience, an interview format is used that draws upon phenomenological methods designed by this writer. The following vignette describes one scenario in which the focus upon positive emotions occurs within the improvisations.

Music Therapy Improvisation and Reflection for Pain Relief

Clinical Vignette

Rose was a 79 year old woman with metastatic bone cancer throughout most of her body. She was admitted to the psychiatric/medical care unit following statements she had made to her son about wanting to end it all, her way. She had two very supportive sons who visited her at home and in the hospital regularly. Rose's chief complaints revolved around the intense pain she felt throughout her body and her depressed and anxious mood. She was often in bed complaining that she was in too much pain to get out and interact with staff, and to engage in the milieu activities and therapies. The treatment team decided to initially deliver services to her in her room with the hope that increased interpersonal stimulation could eventually lead to a reduction in her anxious and depressed mood state. Music therapy began in her roo when she agreed that she could tolerate a brief period of quiet guitar music played by the music therapist. The music therapist chose a soft bossa nova style. Within three fifteen-minute sessions, Rose and the therapist developed a positive relationship. In the second session she slowly raised her left arm while lying in bed and gently rocked it back and forth in half tempo with the music.

She spoke about her brief period of piano lessons as a child and about how much she loved piano music. The music therapist suggested that they walk to the room used for music therapy where the piano was located. With help she was able to make it to the piano bench on the upper register side of the keyboard. The therapist sat on the lower register side of the bench and suggested that she run her fingers over the keys to find some sounds that she liked. She soon created short three and four note motifs, stating that these simple note combinations were beautiful. The therapist encouraged her to continue to explore and concentrate on the sounds that she enjoyed. She raised her left arm and began to gently sway it in an even more expressive manner than she did while lying in bed. The therapist began to provide accompaniment in the lower register with moderately slow arpeggios and chords. One example of a chord progression that was used is: I Major 7, ii7, V7 chord progression. For those wishing to use this progression, a bridge section can be added to reduce repetition.

Rose had her eyes closed during the music and continued to expressively sway her other arm in its own tempo. After three to four minutes she stopped and reported that she forgot about her pain and became tearful. She said the music was beautiful and caused her to feel like she was floating. The therapist encouraged her to further describe the floating. Rose talked about the floating sensation using a calm voice, which seemed relaxed. This was the first time that Rose was able to come out of her room and also the first time she reported any pain relief.

We continued this music making over the next several days. The music therapist checked in with her to schedule a time when they could play music at the piano. During most attempts she felt too weak to stand, but by late morning she was able to attempt to rise up from the bed with assistance and go to the piano. She eventually asked for assistance to walk to the piano at times when the music therapist was not on the unit. It seemed that she was able to achieve similar pain-free states at the piano without the music therapist. When her sons were told of this they offered to acquire a piano for Rose's home where she could be assisted by her home health aide to go to the piano. She was discharged the day after the piano arrived in her home.

Although this may not seem like a formal discharge plan, Rose's discovery of how music therapy could work for her was a lesson for the music therapist on how music-induced positive emotions could lead to a positive disruption of the pain experience. Further work with pain patients led to a format in which a follow-up discussion of the positive emotions and sensations seemed to result in additional relief initiated by an activation of positive emotions music improvisation.

Reflection Interview

The experiencing of music–induced positive emotions can be amplified by structuring a post-music interview using a phenomenological-oriented discussion about the patient's experience in the music. The interview is not meant to acquire data, as in a phenomenological qualitative research method, but to allow the patient full disclosure and expression of his or her subjective experiences. The method is as follows:

The therapist asks "can you tell me about your experiences while playing music? Any thoughts, feelings or awareness's are important to describe." In my experience, patients typically reference one of the realms of music responses, including cognitive, emotional, physical, interpersonal, or spiritual realms or experience that were defined earlier in the chapter. Whichever realm is introduced, the therapist continues to encourage the patient to fully describe his or her experience in that realm without offering a response except to encourage further depth and elaboration. If there is overlap into another of the realms the therapist takes note of the additional realm and continues to encourage expression about the initial realm. For example, if the patient states, "at times I felt a warm feeling in my chest" the therapist encourages full expression of the physical realm. If the patient makes a fleeting reference into another realm, such as "the music sounded joyful" the therapist first encourages any additional physical realm descriptions before stating, "you said that the music sounded joyful. Can you tell me more about that feeling (emotion realm)?"

The emphasis is placed upon full description of each realm that the patient described. The assumption here is that the patient may not know what experiences are relevant to communicate to the therapist. However, full expression about everything of which the patient has experienced from the music elicits a further deepening of non-pain states and increases the likelihood of facilitating positive emotions. When the patient has no more to report about a current realm the therapist returns to the initial request, "can you tell me anything else about what you experienced while playing music?" This question most often elicits a response that links to another full description of experiences from another realm.

As the interview continues, the patient often increases his or her motivation and energy to freely describe sensations, thoughts, and other types of awareness elicited by the music. The therapist does not place value judgments on any of the patient's comments. Nor does the therapist attempt to influence shifts of the discussion into other realms until the patient has no more to report about the current realm. Sometimes, the patient's awareness may only elicit discussion from one or a few of the realms either because of fatigue or because a sense of completion has occurred, at which point the interview is concluded. The therapist may either ask if the patient wishes to play more music or he may decide that the session has produced the maximum benefit and bring the session to a close.

Post Interview: Music Listening
If time and patient interest/energy permit, a music listening of the recorded session can follow the interview. The music listening serves to concretize for the patient the relationship between the positive emotions elicited from the music, with the awareness of a current mood state of well being. The interview may serve as a primer for the patient to again experience positive emotions during the music listening. Often when patients hear the recording of the music that he or she co-created with the therapist, expressions related to a sense of self-efficacy emerge. Patients often experience delight and surprise when listening to the music. The activation of positive moods enhances their memory for the music therapy experience. This can become a subsequent motivator for the effectiveness of the uses of music to alter the pain experience.

Just before the listening begins, the therapist asks that patient if he or she would like to listen to the recording. If the patient agrees the therapist can say, "Try to listen to this with the same words in mind that we wrote down as suggestions of what the music should sound like." After listening a further discussion may take place. The therapist should pay close attention to any patient fatigue and begin to draw the session to a close before the patient becomes uncomfortably tired.

Music and Medicine: Integrative Models in the Treatment of Pain

Prescriptive Uses of Music Therapy
If the therapist has knowledge of impending patient discharge from the hospital he may, before bringing the session to a close, suggest a musical prescription to the patient. This prescription includes encouraging the patient to either take time in the future to conduct his or her own music therapy session. This can include singing alone or singing with preferred recorded music. The prescription can include that the patient plays a musical instrument of which they are familiar, or audiate music (the reproduction of music internally). This should be followed by the therapist's suggestion that the patient concentrate upon the experiencing of beauty from the musical experience, focus upon positive associations or memories elicited by the music, and/or talk about extra musical associations to a friend, family member or care giver. The patient is encouraged to practice this prescription as often as possible. With time, the benefits will occur with less effort.

Clinical Vignette
The following example took place during the earlier stages of the formation of this protocol. As both the music therapist and writer of this chapter, the personal pronoun "I" will be used as we continue.

Ronald is a 44 year old African American male with sickle cell anemia. He lived alone and worked as a part-time security guard. He attended outpatient medical services at a university hospital, and had been hospitalized twice in the last three years. At times he reported the pain from his sickle cell as "something that you can't control, you medicate it." He reported that at times it was unbearable. However, his kalimba playing sometimes lessened the pain.

During his outpatient visits to the hospital Ronald could be seen walking through the hallways playing his kalimba. It seemed that the kalimba was a way for him to reduce the pain. His playing tempo was usually between 110 and 120 beats per minute, with repetitive and subdivided rhythmic groupings without rests. He used a steady moderately loud dynamic range, which caused some calluses on the thumbs of both hands. Upon referral by the unit director he agreed to participate in a single music therapy session as a part of a documentary film.

As the film crew set up their equipment in a makeshift hospital room Ronald and I became acquainted with each other. After a brief orientation to the tenor xylophone, hand percussion instruments and the various kalimbas provided by Ronald and myself, we began to play music together. Our first duet used two kalimbas. I played a steady ostinato figure in response to his kalimba playing. His music was fast, repetitive and with a dance-like feel. It reminded me of West Coast African music from the

Music Therapy Improvisation and Reflection for Pain Relief

Drums of Passion recording by Babatunde Olatunji. Ronald played xylophone set to a dorian scale and I used guitar. I strummed with some melodic motifs using d minor, e minor 7, F major 7, A sus, and A7. The tempo Ronald chose was fast and he played with both hands in a manner similar to someone drumming with hands on a table top while waiting for the automated teller bank machine to complete the transaction. His focus was upon playing repetitive, complex, subdivided rhythms, seemingly, without much conscious thought for melody. Simple, short, repetitive motifs emerged in his playing, organized more so on rhythmic groupings than on melodic characteristic. This style was similar to his solo kalimba playing. The music therapist matched tempo with rhythmic chord strumming while reflecting the most consistent of Ronald's melodic motifs.

The film crew began filming during our first improvisation, yet our focus was fixed to the music. My musical response to Ronald's fast tempo and almost seamless rhythmic groupings was musically demanding. Having to bring instruments to a remote location for the purpose of the filming limited my choice for a chordal instrument to a nylon string guitar. I prefer to use my thumb and fingers because it allows me to play both a harmonic role with bass movement while adding melodies with my first two fingers. I was able to provide a ground and a melodic figural response to Ronald's melodic ideas, however as he was playing loudly and very fast, I was limited in my response to him. At best, I could provide a harmonic and rhythmic response with only limited uses of short motifs. Trying to get as close as I could to Ronald's music, I began to actually feel what his pain must have been like, not on a nociceptive level but within the overall tension and pain experience. It was then that I decided to play in a more relaxed, half tempo, holding, rather than matching, in my approach. I allowed my arms to become more expressive in slow, full strums alternating with melodic motifs that echoed the short melodic contour of his mostly rhythmic motifs.

The improvisation was successful in that Ronald stated that he felt we had really connected and that his music sounded really good with accompaniment. He seemed more relaxed and outgoing as he spoke. His comments were limited to the cognitive realm, mostly in describing how he negotiated the xylophone in relation to the guitar. While he also said that the music had made him feel good, he had very little to say in the physiological, emotional and interpersonal realms. I sensed that what he did not report was significant. He never mentioned pain, nor showed any signs of responding to the joint pain that is typical for people with sickle cell anemia. He made only brief reference to nurses from his inpatient unit. He seemed to be totally involved in an aesthetic experience, in which only his musical perceptions were relevant. I believe that the aesthetic experience when described can draw upon each of the realms in differing amounts, and at different times in the music improvisations.

Ronald's cognitive realm involvement was essentially that of music cognition in working out his rhythms into flowingly symmetrical phrases, fitting accents into the groupings sometimes, seemingly, in response to my guitar playing. He established the necessary physical positioning to maintain tempo, accents and lateral arm movement on the xylophone. Interpersonally, he focused attention in an alternating pattern between his and my music production. Emotionally, he was not distracted by discomfort, yet seemed "at one" with the music. In spite of the presence of the three members of the film crew and the woman who represented hospital media communications, Ronald remained calm, with full attention to the music. It wasn't until after the next improvisation that Ronald began to verbally express in other realms while listening to the recording of our music making.

The final improvisation was arranged by me. I asked for Ronald to return to his kalimba and I sat at the xylophone set to a C major scale, similar to his kalimba tuning. As an induction toward encouraging an experience of positive emotions, I asked him to think of creating a piece of music that could be used for relaxation; a piece of music that could create a sense of peace and beauty. I had intended to begin the piece in order to prime for the mood but Ronald quickly started the music. Again, he played in a fast, subdivided, repetitive manner. One notable difference about this improvisation was the change of the quality in his phrasing. It had shifted to a rolling, rocking feeling set by slight pulsating alterations in his dynamics. I realized that he was attempting to introduce a new option into his music. He had a smile on his face when we caught eye contact with each other.

I hoped that I could musically suggest an additional change in his music now that he seemed less guarded and more open. Since Ronald refrained from taking rests in his playing I wondered if he was also restricting his breathing while playing. Musicians use the saying, "take a breath" as a way to create a sense of separating one musical phrase from another. I wondered if Ronald held his breath as an attempt to block pain. His relentless rhythmic subdivisions may have assisted him, to some degree, in this attempt, but I wondered if doing so also introduced additional tension. I learned from working with an earlier patient that incessant rhythms could be accompanied by interruptions in breathing, resulting in increased physical tension.[10]

I began to play short motif double stops in open intervals as dotted quarter notes in the 12/8 meter, followed by an occasional use of six beats of rests in an attempt to elongate the sense of time. At first, Ronald's dynamics softened, then a brief breath seemed to appear in his phrasing. Our bodies

Music Therapy Improvisation and Reflection for Pain Relief

rocked at the same tempo. I wondered if this was a result of entrainment in response to his meter. The piece came to a mutual close.

I asked Ronald to listen to the recording shortly after we finished the music. I asked him to listen to the music not as a critic, but to focus on the words I used earlier in the induction. I repeated, "allow yourself to let your breathing go freely and see what response you have to it."

As soon as Ronald heard the music his eyes filled with tears and he nodded his head up and down saying, "thank you, thank you" (later he told me that he thanked God for the music experience). From his response it seemed to me that during the final improvisation, there was a tremendous release of energy that he had been holding in, and that this release was very pleasurable for him. It was powerful for him to feel that he was a part of something beautiful. While he was listening to the music and gently weeping I asked him "is that the first time you've listened to yourself in a long time?" He answered, "I guess, yes, and really listened, yes, and with accompaniment it sounded better. It's peace and hopefully someone else can feel that peace."

It seemed that from both the improvisation that was structured to induce positive emotions, and possibly the entirety of all the music we'd played together, Ronald had had positive experiences in each of the realms. He later reported that he was pain free for almost the entire second half of the session.

Conclusion

The protocol described in this chapter is a departure from many other formats of music therapy. It enlists patients into an important and active role in their otherwise passive treatment for pain. It is meant for patients who can tolerate both the playing of instruments and the follow up verbal expression about those responses elicited by playing music. It is clear however, that both increasing the activation of positive emotions through musical expression, and subsequent verbal expressions relevant to the patient's responses to the music, seem to activate neurological gaiting of the patient's pain.

The role of positive emotions as central to the therapy must be maintained, therefore, the therapist does not make references to the patient's pain. Instead, the therapist works on the assumption that the music therapy process attracts healthy responses, which in turn result in a positive change in the pain experience.

This protocol may not be appropriate for all hospitalized patients who are suffering from pain. Serious, acute pain may require a different approach. Future research should include case studies and randomized control trials using mixed methods of quantitative and qualitative designs to further substantiate the use of music therapy in specific contexts.

References

1. Bradt J, Dileo C, Grocke D, Magill L. Music interventions for improving psychological and physical outcomes in cancer patients. Cochrane Database Syst Rev 2011;CD006911.pub2.
2. Lumley MA, Cohen JL, Borszcz GS, et al. Pain and emotion: A biopsychosocial review of recent literature. Jornal of Clinical Psychology. 2011;67:942-968.
3. Finucane A, Dima A, Ferreira N, Halvorsen M. Basic emotion profiles in healthy, chronic pain, depressed and PTSD individuals. Clinical Psych & Psychotherapy. Jan-Feb 2012;19(1):14-24.
4. Mossler K, Assmus J, Heldal TO, Fuchs K, Gold C. Music therapy techniques as predictors of change in mental health care. The Arts in Psychotherapy. September 2012;39(4):333-341.
5. Cepeda MS, Carr, DB, Lau J, Alvarez H. Music for pain relief. Cochrane Database Syst Rev 2006;2:CD004843. 360.
6. Beck C. Education for spirituality. Interchange. June 1986.Toronto. ISSN:0826-4805.
7. Maslow A. Toward a psychology of being. 2nd ed. New York, NY: D. Van Nostrand Co.;1968.
8. Dawson ME, Schell AM, Filion DL. The electrodermal system. In: Cacioppo JT, Tassinary LG, Bernstein GG, eds. Handbook of psychophysiology. New York, NY: Cambridge University Press; 2007:159-181.
9. Thomsen R, Kristine L, H. J, et al. Impact of emotion on consciousness: Positive stimuli enhance conscious reportability. PLosONE. 2011;6(4).
10. Nolan P. Through music to therapeutic attachment: Psychodynamic music therapy with a musician with dysthymic disorder. In: Hadley S, ed. Psychodynamic Music Therapy: Case Studies. Gilsum, NH: Barcelona Publishers;2003.

CHAPTER 7

Music Sedation and Pain

Joanne V. Loewy DA, LCAT, MT-BC

Suffering was the only thing that made me feel I was alive
Thought that's just how much it cost to survive in this world
'Til you showed me how, how to fill my heart with love
How to open up and drink in all that white light
Pouring down from the heavens
Carly Simon & Jacob Brackman

Introduction

Healthcare providers in hospitals are paying increased attention to the administration of care with stronger emphasis on treatment efficacy. There is a current trend of focus that is calling upon hospital teams to reduce a patient's length of stay (LOS). The necessity to identify the source of pain and treat painful symptoms effectively is critical to patients' experience of optimal care, particularly as we seek to reduce their length of stay.

Although one's first thought in aiming to decrease the length of stay might seem to have positive ramifications for patients, particularly those patients experiencing pain. The sooner the pain's etiology is identified, the sooner the discharge. This kind of thinking might implicitly reflect that we are getting better at treating disease ailments more effectively and more quickly, with stronger preventative strategies for homecare. Patients who were one time hospitalized for a week, might perceive a current, shorter stay to mean that they are 'getting better faster.' Another thought is that the impact of the shorter stay will allow patients an opportunity to heal faster because they are thought to fare better in their 'normal' environment.

A recent study[1] addressed length-of-stay efficacy and sought to assess precisely how much cost hospitals actually saved by shortening a patient's length of stay. Interestingly, and perhaps surprisingly, for the majority of the patients studied in this investigation, the costs directly attributable to the last day of their hospital stays were an economically insignificant component of total costs. Reducing the LOS by as much as 1 full day reduced the total cost of care only on average by a marker of 3% or less. This study makes a compelling point and summarizes astutely the idea that physicians and professional caregivers might provide better care, in terms of treatment and cost, if LOS were deemphasized. It implies that our focus, instead, should turn to how we process changes that make better use of *capacity*. There is a marked attention and suggestion here that we alter our care delivery to focus more intently on the early stages of admission, where *diagnosis and assessment* is key, and furthermore where "resource consumption is most intense."[1] Nowhere could this be more important than in the treatment of pain. There is indeed a necessity to diagnose and assess with greater acuity and accuracy, the result of which is thought to yield large cost savings for hospitals and insurance companies. Music therapists can assist in this process in their medical-psychosocial integration strategies and through an evaluation that sets goals to be inclusive of strategies that address pain.

As health care providers in medical settings, music therapists care for patients of all ages and diagnoses, and pain is not uncommon to our assessment of symptomology. Although the evaluation of pain is considered to be vital toward the treatment of a disease, the effects of dis-ease are not always well treated. As reflected in a recent overview in Lancet:

> ...the most notable therapeutic changes have not been the development of novel evidenced-based methods, but rather changing trends in applications and practices within the available clinical armamentarium. We provide a general overview of empirical evidence for the most commonly used interventions in the management of chronic non-cancer pain, including pharmacological, interventional, physical, psychological, rehabilitative, and alternative modalities. Overall, currently available treatments provide modest improvements in pain and minimum improvements in physical and emotional functioning. The quality of evidence is mediocre and has not improved substantially during the past decade. There is a crucial need for assessment of combination treatments, identification of indicators of treatment response, and assessment of the benefit of matching of treatments to patient characteristics.[2]

There are numerous options available for application when considering how to treat pain with music therapy interventions. A music therapy pain assessment will provide critical cues that lead to the most effective treatment plan.[3,4] Recorded music (listening) and active music play (often cited as "distraction")[5-7] are common experiences that are posed as effective interventions in the literature. This may be due to the fact that these options are easily accessible for nurses and doctors to recommend, and may not require advanced training for the practitioner who is offering such an intervention when a music therapist is not on staff.

Release,[3] tonal intervallic synthesis,[8] integration,[3] entrainment,[8] toning and musical visualization[3] are additional viable pain options which are cited and studied less frequently. This chapter will address perhaps one of the most accessible options for treating pain. Sedation, specifically, to assist one's capacity to let go through breath-ing and/or breathing accompanied by a visualization experience, is a useful means of addressing pain, particularly when the a patient expresses anger or exhaustion, and especially in instances where other pain treatment options have been ineffective.

Pain Classification & Etiology

Pain, the most common symptom found in medical settings, can be categorized in a multitude of ways. Although pain is usually identified as a negative perceptual experience, pain is nevertheless, adaptive and is considered to be a useful means of assisting in the evaluation of body function, particularly in the diagnosis and treatment of disease. In this way, it has a unique purpose, or function, even while often presenting as a dysfunction within the continuum of care in a medical setting. One way to understand pain is to look at its effect in the treatment of disease as a symptom related to the etiology of an illness. Pain may be chronic, acute, or exist as the result of a medical procedure. Pain may also be classified as psychosomatic or may present as a secondary response to extreme anxiety. Pain might be adaptive, contributing to survival, or maladaptive.

Maladaptive pain, or "pain as disease"[9] is "uncoupled from a noxious stimulus or healing tissue. Such pain may occur in response to damage to the nervous system (neuropathic pain) or result from abnormal operation of the nervous system (functional pain). Maladaptive pain is the expression of abnormal sensory processing and is usually persistent or recurrent".

Neuropathic pain is considered to be a type of maladaptive pain that results from specific types of pathophysiology. Pathophysiology of neuropathic pain may involve diverse mechanisms dependent on distinct physical symptoms that vary from one patient to the next. Neuropathic, inflammatory or non-inflammatory/non-neuropathic pain can come on suddenly without an apparent source or may be evoked by a specific stimuli. Pain that is caused by a known source may be either allodynic or hyperalgesic. Allodynic pain is when a usual non-painful stimuli is perceived as painful. Hyperalgesic pain is when the occurrence of what might be a usual painful stimulus is perceived as more painful than usual. Wolff classifies pain in four distinct groups and defines its presence according to stimuli[9]:

Nociceptive pain: adaptive transient pain in response to a noxious stimulus (like an alarm that announces the presence of a potentially damaging stimulus).

Inflammatory pain: spontaneous pain and hypersensitivity to pain in response to tissue damage and inflammation. Can be adaptive or maladaptive.

Neuropathic pain: spontaneous pain and hyperalgesia in association with damage to or lesion of the nervous system (like an alarm that is constantly on even though there is no emergency, or gives repeated false alarms). Spontaneous pain and changes in sensitivity to stimuli are fundamental features of maladaptive pain, distinguishing it from nociceptive pain.

Non-imflammatory/non-neuropathic pain ("functional pain"): hypersensitivity to pain resulting from abnormal central processing of normal input (e.g. fibromyalgia, irritable bowel syndrome, tension-type headache, non-cardiac chest pain). Non-inflammatory/non-neuropathic pain is a type of maladaptive pain.

Pain Management

Severe pain, whatever the source, stimulus or etiology, can increase in severity as an illness progresses. Whether pain is a symptom of an acute illness, such as an acute sickle cell pain crisis, a chronic source, such as lower back pain, arthritic pain or recurring migraine headaches, the treatment often involves a plethora of poly pharmacological agents. In recent years we have taken pain more seriously and doctors have been exploring neurotransmitters as the critical mechanism for treating chronic pain.[10] Activated microglia contribute to the maintenance of chronic pain after spinal cord injury.[11]

In current times, the treatment of chronic pain is no longer limited to analgesics such as acetaminophens or opiates. Antidepressants may attend to specific chemicals in the brain that address associative emotions linked to one's perception of pain (see Quentzel, Chapter 1). This is an important development which honors Taber's golden standard definition that pain is not only a nociceptive physical percept of the body, but is inclusive to one's emotional response to that percept.[12]

With advances in MRI imaging, researchers are demonstrating that the changes of percepts in the brain are components that we can track. Increasing use of MRI suggests that subtle changes in the behavioral-affective and senoral-discriminative centers of the brain are more active when there is focus on the pain stimuli.[13] When there is focus on a cognitive task, or the brain engages in an activity that demands alternate neural activity, the pain percept is reduced. We also know that pain, which is not adequately treated, can return.[14]

History of Music Therapy at Beth Israel

The Louis and Lucille Armstrong Music Therapy Program was instituted at Beth Israel in 1994 as part of the Department of Social Work and Home Care services. The program's early focus was on Pediatrics and eventually grew to include a second music therapy line for out patient services, which provided music therapy for children with HIV and their families (see Mondanaro & Vaskas, Chapter 21). In 1996 we became part of the Pain team at Beth Israel and in 2000, we expanded into the Neonatal Intensive Care Unit instituting music therapy services for neonates and their families. In 2001, we grew to serve Oncology, Family Medicine and developed a comprehensive Environmental Music Therapy (EMT) program, for many of our ICUs. In more recent years, music therapy has expanded to the Department of Pain and Palliative Medicine, Pulmonology, Post-Spine Surgery and we have been treating patients within hospice as well.

In 2005, we developed a center and expanded considerably, with several new music therapy positions, a medical director (Stephan Quentzel MD) and the opening of The Louis Armstrong Center for Music and Medicine. We became a department with additional research projects not only in the hospital, but in our outpatient center and in the NYC community as well. Included in our treatment areas was the healthcare and psychotherapy provisions made for musicians, and some of our in-patient programs went community wide, such as our work with children and teens with asthma and adults with COPD. In each and every part of our programmatic expansion, the assessment of pain has been and continues to be a critical part of our treatment.

Philosophy: A Medical Music Psychotherapy Approach to Pain Assessment & Management

The 13 Areas of Inquiry,[4] (Appendix B) are part of the assessment and include: Awareness of Self, others, and the moment, Thematic Expression, Listening, Performing, Collaboration/Relationship, Concentration, Range of Affect, Investment/Motivation, Use of Structure, Integration, Self Esteem, Risk Taking, Independence. Critical information for the therapist, and particularly important in a pain assessment, is the gathering of information related to how the hospitalized patients functioned *prior to the illness/hospitalization*. This is compared to how they are presenting alone and with family within the session. Wellness is an important pre-reference to ego support and emotional supportive development of well-being both in and out of the music therapy sessions. The CAS (Color Analysis Scale, Appendix A) is a usual and customary part of our assessment battery and provides the patient, therapist, doctor and team with integral information that enhances the pain evaluation and designed experiences, which follow.

Since the inception of The Louis Armstrong Music Therapy Program in 1994, our clinical focus viewed the pain experience as an expression of medical and/or emotional symptomology, in virtually each and every assessment undertaken by the music therapists and music therapy interns and fellows. The occurrence of pain, once assessed through verbal and/or musical expression is then, in turn, reported to the attending doctors and residents that are part of our team for input both before (upon referral-discussion of potential options) and after the music therapy intervention. First with our pediatric pain attending doctor Betsy Macgregor MD, where music therapy's presence was evident on the Continuous Quality Improvement's (CQI) hospital-wide pain incentive she conducted, and years later under the direction of Russell Portenoy MD, who afforded us the privilege to institute music therapy in our medical center's pain initiatives. Our assessment and treatment of pain has been acknowledged as an established clinical domain and integrated within the many teams we serve throughout the hospital. Pain and the ramifications of its symptomology is a succinct and distinct area of our focus whether by referral from an attending doctor, nurse, social worker or patient, or as part of a generalized music therapy assessment where we are treating a disease in which pain is not expected to be occurring. Pain is always included as a significant parameter evaluated within our research trials where we are addressing anxiety or another set of symptoms including but not limited to respiratory function, heart rate changes, activity level, activities of daily living, quality of life, psychological and psychosocial function. In fact, the presence of pain can impact any or all of these areas.

Music psychotherapy is a process-oriented approach centered on the dynamic that evolves between the patient/therapist, and the unique relationship that each hold within the music. Issues of historical significance, present status and future possibilities are explored through individual (solo), and collaborative (duet, trio, quartet, ensemble) music experiences. Music psychotherapy includes the identification of themes (music/emotional) in a clinical context. Through repetition of what is known (review, orientation) and/or the development of what is unfamiliar (creative, improvisational) the music psychotherapeutic relationship provides insight and a mechanism for constructing meaning and understanding action. This construction may occur through exploration and integration of sounds and silences through vocalization, song and/or verbalization and through the use of musical instruments.[4]

The philosophy and training within The Louis Armstrong Music Therapy Training Model is based on a psychotherapy orientation. The therapist uses music psychotherapy principles (www.musicandmedicine.org) to achieve body-mind resonance. The development of an Integrative Medical

Music Psychotherapy Model as it is practiced with infants, children, teens and adults of varying medical diagnoses is depicted in Figure 2 on page 156 of Chapter 10. Aspects of music are correlated with aspects of medical need. Outlined are four essential areas of treatment that integrate the musical and medical components and serve to provide optimal levels of care, blending mind, body and spirit.

Music Psychotherapy Assumptions

I have built my clinical practice on the philosophy outlined by the following Music Psychotherapy Assumptions, which are critical to consider in medical settings, and most particularly when treating pain:

1. A complete medical music psychotherapy assessment will offer a hypothesis on how the mind is affecting the body and vice versa.
2. A person's psychological coping mechanisms may be enhanced through music therapy. This has been shown to alter the immune system's receptivity to healing and can enhance the body's capacity to recover from pain crisis related to illness.[15]
3. Effective medical music therapy involves treating the rhythms, resonances, tones and timbres of the body in an effort to stimulate harmonic balance.
4. Pre-composed, as well as improvisatory chants may contain, sedate, and/or relax patients of any age, race or gender.
5. Live music making and visualization can relax the body by reducing the systolic blood pressure, regulating HR & respiratory function which may be particularly helpful and/or necessary before, during or post surgery; or during times of anxiety or painful crisis.
6. Native African drumming, toning, and other release oriented music making experiences can reduce the body's perception of pain.
7. Singing and wind playing in a music therapy context can deepen the level of breath in acute asthmatics and adults with COPD expressed in: lung volume capacity, emotional incentive, and motivational realms.
8. The use of passive music (e.g. listening to recordings) though often therapeutic, is not in and of itself, music therapy. Entrainment principles applied actively in experiences of live music application can promote a healing effect conducive to a medical music therapy intervention whereby physical symptoms and emotional experiences can be dynamically sensed by the therapist and the patient in the moment of exchange.

Music Therapy in Treatment

Music Sedation as a Treatment Option
Music Sedation is an essential and viable treatment option for patients of all ages and diagnoses. Sleep may serve as a critical function necessary in the treatment of any disease, and sleep is also critical for the maintenance of usual health and wellness, particularly in recovery or in patients that are susceptible to recurrence of disease. In many instances, pain can be suppressed or the perception of pain can be softened, if the body is able to sleep because during rest and particularly in deep sleep, the mind's perceptions can be deactivated so that the cycle of pain response is shut off. Notably, an effective evaluation and assessment session are necessary in order to build the trust it will require for a patient to be able to transition from wake to sleep, in the presence of a therapist who is singing and/or providing live instrumental music.

Sleep/Sedation in Neonates and Infants
When an infant is in discomfort, irritability may be expressed through a high-pitched scream. The meningeal cry and the cri du chat are actual types of crying sounds that assist in the identification of specific diseases in infants [16]. The music therapist may frame a cry response to an assumed root or tonic tone of the infant's cry, on a perfect 5th or on a Major or Minor 3rd. These are the actual components of 'the child's theme'-which is common to lullabies around the world and has been for so for generations. Eventually the tone can be pulsed. It begins after an audible breathing sound is presented, and the tone begins only as the infant commences and ceases when she/he ceases to cry. The infant is the conductor. The therapist entrains to the breath of the cry and eventually, the therapist and infant release the vocal tone naturally, at the exact same time. As the scream softens and ritards, the therapist can pulse a triplet meter to create a feeling of motion for the infant, exactly during the release of the infant's cry.

In this way, the sound is surrounding and holding the infant, creating a feeling of balance and also one of being heard and supported. The cry will often then eventually become less accented, less pronounced, and less severe.

To assist an infant in releasing a cry, when she/he is observably uncomfortable, but observed to be holding in, or holding on to tension, the therapist may want to provide a one note 'blanket of tone' on a vowel sound. Tonal vocal holding[17-19] provides comfort and reassurance to the infant that someone is present and furthermore, that a release of tension through sound may be natural.

Music Sedation and Pain

Song of Kin/ Lullabies for Sleep/Sedation
Developing a musical ritual for the most difficult of separations for babies can be useful. Encouraging a caregiver to identify either a song from their past, a song of kin[20] may be assuring for all populations, both with children and adults particularly because it is apt to hold one's tradition, culture and/or family history and values.[21] There is also a pride, which comes in the familiarity and the strength that caregivers seem to imbue when song of kin is used. Loewy[22,23] developed a method for using song of kin to sedate. Encouraging caregivers to sing to their family members in illness and in wellness, within active and interactive circumstances and particularly during moments right before sleep times may be the most important means of providing assurances that music may be a critical threadline between activity and sleep. In this way, it can be a safety net and used purposefully and pharmaceutically as a non-invasive method for sedation and sleep, which is integral toward the healing process of a disease and the maintenance of health in wellness.

Music psychotherapy and the therapist's role can distinctly address ways in which the music can become an active and actualized agent of connectedness from the patient perspective. Music and its capacity to provide mechanisms of affectual and purposeful integration within the body-mind trajectory, and as a part of the relationship that music can afford between patient and staff recognizably offer unique hosts of opportunity for a broad range of treatment strategies.

Music as Sedation
There is strong evidence that music can 'soothe the savage breast.' At The Louis Armstrong Center for Music & Medicine at Beth Israel Medical Center, music therapy is a well-utilized option for patient referrals of all kinds of pain and for all ages-from NICU through end of life. In 2005, our Pediatric team investigated the effects of chloral hydrate when compared to music therapy for sedating babies and toddlers for medical testing.

We found that the use of live music, lullabies sung by a parent who was supervised, and/or music therapist was overwhelmingly more effective than the pharmacological agent of choice, which at that time was chloral hydrate. As we studied the 60 children who were randomized into drug or music groups and matched for age and diagnosis, we learned about emergence delirium.[20] Several of the subjects in the pharmacologically sedated group had a response to the chloral hydrate where an opposite undesirable effect took place-called 'emergence delirium.' At other times pharmacological sedation kept children asleep for hours, where when music was used, children would often awaken shortly after the test was complete. Through our research, we showed that music therapy is a viable option that doctors should consider, particularly for medical tests. This is not to suggest that it necessarily be used as a replacement for a pharmacological agent, but perhaps under specific conditions this might prove useful. At other times music may complement a sedative, because when tendered therapeutically, by a music therapist, it might relax the patient thus allowing a sedative to work more quickly and with greater effectiveness and this can reduce both use and cost.

The fact that the process of sedation might include a parent may be comforting to an infant or young child. It may also be comforting to a parent who otherwise might feel threatened or helpless. This is particularly true for parents of infants in the NICU.[21-23] In best practices, family-centered care provides a basis of 'normalcy', trust and compliance for treatment.[24] As music may be a part of a child's usual routine when s/he is well, its effectiveness for use within aspects of critical care should not be overlooked, particularly with critical care pediatric populations.[25] Music therapists are certified and trained to work with developmental aspects of care particularly when children are faced with stressful challenges. In music psychotherapy, the musical relationship between child and therapist can enhance feelings of comfort and support during treatment. Music interventions directly affect treatment issues which can become prevalent as families face new diagnoses, uncomfortable procedures, and/or frightening hospital stays where thoughts about school, events and routine sports or other activities are missed and replaced with fears and nightmares about not only dread of what might come next, but a loss in recovery of their current 'status' in the classroom, on the sports team or within their achieved placement in a music, art or drama group.

Community Jam: A Symphony of Sounds
Each week on most of our hospital's units, we have a Community Jam. Patients, families, and staff of all disciplines, gather in a communal place; the family lounge, playroom, or even in a hallway or indoor bridge to play music together. The playing of musical instruments that can provide a creative soundscape aurally and visually can connect members of the hospital community together in equal measure. Patients' instrumental play may be drawn to 'groove' with other patients' providing a network of attentive support that is playful and fun.[26] Favorite songs might link parents of patients to other parents or staff, where they might share potent memories of their respective worlds outside of the hospital. Fill in songs, such as blues or reggae can pull the community into artistically and dynamically expressing their wishes, intentions, or frustrations. The jam provides the means for hospital roles to be forgotten and individual expression to enhance community.

Environmental Music Therapy (EMT)
EMT is another useful group modality for hospitals, particularly chemotherapy and waiting rooms,[27] (see Rossetti & Canga, Chapter 16) where the pain experience is lessened, and where patients, especially elders, and babies and toddlers may feel trust enough to doze off or sleep. Perhaps surprisingly, such patients might relinquish the control to their environment more in a music group, than when they are in their own hospital room where others are not present and where loneliness and/or fearfulness may be heightened.

Clinical Work

The following vignettes include brief snapshots of actual pain treatment sessions, which involved sleep-sedation. They are taken from actual assessments and chart notes of past sessions.

Chronic Pain

Musical Sedation and Nurturance leads to 'Dear Prudence'
We think of chronic pain as the occurrence of discomfort that lasts beyond an expected disease recovery period. Chronic pain is hurt that endures and it challenges patients of all ages, and particularly children, and their parents.
     Singing is a useful modality in music therapy as the voice is the only musical instrument that is housed inside the body. And as such, it can provide for a myriad of sensory experiences that are distinctly intertwined with neurological and cognitive function. When the voice sings, pulmonary and cardiac function resonate, because breathing takes effort and although respiration is an involuntary function in non-music moments, meaning, we breathe automatically; in singing we actually choose how much effort, or how deeply we would like to breathe to express ourselves.[28]
     For a patient experiencing pain, singing can be a containing experience whereby 'toning' areas of the body, or 'chakras' may be synthesized to blend and soothe. Particular regions of pain in the body may be activated, and blood may flow more easily with live singing, especially if the therapist is elongating tones that a patient is singing with consonant intervals sung on vowel sounds.[8] This can be a wonderful precursor to sleep.
     Songwriting can be quite effective to utilize in music psychotherapy, to address embedded anger related to hostility that may be stimulated at the onset of when chronic pain seems everlasting or when medications do not seem to be taking effect.

Music and Medicine: Integrative Models in the Treatment of Pain

Case Vignette: James
James, a 17- year- old boy from India was having pain of an unknown origin. Although he thought his discomfort was from eating "bad chicken"-after a two week hospitalization food poisoning was not in question. The doctors were testing for abdominal sarcoma-cancer. Two weeks had begun to feel like "two years" to James and one day I convinced him to put his ipod away. I rarely ask teens to do this, because learning their music can be critical in establishing a connection. James loved the Beatles. We had listened through an ipod station to 'As My Guitar Gently Weeps' 'Blackbird' 'Barbara Ann' and 'Yesterday.' In his second session, after listening to 'Yesterday'-we delved into how he came to learn the Beatles-through a close relationship with his Uncle, who was in India, and whom he had visited last Christmas. We talked about the lyrics and James knew all about Paul McCartney's relationship with Linda. He also knew that she died of breast cancer at 56. James told me he had had a girlfriend for 2 years. In his first session, James was reportedly in pain, in his stomach and the prescribed medications were, as he put it not "working." As we listened to his favorite music, his trust with me built and we ended this session with his request that I play and sing "Blackbird"-I sang it for a while extending the "fly" over and over until he fell into a deep sleep.

    I remember recalling how sweet it felt that this mature teen from a foreign land, had clearly trusted me, so much so, that he was able to ask for the song he wanted, and under the conditions he desired-which was to be nurtured by my voice and the music until he could fall away to sleep.

    In the session to follow, my plan was to work with his fear and to address his pain that was apparently not subsiding easily and which doctors said may be continuing for quite some time, although medications were "helping somewhat" at that time. James professed his favorite Beatle's song of all time" at this next session to be 'Dear Prudence.'

    I tuned a guitar for James in an open a tuning and asked him to strum. He made a hidden grimace, at first, but did so. My thinking was that the guitar was gentle and he could hold it next to his abdomen and feel the vibration.

    I played consonant chords on my guitar in an open C tuning and sang 'Dear Prudence' - but realizing I was unfamiliar with the lyrics, I asked him to sing, and to my surprise he did. I sang "ahs" on harmony, knowing well, the melody of the tune. After a few times through - I sang "Dear..." and left a space. Silence. I asked James about his girlfriend in the melody...first, upon hearing her name was Judy, I sang a recitative (verse), which was an inquiry: "If you could sing this for Judy...what would you say...?" "Dear Judy..." and I left a space...James sang "I'll ask you to stay...even though we don't know what's coming, even though we both have to pay...dear Judy."

James' spontaneous and self-composed lyrics and singing went on and on - I was holding the harmonic structure on my guitar. His words relayed his fear of losing Judy as the result of this time that he was spending away from her. I related this to his own loss and fear of losing himself to a potentially fatal diagnosis.

As in this circumstance, listening, sedating-or putting to sleep with musical nurturance once trust was built, and then the next session's song writing and singing together, provided a poignant and physically comforting and cognitively grounding experience for the containment and expression of pain. Always related to an inter-connection between the mind-body and spirit, music can access any one of these three domains, or all three at one moment in time. Music making with another person happens at the same time, in the moment of play in a uniquely dynamic context. 'Dear Prudence' served as an important theme throughout James trajectory of treatments over the next several months.

Acute Pain

Release toward Relinquishing- 'Chitty Chitty Bang Bang'
Procedures can be scary for children of all ages because they often feel as though it is something done "to them" rather than "with them." At times, doctors or residents in a hurry might be apt to perform a procedure at bedside, which is not best practice. The treatment room is designated as a space where procedures should occur, whereas a bed is perceived as a safe place for children, and should be reserved as such.

Acute pain, or pain brought on by needles (veni-punctures) can be frightening and a therapist cannot have enough instruments and/or creative ideas on hand.[29] In general, procedures, particularly for young children can move along with minimal interference if there are activities where the children can play and feel in control of the situation. I have witnessed procedures where children were manipulated to look away or be "distracted" by staff, or in other cases held down by staff until the puncture was completed. This is not recommended. Music that moves and is productive, where a child can beat a drum with a free hand and elicit a "stop" and "go" from doctors in a musical context guided by the therapist takes very little time.

Case Vignette: Audrey
Audrey was a 5 year-old girl admitted for dehydration, and who hated to have her blood drawn. I noticed a "Chitty Chitty Bang Bang" pillow that her father said he had purchased when they had seen their favorite Broadway

show together. Audrey did not speak to me, and kept her thumb in her mouth most of the time, though she did nod "yes" and "no" while hugging her pillow. Her father was quite nervous about her blood draw because in the ER he had watched her "freak out" when the nurse tried to place her IV.

Upon permission from Dr. Heaton and having assessed Audrey, I knew that having her father in the room during the blood draw might not be the best idea. He presented as quite emotional and Audrey seemed to be cued to fear by his tension, though he was unaware of this and had the best intentions.

Upon father's approval and the doctor's referral, I accompanied Audrey with her pillow and with a cymbal and snare into the treatment room. We explained the procedure to Audrey and told her she could count off before Dr Heaton would stick her. We told her we would drum until the 'stick' would happen and then make a cymbal for the needle to go in and for 'Chitty' to fly fly fly, in the sky-at which point I would sing out: "your un-categorical, a fuel burning oracle…etc (the lyrics to Chitty).

There was no angst, no stress, no tears - no one even thought about it. We called the procedure what it was - a "blood draw" and Audrey did not seem bothered by it. Father was standing outside the treatment room, listening. The veni-puncture occurred in one stick, and future blood draws were reported by her Dad as "painless."

After the puncture was completed and the blood was successfully drawn, Audrey and I moved the session to her bed. She was still holding her pillow and I made some' flying variations on the 'Chitty" theme as her father 'flew' her back to her hospital room and bed. He sat next to her rubbing her head and I moved into 'Hush-a-bye Mountain', initially using my voice humming and eventually a metal slide whistle which I entrained to her breathing. She was soon asleep. The music therapy in this case served as procedural support and then reconstitution, where she was brought back to her father and a safe, contained place (bed) with a lullaby of familiarity.

Conclusion

Music sedation involving psychotherapeutic interventions that occur in consultation with the medical team and through careful assessment practices may offer infants, children, teens and adults a physical and emotional means of support. This is especially important during hospital stays where the onset or reoccurrence of chronic, acute or terminal pain may place a risk in patients' perception of safety. Assessing pain with creative tools and treating its symptoms physically and psychotherapeutically, through vibration or toning, releasing tension in music play, or metaphorically, and through incorporation of music experientials such as musical nurturance, song writing and music listening, may be a critical link toward trust and safety-both of which are essential elements in the process toward healing and recovery.

This chapter began with the classification and etiology of pain and some distinct qualifiers of how pain management has been addressed in a clinical music therapy context. There was discussion of the unique aspects of hospital work and how delicate the treatment of pain and its contributing factors become within the context of a medical music psychotherapy approach. The particulars of how we approach patients that are inclusive of accepting resistance are a critical factor. Finally, music sedation was outlined as a viable treatment option for patients of all diagnoses. Its clinical use as a means for assisting in pain management and/or within a procedure regimen or for enhancing intimacy and a feeling of comfort particularly during stays that are accompanied by painful episodes should not be overlooked. Music sedation can be nurturing and used for transitions, from wake to sleep temporarily, during chemotherapy or radiation, or as an accompaniment to pharmacological treatments pre-surgery. Music sedation can assist in the transition from life to death, and has helped many patients and families let go of the anxiety that accompanied the pain of disease symptoms or unknowns that escalated or contributed to mistrust in their care or treatment.

It is hoped that the use of music in pain and sedation will continue to grow as our allied medical team members increasingly recognize the important role that music therapy may play in sedation. In this way our referrals will increase and music therapy will continue to be implemented as a viable option for patients experiencing pain.

References

1. Yu, H., Wier, L., Elixhauser, H, (2011). HEALTHCARE COST AND UTILIZATION PROJECT, Statistical Brief 118, Agency for Healthcare Research and Quality Hospital Stays for Children, 2009.
2. Turk, D., Wilson, H.,Cahana, A. The Lancet, Volume 377, Issue 9784, Pages 2226-2235, 2, June 2011.
3. Loewy, J .Music psychotherapy assessment. *Music Therapy Perspectives*. 2000;Vol. 18(1), 47–58.
4. Loewy, J.V.. Music psychotherapy assessment in pediatric pain. In C. Dileo (Ed.),*Applications of music in medicine vol. II: Theoretical and clinical perspectives*. 1999; Silver Spring, Maryland: AMTA.
5. Magill-Levreault, L., Music therapy in pain and symptom management. Journal of Palliative Care, Vol 9(4), 1993, 42-48.
6. Skevington, S.M. 'Investigating the Relationship between Pain and Discomfor and Quality of Life, Using the WHOQOL'. 1998; Pain 76(3): 395–406.

7. Thaut, M.H and Davis, W.B. 'The Influence of Subject-Selected versus Experimenter Chosen Music on Affect, Anxiety and Relaxation', Journal of Music Therapy. 1993; 30(4): 210–23.
8. Loewy, J. Tonal intervallic synthesis as integration in medical music therapy, Baker, F. & Uhlig, S. (Eds), Voicework in Music Therapy London: Jessica Kingsley Publishers; 2011; 253-266.
9. Woolf C. Pain: moving from symptom control toward mechanism-specific pharmacologic management. *Ann Intern Med* 2004;140:441-451.
10. Willis, W., Role of neurotransmitters in sensitization of pain responses, Ann N Y Acad Sci. 2001 Mar;933:142-56.
11. Hains, B. C. & Waxman, S. G. Activated microglia contribute to the maintenance of chronic pain after spinal cord injury. J.Neurosci. 2006; 26, 4308-4317.
12. http://www.tabers.com/tabersonline/ub/view/Tabers/144811/0/PAIN
13. Bantick, S., Wise, R., Ploghaus, A., Smith, S., and Tracey, I. Imaging how attention modulates pain in humans using functional MRI. Brain, A Journal of Neurology. 2008; Vol 125, 2; 310-319.
14. Curr, Med Res Opin, Portenoy, R, Messina J, Xie F, Peppin J. Fentanyl buccaltablet (FBT) for relief of breakthrough pain in opioid-treated patients with chronic low back pain: a random-ized, placebo-controlled study, 2007 Jan;23(1):223-33.
15. Pert CB, Ruff MR, Weber RJ, Herkenham M. Neuropeptides and their receptors: a psychosomatic network. J Immunology; 1985; Aug;135 (2 Suppl) :820s-826s.
16. Loewy, J. Tonal Intervallic Synthesis in Medical Music Therapy in Baker, F. & Ulig, S. (Eds) Voicework in Music Therapy. London, Jessica Kingsley Publishers. 2011; 242-263
17. Loewy, J. V. The musical stages of speech: a developmental model of pre-verbal sound making. *Music Therapy*. 1995;13 (1), 47-73.
18. Loewy, J. Music therapy for hospitalized infants and their parents in Edwards, J. (Ed) *Music Therapy and Parent-Infant Bonding*, London: Oxford University Press. 2011; Chapter 12; 73-85.
19. Loewy, J. Integrating music, language and the voice in music therapy. *Voices: A world forum for music therapy, Vol 4(1)*. 2004. Retrieved December 13, 2012 from http://www.voices.no/mainissues/mi40004000140.html
20. Loewy, J. Hallan, C., Friedman, E. & Martinez, C. Sleep/Sedation in children undergoing EEG testing: A comparison of chloral hydrate and music therapy. *Journal of Perianesthesia Nursing, 2005, 20(5), 323-31.*

21. Loewy, J., Stewart, K., Dassler, A., Telsey, A. MD, Homel, P. The Effects of Music Therapy on Vitals, Feeding, and Sleep in Premature Infants, Pediatrics, 2013.
22. Loewy, J.V., Azoulay, R., Harris, B., & Rondina, E. Clinical improvisation with winds: Enhancing breath in music therapy. In R. Azoulay & J. V. Loewy, eds. Music, the Breath & Health: Advances in integrative music therapy New York: Satchnote Press; 2009; pp. 87-102.
23. Loewy, J. Music Psychotherapy Approaches for Infants & Children Experiencing Pain, Painvew: American Society of Pain Educators, 2013; Vol. 8, No. 3.
24. Abromeit, D., Shoemark, H, & Loewy, J. *Music therapy with Pediatric Units: NICU in Medical Music Therapy for Pediatrics in Hospital Settings,* Albromeit, D. & Colwell, C. (Eds). Silver Spring, MD: AMTA. 2008: pp.87-102.
25. Mondanaro, J. Music therapy in the psychosocial care of pediatric patients with epilepsy. *Music Therapy Perspectives*. 2008; 26(2), 99-26.
26. Jampel, P. Performances in Music Therapy: Experiences in Five Dimensions, Voices: A World Forum for Music Therapy, Vol 11, No 1, 2011, normt.uib.no/index.php/voices/article/viewArticle/275/440 retieved January13, 2013.
27. Canga, B. Hahm, C., Grossbard, M., Lucido, D., Loewy, J. Environmental Music Therapy: A Pilot Study on the Effects of Music Therapy in a Chemotherapy Infusion Suite; 2012; 4, 4, 221-230.
28. Loewy, J. Children with Respiratory Diseases in Bradt, J. NH: Barcelona Publishers. 2013.
29. Loewy, J., MacGregor, B. Richards, K, Rodriguez. Music therapy in Pediatric pain management: Assessing and attending to the sound of hurt, fear, and anxiety. In Music therapy in pediatric pain, Loewy, J. (Ed). Cherry Hill, NJ: Jeffrey Books. 2012; p. 45-66.

Music and Medicine: Integrative Models in the Treatment of Pain

APPENDIX A

CAS (Color Analysis Scale) Please color to indicate the location of your pain(s), its intensity on the figure below.(red, blue, green and yellow crayons provided)

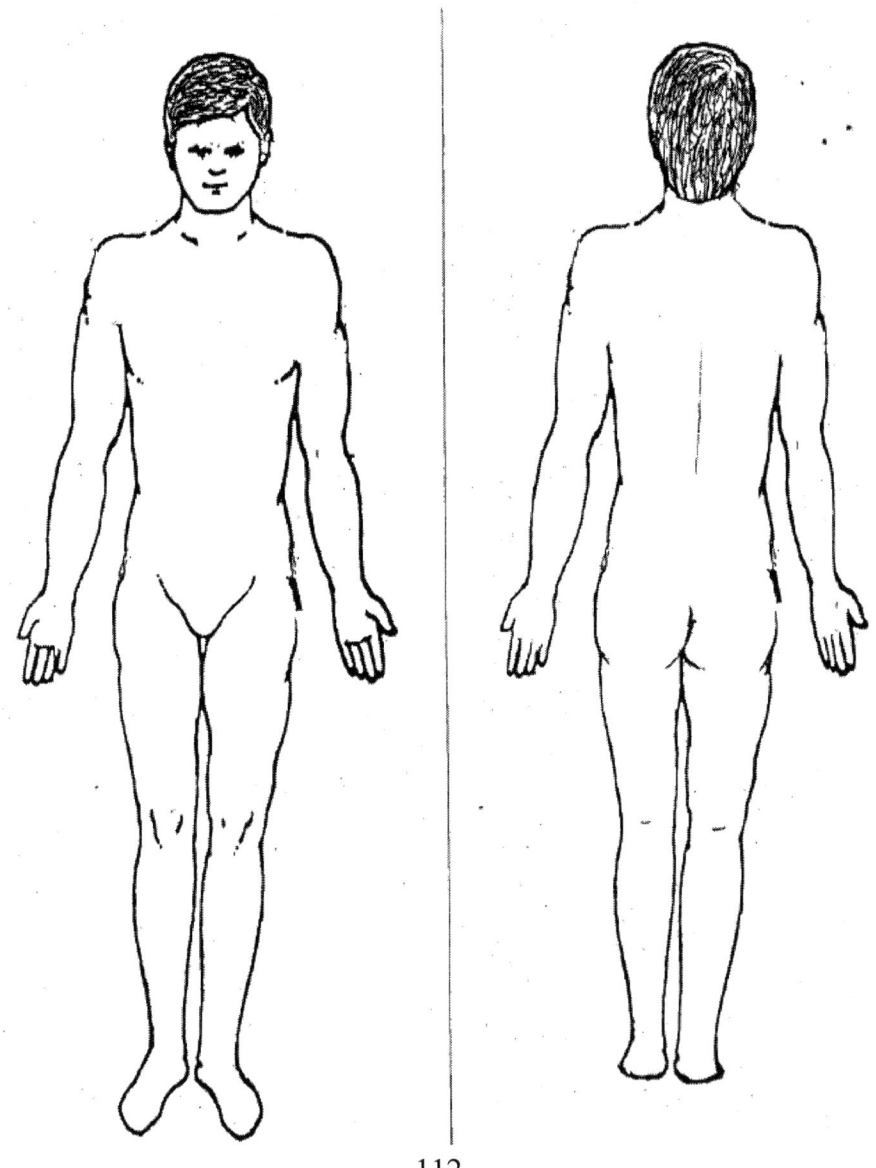

APPENDIX B

Loewy, J. Music psychotherapy assessment. *Music therapy perspectives.* 18(1): 47-58.

Table 1

13 Areas of Inquiry

Areas of Inquiry	Qualitative Means
1. Awareness of self, others & of the moment	Musical, verbal, nonverbal reflection
2. Thematic Expression	Instrument, song choice, quality & style of singing and playing
3. Listening	Receptivity, ability to hear others
4. Performing	Speaking, playing, singing alone
5. Collaboration/Relationship	Willingness to interact in activity together, quality of expressing with others
6. Concentration	Ability to focus in and out of the music
7. Range of Affect	Qualities of expression, variety of moods & themes, dynamic variance
8. Investment/Motivation	Willingness to build musical experience or conversation, sustaining involvement in the musical-verbal dialogue
9. Use of Structure	Reaction to space-boundaries, adherence,/resistance to formatted themes vs. free improvisation
10. Integration	How forms (music, words, feelings, songs, thoughts) are put together
11. Self Esteem	Evaluation of the created themes-taping
12. Risk Taking	Experimenting, trying something new, playing alone & together with others
13. Independence	Ability to separate self/others musically & verbally

Music and Medicine: Integrative Models in the Treatment of Pain

CHAPTER 8

Finding Relief from Pain through the Use of Music: A Gestalt Therapy Approach

Frank Bosco MA, MT-BC, LMT, RPP, SEP, LCAT

*"It is good to have an end to journey towards;
but it's the journey that matters in the end."*
Ursula K. LeGuin

Introduction

The experience we call "pain" often involves what might be considered a vacillating process from the functional to the dysfunctional. In terms of being a call to action, our experience of pain can run from the subtle to the most extreme degrees of human experience. We might experience pain as something of a benign motivation to subtly shift our posture one millimeter in the direction of greater comfort when sitting or standing, to pain that signals us to do something to save our lives, as in seeking medical attention. On the other hand, there is pain that we simply put up with and do nothing about either, because we choose to ignore it- perhaps seeing it as inconsequential, or, because we believe that we cannot do anything about it even when it may limit or even lead to the end of our life.

Clearly pain has a purpose as it signals direction for the volitional controls that we may have access to with any given incident that avails us a choice to respond to this pain in the most favorable way. Anticipated pain, such as a surgical procedure for instance, can often be averted with the use of modern anesthesia. On the other hand, pain due to some sort of accident— e.g., stubbing a toe, poking an eye, pricking a finger, suffering a fall, etc., tends to create a sharp reaction as a standard alarm response is carried out by the sympathetic nervous system. This experience of pain alerts us to a given situation in the moment, that requires our immediate attention. As we orient to the situation in this moment we can then hopefully assess the situation and take appropriate actions. Once these actions take place and all the necessary or possible steps or interventions have taken place we may no longer have need for the pain--in general. However, 'the body' does not always agree with this. Physical and behavioral responses continue in some fixed pattern that remains somewhat separate from reason. Some other response to this situation is needed in order to alter the repetition of this pain pattern.

Music and Medicine: Integrative Models in the Treatment of Pain

This chapter is mostly about what happens when pain persists and in essence, some part of our being does not get the message that this pain experience is no longer serving the greater good of our whole being. In the language of gestalt therapy theory we could say that this type of pain has become an annoying figure disrupting our lives as it continues to emerge from background to foreground. As a background figure, pain can be a reminder that no matter what else is good with life "all" is not well as we are occasionally distracted by the fact that something does not feel right. When pain is a figure in our foreground of awareness, we can no longer distract ourselves from the power pain can have to dominate our conscious mind, often to a debilitating degree.

In my private therapy practice of well over 30 years now, I have addressed a wide variety of physical and psychological pain scenarios including such things as for instance, the results of medical mishaps, victimization and abuse, severe trauma from war, car accidents, falls, etc., genetic deformation, and diseases of most every kind. I have studied and practiced a wide range of theories and techniques to help people in many areas of life's struggles and in this chapter we are focusing on how to deal directly with the pain process. In order to exemplify the synthesis of physiological and psychological understandings that my work engenders, I will now discuss what I feel is the most common and somewhat ubiquitous form of pain that every human being can relate to. I will later describe my specialty in working with music and gestalt therapy for this type of pain as it will hopefully inform others as to how to apply such an approach with most *any kind* of pain.

The Most Common Pain

The variety and degrees of debilitation we can experience as a result of pain is in itself a remarkable aspect of pain. When considering that most any pain, be it physical or emotional, tends to always be accompanied by or perhaps even, stemming from muscular tension, it is easy to imagine that the most prevalent pain we encounter in life would be *myofascial pain*. In essence, "Myofascial pain is the pain that is generated by hyperactive focal areas of irritability in muscle or its associated fascia that are called myofascial trigger points."[1] Pain due to active *myofascial trigger points*[2] for instance, can range from a mild stiffness that only hurts when movement causes these muscles to be stretched, to excruciating symptoms that keep people from being able to work or even just get out of bed. Also, these trigger points are known to keep people from sleeping soundly due to a low-grade disturbance they produce throughout the night causing muscles to contract and leaving us achy and sleep deprived in the morning as they can keep us tossing and turning in a restless sleep.

These irritating trigger points may, in some cases, not be so severe as to distract us from the busy details of our day. So we might then push through the "manageable" pain and fatigue they leave us with in the morning in order to get on with our daily activities. In fact, this level of pain may naturally slip into the background and perhaps "go away" altogether for the better part of the day. What tends to be happening in these cases is that tight muscles, in the back, for instance, are being called into action just enough to get the circulation through movement that they need to feel a bit better. Furthermore, by focusing on other things in the moment we are *not* giving attention to this physical sensation in a way that would only exacerbate the issue instead of solving it.

However, an unfortunate pattern develops here. This becomes only a temporary solution as, we have still not dealt with the causative features of this problem—and so, the problem persists. The trigger points are still in some semi-active state ready to call out for attention as soon as things get quiet again. Feeling exhausted, we collapse into bed at night only to be again disturbed later on that night after we've fallen asleep and the low-level distress signals from these trigger points calls our sleeping muscles into (contraction) action, thus, perpetuating the syndrome.

Trigger points are indeed an unwieldy system to treat. Their insidious and pervasive nature causes much confusion about how they function to proliferate pain symptoms in the body. To my experience this is rarely well understood and therefore, mostly ignored or marginalized by the medical community even though the work was pioneered back in the 1940's by the late Dr. Janet Travell and has been embraced by many massage and physical therapy professionals in recent years. A welcomed exception to this is Hal Blatman, MD, who I had the good fortune to meet recently. In his book on the subject of pain relief, Blatman, initially trained in orthopedic surgery, describes how he first came to hear about and explore this idea of myofascial trigger points in the early 1980's.[1] He describes how this work was totally new to him and radically changed his thinking about conventional diagnostic conditions and their origins. A new world seemed to open up for him as he went on to study and practice medicine using this "myofascial pain" model. Later he even had the opportunity to actually study with Dr. Travell and now, continues to *preach and teach* this work to medical professionals.

This all relates to my own story of how I came to understand and work with pain in general. After several years of practicing techniques of medical massage and shiatsu I took a seminar in the study of trigger points in 1981 with a chiropractic physician, Dr. John Kasler and similar to Dr. Blatman's story, this changed my practice profoundly. I began working with my massage therapy clients in a much more medically oriented way as I could now offer them a much clearer way of understanding and relieving all kinds of pain symptoms. I developed and experimented with many ways of working manually with trigger points--short of using needles and drugs as a medical doctor might. Additionally, I emphasized a dialogical educative process to give people a better sense of how they could have an active role in getting pain relief as needed and an overall sense of self responsibility in the process. An important step in pain management is feeling like we are responding in a helpful way. A simple illustration of how I might approach this work follows.

A Typical Case of Active Trigger Point Pain

When addressing pain due to myofascial trigger points a paradoxical conundrum arises. Question: What does it feel like to have someone pressing a point on a contracted muscle that is already causing pain? Answer: worse and, in a way, better! Even though there is a heightened degree of sensation in the moment, the sense of relief seems to counterbalance the sense of pain—to some degree. This can then be termed, "good pain" as it is part of the process of attending to and hopefully relieving the overall suffering from the condition. With proper intervention at this point, it is helpful to build on this theme and sustain the sense of on-going relief. By offering people ways of managing strong sensation in a more self motivated and autonomous manner they can not only find relief from suffering but also, they can learn a new way of being in relation to their body, other people and the world at large. Ultimately, this can lead to influencing change in the way in which people perceive and respond to many aspects of life as this work can expand into a whole course of psychotherapy.

    For our purposes here, I am interested in introducing people to how I work with presenting symptoms of pain in a manner that teaches people that with the help of music they can redirect their focus to relieve themselves from the sense of pain. As I was my own "lab rat" in developing this approach I can personally attest to its effectiveness. I have had many dental (root canal) procedures using this approach where I successfully nullified the strong sensations involved in extracting a live nerve with the use of this focusing approach. I have written about this in some detail before so, suffice to say, I did not use any drugs whatsoever in these procedures and I did not suffer any pain,[3] I did however, have a very enjoyable experience of listening to classical music on my ipod.

    In my practice as a body-oriented music psychotherapist I usually offer hands-on bodywork for pain relief to anyone in my practice who needs it. I use a variety of approaches but when my work involves pressing trigger

A Gestalt Therapy Approach to Using Music for Pain Relief

points I almost always try to educate people as to how to visualize the sensation of pain and to work with musical stimuli. I have a specially designed bodywork table for this purpose with speakers that project music directly into the body in stereo.

Consider a typical session addressing trigger points that are activated in the neck and shoulder and causing some degree of associated pain in the left forehead. Trigger points often have a direct connection to sensations some distance from the points themselves. This is known as "referred pain", and when it is located in the head area this presents a particularly common "headache".

I might begin by having a person lay face-up on the table, giving them some time and support with any combination of words/touch/music to help them to settle and orient to being on the table. Next, I could begin pressing (or squeezing) points in the left sternocleidomastoid muscle (the muscle running from the top of the breastbone area to the area behind the ear) as the left forehead is a "target area" for referred pain from this muscle. A dialog would ensue:

Me: I'm looking (palpating) for a sensitive point here. How does this one feel?
Patient: Well, that's a little sensitive, but not too bad.
Me: OK, but we need to find a really **good** sensitive point to work with here so, now,(moving to the center of a trigger point) how's this one?
Patient: Now that hurts, that's a point, I feel that over my left eye!
Me: OK, so that's a *good* point then?
Patient: Yeah...that's a *good* one!
(The subtle reframing of the trigger point to something of a "good" hurt helps relieve anxiety.)
Me: OK, good. So take a good deep breath and tell me if you can relax into that level of sensation or should I lighten up the pressure a bit?
Patient: No, it's ok, I can handle it.
(As I notice some bodily movement I begin to wonder how they are "handling it"? Are they thinking of the "no pain, no gain" principle?)
Me: OK, but I notice your foot is moving a bit and I'm wondering if you are relaxing enough with this. How would you rate your pain on a scale from 1 to 10 where 10 would be excruciating pain?
Patient: Well, it's about an 8.
Me: Humm..? That might be a bit too much. I want to help you stay more comfortable than that, say maybe about a 5, and then we can bring it down to about a 2. Try that deep breath again.

At this point I might suggest some visualization techniques along with the reminder to be constantly conscious of their breathing. I might also adjust my touch to get the level down to a 5 or so. The ideal here is to be able to press harder into the trigger point as the muscle relaxes. With less resistance there is less pain even though I am pressing deeper into the muscle! The approach here is gentle and relational. As people relax they can feel more in control of their pain and this in turn allows for greater relaxation, which again, leads to more of this sense of control in response to the pain until it becomes an emotionally neutral sensation. The situation can then be devoid of any call for action; the only thing one needs to do at that point is stay aware of incoming signals to the nervous system and monitor any unnecessary responses in the body so as not to let muscular contractions create a distraction from feeling the center of the primary pain.

From my experience, both personal and professional, I understand this as a process of increasing awareness. As we practice being aware of such things as events in our body and being, we become more adept at handling the physical and emotional influences that we encounter in life in general. This is the kind of growth process that we should expect from any successful therapy.

What Really is a Pain in the Neck/Ass?

I have often made the point that colloquial expressions are born out of the time-honored observations that have received consensual societal validation. We use such language with knowing that their validity comes from the real life experiences that they refer to. In regards to pain, common expressions point to the truth that there is a bridge between the physical and the psychological.

The perception of pain (nociception) obviously serves a purpose. But, what do we do when pain is not something we really need to be aware of and it functions only as a nuisance (in the vernacular: a pain in the neck/ass) or perhaps even something akin to torture? What can we do to alter the experience in order to nullify its noxious and unneeded effects or perhaps, even better, to adapt to the experience in a way that shifts it towards something positive such as relaxation? Something must shift in terms of our focus in order to increase some awareness of our condition.

Paradoxically, increased awareness with regards to nociception can *lessen* the immediacy towards taking distracting or annihilating actions (e.g., pain "killing" or numbing drugs) in favor of relegating awareness of that sensation to the background of a more rewarding experience such as music. One might think that focusing directly on a painful sensation would only increase its sensitivity but in actuality this can lead to a minimizing of the urgency of the call and therefore a diminished sensation. This is not unlike when babies who might sit whining about something they want in the moment and then, failing to get their parent's attention, they resort to louder cries or hysterics to get something—like their diaper changed, for instance. With the proper attention the child's cries settle as its focus changes to the caretaking activities of the moment. We can consciously and autonomously regulate our experience of pain in much the same way. Focusing directly on the sensation in the moment functions as a way of paying attention to an emergent event. When done effectively, the heightened awareness can circumvent the need to escalate the call to emergency status. Gestalt therapy[4] offers some insight as to how we can experiment with a shifting focus in a way that can give us the sense of autonomy to regulate the perception of pain by addressing it as an emergent figure from our nervous system.

GESTALT = THE WHOLE FIGURE/GROUND EXPERIENCE

Gestalt therapy has its roots in Gestalt psychology[5] that gave us the notion of the figure/ground experience of perception. In essence, this expresses that we see whole things as they are identified as a figure being in relation to a background or we might say a "ground" of the experience. The whole of the experience is then more than just one or the other as we might try to see them separately. Instead, as we must perceive the two in relation to each other we can be aware of more than just the separate parts as we notice how one relates to the other. A simple example of this to consider is how we might try to find just the right frame that brings out the best in a picture, to be hung in just the right place, etc. Our eyes can perceive the whole thing hung on the wall even as we might focus on some individual feature within the picture. As we gather the information in the picture, say a painting of some sort, we can have an experience of appreciation for the beauty, taste, skill, thoughtfulness, poignancy, etc., of not only the image and its artistry but, for the framing and setting in which it was hung.

In the classic image below we can be entertained by the phenomenon of being able to shift our focus back and forth between two distinct mental images of this single picture. Either we see a vase or we see the two matching faces that otherwise function to outline the vase. It can be argued that as fast as we may be able to switch from one image to the other, our brains are such that we do not actually "see" or, hold the mental images of both things at the exact same moment. However, as we become more familiar with the overall image—i.e., the whole 'gestalt', it can begin to take on another meaning as an image. In this case, it tends to be associated with gestalt therapy itself and in a sense is often used as an unofficial logo referencing anything having to do with 'gestalt...' An interesting phenomenon occurs here. In the instant that this image registers in our brain as a logo it is no longer perceived as either a vase or two faces but instead it is this new third image. We can immediately recognize that this overall picture represents something more than that which meets the eye. Thus, as it is commonly understood in the practice of gestalt therapy, the whole thing is greater than just the sum of its parts.

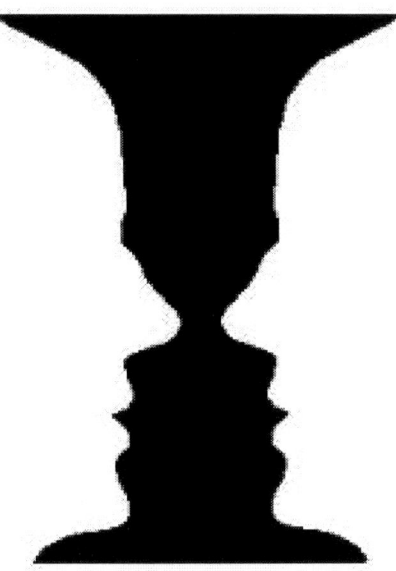

Gestalt therapy emphasizes focusing on awareness of what is happening in the present moment and so attention to one's physical processes (e.g. breath, sensations, movements, etc.) is an essential part of the therapy process. The primary focus of this work involves the elimination of interruptions to clear, flowing and graceful contact with self, other, or the environment. The practice of gestalt therapy accomplishes this task as it constantly attends to the interaction between thought and sensation in a person's process. By attending to the sense of how these interruptions effectively limit contact we can make choices as to how to alter this personal adaptation to the world in favor of another kind of adjustment to ourselves, others, or the environment that affords us a more desirable quality of contact.

We assert that the nature of contact is such that it is that what occurs at, and, with our sense of boundaries with self, other, or environment. Therefore, in examining our relationship to an experience of pain we may focus on the internal process within our body (e.g., sensations, like the degree of comfort/distress), other people influencing our pain (e.g., if it is a medical procedure, do we trust the doctor, nurse, family member, etc., involved? How does this affect our ability to deal with the pain?) or, the environmental circumstances (e.g., do we have any control over the environmental conditions such as, temperature, noise, cleanliness, etc.?).

GESTALT THERAPY Experiments

In gestalt therapy, experiments are designed and enacted by the therapist and/or the patient for the purpose of exploring something in a new way. In doing gestalt experiments we have access to "real time" behavioral tendencies. One imagines a scenario as the body actually adjusts to it dynamically, that is, complete with sensorial aspects that are present in the moment. In these experiments, careful attention must be paid to the presence or absence of:

1. **Support**—needed to provide a ground of opportunity for new behaviors and feelings to emerge. Adequate support for an experience may already exist within a patient's own sense of self. If not the therapist must provide the needed support through their own presence or perhaps by adding supportive elements to the design of the experiment.
2. **Congruence or incongruence of vocal or instrumental expression**—whatever the patient expresses must be evaluated for its authenticity in the moment. Any form of expression in the process of the experiment is, in effect, a result of the experiment already and must be treated as such. A common example of this might be when someone speaks words but does not seem to communicate them with appropriate feeling. We may need to reserve judgment in the moment in order to understand the greater context of their expression. As we let the experiment unfold the patient may discover this incongruence on his/her own and possibly, even arrive at some resolution or helpful adjustment to this. If not, the therapist may be able to point it out in some appropriate and well-supported manner yielding either a result for what was completed or a suggestion for further experimentation.
3. **Patterns that suggest forms of holding back, such as slowing down, stopping, or any form of interruption to the flow of expression**—such patterns need to be understood and reconciled for what they are in the context of the experiment. There are many ways and many reasons that people hold back expression in general and this type of behavior can be a functional part of a person's communicative style. In experiments therapists have to determine with skillful discernment what aspects of the patient's communication might yield a valuable exploration.

Going back to the typical case example presented earlier, let's consider what might be a good experiment based on what has happened thus far. For instance, if I was correct in detecting a "no pain, no gain" type of attitude—and I can think of many times when I was—I might be inclined to explore the background to this as it presents as a counter-productive stance to what I am attempting to do. This would in effect be what we might call a "fixed gestalt" that is contrary to sensing a more present and fluid involvement with the experience of pain. Suppose for instance, that this person's response to my last comment was:

Patient: No don't stop. I can handle it! (and, with an even more emphatic tone…) I'm used to pain!
Me: Well, ok, I realize you are but, I'm wondering, what kind of relationship you have with your pain? Sometimes when we get too used to having something we tend to ignore certain aspects of it. Like, when you're in a relationship with someone and not really expressing your feelings to each other.
Patient: So what do you want me to do? I can't talk to my pain, can I?
Me: Well, actually that might be an interesting thing to find out. Do you want to try an experiment where you have a conversation with your pain?
Patient: Uhhh…? Sure. (?)
Me: Ok, just imagine that fan up there on the ceiling is your pain. I'll keep pressing into your neck muscles here to help keep you in touch with who you are talking to. Ask it questions, anything you want to know about it.
Patient: OK. "What are you doing to me?"
Me: Good and, feeling into that question how about also telling it what you feel it's doing to you?
Patient: It just bothers me all the time.
Me: Ok, just try saying that directly to it like it's a person here with you.
Patient: You're just such a bother, you're always distracting me…getting in my way so I can't get any work done.
Me: Ok now…can you speak as if you are your pain…talking back in response to you?
Patient: I just want your attention.
(*As this patient pauses I notice a change of expression and I ask what's happening…*)
Patient: Well, I'm thinking of this lady in my office, who just constantly comes up to me and just starts talking. She drives me crazy…she drives everybody crazy!
Me: I see. So you might say she's a real pain in the neck?
Patient: Right, but I can't do anything about it because she's the boss' personal secretary and I need to stay on her good side because she can make

life very difficult for me if say anything that upsets her. So I just have to put up with it

So at this point the experiment has just confirmed that the patient's "pain in the neck" or, "headache" could be related to a real person who cannot then be confronted due to some fixed gestalt having to do with a fixed notion of how we just have to tough it out just put up with things. There is plenty of room here for further exploration through gestalt experimentation. I can immediately think of many sessions where this kind of attitudinal posturing has been fixed since a person's childhood where for instance, they may have had to keep quiet and not complain about a sibling for fear of upsetting parents who tended to be unsympathetic or even violently reactive.

I once worked with a woman who grew up being sexually abused by her older brother and felt she could never say anything, believing that if her alcoholic father found out he would badly beat her brother. She told me she didn't know what would be worse, if her father beat her brother to death and she had to live with the guilt or, if the brother survived the punishment but, then found a way to get back at her for saying something.

The beauty of experiments is that we get to experience something that we never actually did in life. We can do this by altering the imaginary circumstances to fit the needs of the patient with whom we are working. In working with this woman over time, she finally came up with the idea of the comic book figure "Wonder Woman" as a *resource*[6] to accompany her in an experiment that started while I was pressing into some tender points in her forearms (i.e., the finger and wrist muscles). This work occurred during an Elemental Music Alignment—a body-oriented music approach[7]--session. We were working with Wagner's "Overture to Tanhauser" a piece of music that builds slowly as it develops its themes to a bold and valiant stature. As she later reported to me, the work on her forearms in the beginning of the piece made her think of Wonder Woman's magic wrist cuffs that were known to deflect bullets and such things. Later in the piece, the string section produces swirling descending lines that she equated with Wonder Woman's powerful lasso. As the music was building into a very powerful climax, she imagined herself confronting both her brother and father, and containing their attempts at violent transgressions with Wonder Woman's powerful tools—her lasso and her magic wrist cuffs.

Much has been written on the topic of gestalt experiments. In his most seminal work originally published in 1951, Fritz Perls is credited with being responsible for devoting what was meant to be the second half of the book to the work of experiments.[4] Let it suffice to say, that as a gestalt therapist anything I would do in regards to taking someone through some process of pain alleviation, would be done in the spirit of a gestalt experiment where attention is given to emergent events as they are presently

Three Steps for Handling Pain

In addition to using gestalt experiments as part of a psychotherapy process to dialog with one's pain either verbally or, as in my practice, musically,[8] I will often, as a practical measure, teach people how to explore handling pain on their own. My approach to doing this is threefold:
(1) use a focusing technique to minimize pain related sensory stimulation and mental/emotional distraction. By focusing on the center of the sensation and actively making the effort to find this pin-pointed focal point in the midst of a larger area of sensation we are limiting the scope of sensation while still intensely paying attention to it.
(2) encouraging relaxation and awareness throughout the entire body utilizing conscious diaphragmatic breathing in the interest of letting go of tension and pain, and
(3) providing the proper music to help deprioritize the sensory stimuli from pain in favor of auditory stimuli from the music.

Any one of these three techniques could be used exclusively, and perhaps effectively. However, I find that used in combination the results tend to be more profound and perhaps more importantly, enduring.

Pain and Trauma Related Emotions

An important consideration for working with pain symptoms is how it might be related to trauma. When pain is a result of trauma and, *pain is always found in some form with trauma*, the memory of the original occurrence or the ensuing pain pattern is coupled with an emotional mindset, a *thought pattern* that is emotionally bound.

Such related emotions need to be processed so as to become uncoupled from the physical pain as we investigate experiences of pain in a holistic manner (as in a gestalt approach). Parsing out the emotional content of the pain leaves the purely physical aspects of the pain available to be met with an accordingly appropriate physical response. For example, *if* there is nothing to *do* physically in the moment to adjust to a painful sensation, the primary directive to all the skeletal muscles in the body should be to *do* nothing in the moment, in other words, *relax*! As we relax tension in the body that was caused by the experience of pain, we begin to have access to our ability to change how we relate to this pain. In this way we can uncouple sensation from an undesirable behavioral response—that of tightening muscles. The end result of this uncoupling is for pain to become an experience of strong sensation that signals us to relax into an overall sense of our body.

Bringing awareness to the specific nature of this coupling we can begin to unravel some of the mysterious aspects of why a pain persists. We can at some point realize that a pain, having 'served it's purpose' is perhaps, no longer functional and therefore has no need to be emotionally bound to the individual's experience. It can then be relegated to a more appropriate place in the brain/body as a memory of something in the past--happily forgotten pain.

In order for this to happen, **secondary gains** (e.g., getting special attention from loved ones) and issues involving **'retroflection'**[4] (e.g., putting up with pain as a form of punishing, abusing, or neglecting oneself instead of having a releasing or externalized response) must be examined and processed. Such systems of rewards and punishments need to be moved out of the way in order to allow for a rechanneling of one's focus to an emerging sense of relief, a pain free recovery.

"Mindfulness" and other forms of meditation and awareness building techniques can all be employed to manage pain with one common goal: to find peace in the body/mind. This would mean a relief from or absence of pain—not necessarily a condition of total health, but certainly a condition of greater ease leading to greater health and the absence of "dis-ease".

Music Alleviates Fear

When it comes to the emotion of fear, music can save the day like a hero that gets our attention saying, "Have no fear, Music is here!" I would not overstate this, however, as we all know from any scary movie, music can certainly be used to induce a sense of fear for what is about to happen. Since music is a purely physical phenomenon in and of itself, it requires human interpretation to still our emotions in any way. This is utterly dependent on the manner and the context of the listening experience. Music has the capacity to occupy the anticipatory function of the brain. By focusing on the incoming stimulus that music is to us we can practice hearing each note of it as it enters our central nervous system. And then by keeping ourselves actively and happily anticipating the next note to be heard, we can neutralize any feelings of fear and dread. We can essentially re-direct our thought process towards a more desirable state of anticipatory function by this method of listening to the music.

The forward thinking process actually keeps us present with the 'here and now' processing of moment-to-moment, and note-to-note changes.

In gestalt theory we could describe this as an awareness of the nuance of the emergent figure of sound, i.e., the next note or musical event. Theoretically, all sound has been preceded by other sounds since the beginning of time and all sound emerges from and returns to a *ground* of silence. However, in listening to a piece of music we can consider the immediate context of sound to be the ground for the next musical figure of sound to emerge. With this focused listening we can begin to alleviate pain by letting go of the distracting elements of tension.

Tension in the body is competing for our *attention*. Tension by its very nature needs our *attention* as it seeks some form of relief. On its own it is often a painful reminder that something is going on that we must deal with. Tension can be likened to a small child in this way. Picture this child left in a bathtub as it is filling up and calling out, "Mommy! Mommy!" fearing the water is getting too high. We might say that "tension mounts" quite literally in this kind of situation as it is equated with increased anxiety in the moment. Relaxing this tension naturally lowers the level of anxiety.

Music as a Preferred Sensation

The appropriate selection of, and, active listening to music can then provide a ground for experimenting with new and preferred patterns of focusing on moment-to-moment incoming sensory stimulation. Pleasing and mentally engaging, what I like to call, "busy" music[3] can be employed to help mitigate unnecessary emotional and cognitive responses to strong sensations. This mitigation allows for an increased sense of the body and the ability to simply relax in response to such strong somatic stimuli so that it can dissipate peacefully.

Picking up where we left off with this typical pain patient, let's consider another possible outcome. If we choose not to go in the direction of more dialogical experiments we might say something like:

Me: So you really feel there's nothing you can do here and you just have to put up with this annoyance?
Patient: Yeah, I just have to suck it up…you know get over it.
Me: Well, how are you going to do that?
Patient: I don't know.
Me: May I suggest something then?
Patient: Please…
Me: How about imagining that this woman is here with us literally in the form of these painful trigger points? You would want to let go of them and relax, true?
Patient: Yes, of course.

A Gestalt Therapy Approach to Using Music for Pain Relief

Me: OK, so focus on the center of these points as I press into them, see them as little targets that expand as you breathe into them. Breathe into the bull's-eye of the target and imagine it blowing up as it becomes a target itself with concentric circles and see another tiny bull's-eye in its center. See the center of that bulls-eye as you feel a sense of relaxation throughout your body, take a deep breath taking inventory of any tension you might feel and letting it go now as you exhale. Now how would you rate your pain?

Patient: It's down to about a 3 or 4.

Me: Good. Now, (putting on Bach's "Brandenburg Concertos") I want you to listen to this music picking out any of the various melodic lines you are drawn to and…while continuing to breath into and let go, relaxing around the sensations in your body, listen for the next note that is about to happen in the melody line you are focusing on in the moment. Keep listening for the very next note. Feel the excitement now as you anticipate the next note, and then the next note…and then…?

At this point the music becomes much more central to our experience. The pain, pales in importance and simply recedes to the background allowing us to relax and enjoy the musical ride.

Conclusion:
Some Problems with this Approach

In conclusion, I would like to add that while this approach can be somewhat simple, there are some factors preventing or limiting someone from focusing on the issue of pain. For instance, sometimes pain can be overwhelming and not matched with the person's ability or understanding of the process we would be introducing them to--including: how to do such a process or how it could or would work for them. Therefore, they may not be convinced they should even try it.

Someone might have a lack of interest, willingness, desire, or commitment to learning, practicing, or staying with this approach. Often people are so uninterested in getting closer to their pain experience that they treat it like a partner with whom, out of anger and frustration, they refuse to speak to. Instead of having a sense of being in contact with their pain or considering their relationship to it, they might just prefer to simply take, or try out various medications--sometimes at considerable risk. While I recognize that is in many cases the right and perhaps the only thing for a person to do, I would like to assert whenever it is appropriate the idea that…

Pain is a messenger. We do not need to kill the messenger…just listen it and then, let it go.

Music and Medicine: Integrative Models in the Treatment of Pain

A great teacher, the late Richard Kitzler, used to remind us all at meetings of the New York Institute for Gestalt Therapy that some things in life are *simple*...but not *easy*. This fundamental concept clearly applies to my approach here. A certain mental and emotional fortitude is often needed to change our instinctive response of tightening muscles and feeling fear or frustration in reaction to painful sensations. For some people this is quite natural as they may be extremely open to new ideas and change in general and/or very disciplined in their approach to facing new challenges. Then again, for many people that I have worked with it has not at all been easy for them to change such deeply engrained conditioned and habitual patterns of behavior in favor of this more *mindful* approach that requires them to "simply" relax!

I acknowledge that with regards to the practice of this approach, it is indeed, 'easier said than done'. However, with constant monitoring and support in the process I have successfully taught a multitude of people over the years a method for finding peace through their pain. Eventually, by allowing physical sensations to dissipate into a background of relaxation throughout their body, they have learned to experience a foreground of lively anticipation focused on each new aural sensation emerging from a piece of music like being on a wonderful journey.

"Happiness is a journey, not a destination..."
--Souza

References

1. Blatman H, Ekvall B. The art of body maintenence: Winner's guide to pain relief. Concinatti, OH: Danua Press; 2002.
2. Travell J, Simons D. Myofascial pain and dysfunction: The trigger point manual. Baltimore, MD: Williams & Wilkins; 1983.
3. Bosco F. Sensing and resonating with pain: A process-oriented approach to focusing the body/mind using music therapy. In: Loewy JV, ed. Music Therapy and Pediatric Pain. Cherry Hill, NJ: Jeffrey Books; 1997:7-21.
4. Perls F, Hefferline R, Goodman P. Gestalt therapy: Excitement and growth in the human personality. Highland, NY: The Gestalt Journal Press, Inc.; 1994.
5. Kohler W. Gestalt Psychology. New York, NY: Liveright Publishing Corporation; 1947.
6. Bosco F. Daring, dread, discharge, and delight. In: Loewy JV, Frisch A, eds. Caring for the caregiver: The use of music and music therapy in grief and trauma. Silver Spring, MD: AMTA; 2002:71-79, 176.

7. Bosco F. The use of elemental music alignment in the journey from singer to healer/therapist. In: Meadows A, ed. Developments in music therapy practice: Case study perspectives. Gilsum, NH: Barcelona Publishers; 2011:470-485.

8. Bosco F. Translating Somatic Experiencing and Gestalt Therapy for Trauma Resolution into Medical Music Therapy Practice with Adults. In: Stewart K, ed. Music therapy and trauma: Bridging theory and clinical practice. New York, NY: Satchnote Press; 2010:58-73.

Music and Medicine: Integrative Models in the Treatment of Pain

CHAPTER 9

Music Therapy Based Release Strategies for Acute and Chronic Pain: An Individualized Approach

John F. Mondanaro MA, LCAT, MT-BC, CCLS

"There is nothing that can stop the creative. If life is full of joy, joy feeds the creative process. If life is full of grief, grief feeds the creative process…We have seen again and again how immense can be the power of limits, the power of circumstance, the power of life's pull in generating original breakthroughs of mind and heart, spirit and matter."
Stephen Nachmanovitch

Introduction

The emerging paradigm of healthcare is one that is changing to meet a growing world consciousness and demand for the availability of integrative treatment options. Exposure and awareness of the many holistic therapies and life practices ensuing from a preventative philosophy in regard to illness mandates that providers be integrative of non-pharmacological treatments such as music therapy. Certainly in the treatment of pain as a symptom of illness or injury, medical music therapy as both a form of psychotherapy and an intervention for the psychoemotional and physiological responses to pain holds a unique position among other integrative therapies. Its potential to function at all stages of life, consciousness, and across cultural groups, positions it strategically as integral to an interdisciplinary team approach.

For the sake of brevity, this chapter will focus on music therapy based release strategies in the context of acute pain episodes that occur across a range of diagnoses and conditions. Focusing on the release of tension contributing to, or ensuing from the experience of pain, music therapy assessment of patients across multiple domains of the human experience can contribute richly to the treatment dialogue at a pragmatic level. It offers nonpharmacological options in the treatment of physiological responses to physical pain while offering rich possibilities for addressing the psychoemotional aspects of the pain experience as well. Several cases will be presented here within the context of patient and family-centered care to elucidate an efficacious use of music therapy based release strategies in the treatment of pain.

Music and Medicine: Integrative Models in the Treatment of Pain

The Traumatization of Diagnosis

In my experience working in the medical model, I have bore witness to the impact that acute pain can have on the resilience and coping ability of an individual. The many layers of loss that can present across diagnosis and condition contribute to the experience of pain by impacting one's sense of control and autonomy. Loss as a theme, presents in varying degrees, and indiscriminately regardless of the nature of the condition. Whether resulting from an elective intervention with a short-term recovery prognosis as in orthopedic surgery, or the residual pain episodes attributable to a chronic illness such as cancer or HIV/AIDS, the pain experience can elicit varying degrees of traumatic response. The interruption in one's ability to participate fully in life can prove not only defeating to the individual, but impacting on the family system of that individual as well. Understanding this reality is crucial to maximizing the effects of music therapy intervention.

The onset of symptoms leading to diagnosis may seem sudden, random, and certainly indiscriminate, and the individual's response may elicit traumatic mechanisms, such as a range of fight or flight responses. Such responses can give rise to secondary responses by the individual's caregivers as competition for ownership of the role of 'best caregiver' presents. The stress and anxiety of diagnosis may also elicit a range of responses in the patient and caregivers alike. Competition versus cooperation with professional and personal caregivers on behalf of the patient can become a dynamic force requiring sensitive negotiation by the interdisciplinary team. Additionally, assertiveness in the form of goal attachment can shift to adaptation, or a surrendering of such goals to align with the trusted caregiver.[1] These changing dynamics are wisely considered by a care team, defining a treatment plan for an individual who may be too overwhelmed to fully process the information being given.

Physicians and other providers of care recognize that the patient's experience is a layered one in which the manifestation of physical symptoms from illness may be rivaled by the many levels of psychosocial loss.[2] Loss of basic routine, role in family, ability to work, spiritual meaning, and certainly a sense of losing control may all contribute to a general loss of self-esteem for the individual. The integration of psychosocial and spiritual support services such as music therapy, social work and chaplaincy, assist in addressing the comprehensive needs of the hospitalized individual. This personal approach informs the care in a manner that indisputably places the patient at the center of care. The foundation of such personalized care serves the assessment and treatment of symptoms that may ensue from a given diagnosis. For example, dyspnea, or shortness of breath, labored respiration, pain, and the ensuing anxiety that these symptoms may cause, can impede the individual's ability to integrate an understanding of not only various treatments, but of the diagnosis itself.

Accurate assessment of pain is perhaps the greatest challenge to physicians because of the complexity and subjectivity of pain itself. The patient's report is maintained as the "golden standard"[2] of pain assessment, and in cases where assessment fails to identify the physiological genesis of the individual's pain, it is more common to address the report from an integrative approach. The role of psychosocial staff is essential to this level of treatment because the forums provided during such therapy can provide invaluable insight for the interdisciplinary team as to patient's process with the illness and the treatment. Music therapy is perhaps uniquely positioned to provide such insight because of music's capacity to connect physical, spiritual, emotional, and psychological domains. This philosophy finds its way into the pledge that Beth Israel Medical Center makes to its patients, "…to treat all individuals with dignity and respect, while working to restore and maintain the health of their mind, body and spirit".[3]

Simultaneous to consideration of the patient's needs, the integrative team also illustrates recognition of the individual's personal caregiver(s) and the role of any children who may be involved. Communication is vital, and whether or not elements of traumatic response are visible, the individual(s) may benefit from repetition and review of the facts and sequence of events that led to the current time and space. The following example illustrates this idea.

Case Vignette: Leslie

One particular case involving Leslie, a twenty-six year old woman diagnosed with Acute Myeloid Leukemia (AML), required numerous dialogues with the medical team to dispel misconceptions of which she was holding on to tenaciously.

Leslie had been admitted to the Emergency Room for the evaluation of symptoms mimicking food poisoning. Her work up revealed that she actually had AML in addition to hepatitis C. Her coping mechanism with this overwhelming news was denial. She continued to talk about her food poisoning, and repeatedly said she had eaten raw seafood, ignoring that she had been diagnosed with a deadly leukemia that required immediate intervention of intensive chemotherapy.

While a treatment plan was initiated, her ongoing denial and focus on the food poisoning story created a barrier to her ability to fully integrate herself into her care. As a therapist my priority was to create a space for connection and process in which Leslie could reconcile the truth of her diagnosis with the less-threatening narrative she was sustaining. My advocacy for the medical team's patient repetition of diagnostic information allowed

Leslie to eventually integrate an understanding of her illness, and to optimally participate in her care.

Music therapy focusing on music that was thematic across the vicissitudes of her care provided Leslie and her family a context in which to find meaning and aesthetic sensibility during a frightening time. Today Leslie is in complete remission. There cannot be too much time allotted to communication that ultimately empowers patients' process with understanding diagnosis and treatment options. Good care is individualized care.

Integrative Treatment Planning

Family Centered Care

The World Health Organization endorses a care approach that features the tenets of interdisciplinary and family centered care. The latter, aims to integrate emotional and developmental needs into the practice of medicine, and sees family involvement as essential to care but also looks to develop a treatment plan specific to each family.[4] The professional caregiver looks at the patient and the illness within the context of the various systems in which they both exist and attempts to identify the biopsychosocial-spiritual aspects of the family's experience, while exploring the culture and beliefs of the family, as well as the strengths of each member of the family system, and the resources available.[5] Evolving from Family Systems Psychology, family-centered care looks at illness as the experience of the entire family unit and highlights the important role that families play in ensuring the health and well being of the individual who is ill.[6]

The evolution of Palliative Care as a distinct discipline, and one that has achieved independence from it's long held affiliation with Hospice Care is significant. Unlike Hospice Care, which focuses on comfort care for the imminently dying, Palliative Care has centered its focus on the individual's quality of life by giving forum to the psychosocial, emotional, and spiritual needs of the patient.[2]

A conscientious assessment of the various relationships in the family system can identify patterns of communication and areas of conflict as well as to acknowledge existing strengths. This approach strives to identify and reinforce healthier patterns of communication by understanding the degree to which the family system has been disrupted by the presenting illness.[4,5]

Music Therapy and Pain: Body, Mind, and Spirit Integration

The effects of music on the body have been studied specifically in the areas of acute pain[7-9]; post-surgical stress[10-12]; cancer[10,13]; procedural support[14]; and on depression and mood disturbance due to chronic pain.[15,16] The theoretical orientation of the Louis Armstrong Center for Music and Medicine centers on a valuing of this integration and acknowledgement of the effects that the body can have on the mind and the mind on the body. The assessment[17] of this interplay of mechanisms divulges therapeutic entry-points by which the therapist can optimally support the individual experiencing pain, illness, and hospitalization.

An understanding of the Gate Theory of pain and the neurological effects of music,[18] as well as the principles of entrainment,[19] inform the music therapist's interventions when addressing an individual's pain, but perhaps an even greater point of emphasis in the work is the use of visualization and breath work that is personal to the individual. Such intervention provides opportunity for the individual to escape the immediate environment though the imagination, and yet still be connected to the circumstances that are unique to his or her pain. This is achieved by way of an effective therapeutic alliance in which an individual's sense of control and mastery of their experience is reinforced by the therapist. Within this alliance, psychoeducation about the use of breath work empowers the patient in reconnecting to mindful breathing as a resource. Direct guidance by the therapist, is gradually minimized as greater emphasis is placed on supporting the individual's autonomy and reclaimed connection to his or her vitality or resilience. Breath as a resource, when clearly understood and accepted by the patient, can optimally contribute to the efficacy of music therapy in the treatment of pain.

Release Strategies in the Treatment of Acute and Chronic Pain

The idea that tension in the body occurs in response to pain is one that most of us can easily relate to, with reflection on such moments in our lives. Stubbing one's toe on the leg of a chair for instance, can cause an immediate cry or shout in most people. In the preceding moments however, there mounts a profound tension or holding that occurs before the release. In less immediate circumstances, the impulse to hold or tense-up to avoid further trauma or a painful spasm, can result in mounting tension. This holding creates tension on both conscious and unconscious levels that can result in shallowed breathing and tightened muscles throughout the body. This general response to the experience of pain, regardless of origin, continues to mount in intensity if left unresolved. Tension release will occur naturally to some degree when either the body exhausts itself from the holding, or when the patient's threshold for coping increases, resulting in the time needed for the body to adjust. The use of harmonics, tempo, volume, or rhythm through drumming[20] to mirror the process of tension resolution naturally occurring in the body is effective and can be used on an individual basis, and certainly according to the patient's preference.[21]

As a caring husband and overzealous music therapist, I accompanied my wife's contractions when she was in labor with our son. Creating musical tension on my guitar at the peak of the contractions, and then resolving the tension as the contraction subsided was my intention. Interestingly, the use of volume and tempo, evoked extreme agitation in my wife, and almost got me thrown out of her room. However, when I quickly reverted back to a chord progression based on a partial circle of fifths, I found that this intervention provided release and resolution more subtly. More importantly, my wife found this harmonic approach more tolerable, and actually found it supportive of her own cycles of focusing and breathing. I have tended toward the use of harmonic tension resolution ever since.

Tension Release through Harmonics: Case Vignette
The following case presentation is that of Huan, a Chinese-American man diagnosed at the age of 40 with end-stage, metastatic lung cancer. His immediate family consisted of a wife, two sons ages 5 and 8, a 15 year-old nephew, and an elderly patriarch of the family whose identity was not fully clarified. Huan had been active in physical work, and was in optimal physical condition, which partially explained his succumbing to his illness very late in its development. His wife appeared to be devoted and loyal as per tradition, and graciously attended to her husband's needs. The two younger boys, again aged 5 and 8 were developmentally appropriate in their disparate displays of affect. Finally, it was the 15 year-old nephew of the patient who made an indelible contribution to the dynamics of the family. Having realized early on that this teenager was the only English-speaking member of the family, allowed the team to understand more fully the pressure he was under in the moment.

Preliminary psychosocial assessment and care for the patient had been provided by a Chinese social worker in collaboration with the palliative team's social work coordinator/clinician. The patient's pain was being fairly well managed through pharmacological means, but a primary stressor for the patient and his wife was the subject of their children. Culturally, it was not the norm to include children in the ongoing events of the patient's care. The idea that the children would see their father in a weakened state was an obstacle to their initial acceptance of a plan that would bridge the communication gap that was widening as the patient was imminently dying. As the level of emotional stress began to deepen for the couple, they became increasingly receptive to learning more about how the team could address the needs of the children and ultimately the entire family. Music therapy was identified as a service that might be effective in providing a forum for both the children's process and an additional intervention to address the patient's pain experience. The music therapist initially explained the services in terms of addressing the patient's pain through tension release and breath work. Also emphasized was the possibility that the needs of the children had been overlooked, and that in the absence of developmentally appropriate and accurate information, there could exist the potential for distorted versions of what was happening to their father. The importance of providing the children with a foundational understanding of what was actually happening in their father's care was cardinal to supporting a culture of inclusion within the family unit. The timing of the referral however rendered it impossible to approach the work with the children in the most ideal of ways. Timing did not afford opportunity to prepare the children for what they might expect, see, and hear in the hospital room with their father, nor was their time to gather their narrative of the events leading to the patient's current hospitalization. The work that could take place was ultimately purposeful and certainly important in the trajectory of events that were to occur.

Prior to the arrival of the children, I had arranged large panels of white paper and markers on an empty space in the room, upon which the children could express their feelings in color or symbol, when their threshold for music was exhausted. Once in place, I created on the guitar, a steady soundscape of tension-release chording that cycled over a partial circle of fifths. Huan had declined active engagement in the music, but was receptive to holding a set of Baoding balls, commonly known as Chinese Stress Balls. Believed to have originated in Baoding, China, a small town in the Heibei province, during the reign of the Ming Dynasty, the chrome plated balls were light enough for the patient to hold and move. Perhaps even more important, was their capacity to remain cool to the touch, which was an unexpected benefit given the Huan's difficulty maintaining a comfortable body temperature. While his wife would periodically run a cool wet cloth over his torso, Huan would stretch his arms upward to the ceiling in a type of Tai Chi motion. His graceful efforts seemed to increase in strength, as I mirrored his fluid motion.

The arrival of the children and their subsequent exploration of the various instruments seemed to bring lightness to the room. The mother's facial expressions softened into smiling, and Huan's own physical presentation appeared invigorated. Perhaps he was truly transcending the physical pain of his illness through the embodiment of the music and expression of Tai Chi, or perhaps he was internally driven to present a strong paternal image by which his children could remember their father. From a theoretical perspective, the session seemed to defy a commonly held notion that music therapy at the end of life must adhere to the provision of a soundscape of celestial sounds to ease the transition. Here, the creation of music that supported this man's engagement with his environment, in spite of the effects of his illness, illustrates music therapy as an embodied experience that can call one into life itself.

During this session, I focused on the creation of a non-threatening environment in which the children could visit their father. The ensuing space allowed the family to be united within a context that could momentarily shift the focus from being overwhelmingly medical to one of shared creativity and aesthetic experiencing. Certainly, the roles of creating something pleasing for their father, gave the children a sense of empowerment and control, and for the wife, a sharing of a loving space in which her family could find meaning.

The 5 year-old presented as playful, and egocentric in what appeared to be his synthesis of the music space that was created. He explored the instruments and played each one with abandon, occasionally referencing his father and mother for approval. The 8 year-old, engaged with greater reserve, as if negotiating feelings of playfulness with recognition of the seriousness of the situation. During the session, he often turned his attention to his younger sibling, in vacillating displays of encouragement and displeasure of his expressive play.

The 15 year-old nephew remained stoic yet engaged in the session, claiming the rain stick as his instrument, and sensitively offered its sound intermittently. Amidst the music making of the younger boys and the therapist's guitar, this young man offered an unspoken strength that elicited the respect of the family and of the therapist. Also present in his demeanor was what I perceived as scrutiny of the involvement of those outside the immediate family, and this was to be outwardly expressed in the next and final session.

I returned the following afternoon as promised and found Huan semi-alert, attended at the bedside by his nephew. The wall was adorned with the drawings and sentiments expressed in Chinese lettering created by the children after I had left the day prior. The wife was in a consult room with the social workers at the time of the visit. Upon entering the room, the patient appeared to acknowledge me and nodded affirmatively to my gesture to provide soft music. The nephew interceded however, stating that he did not feel that "music therapy was necessary". Recognizing the nephew's position in the family, I felt conflicted in the ethical obligation to honor Huan's request while also honoring the nephew's assertion of power. I excused myself momentarily to check-in with Huan's wife as to her prior request for music therapy. Returning to the room, I respectfully reflected to the nephew, that I would defer to Huan's wish as well as the wife's prior request for music therapy by providing a brief session of tranquil music. Huan was visibly weaker and expressed no wish to actively participate as in the prior day. Recognizing this shift, I again created a cycle of tension resolution chording, integrative of musical motifs introduced in the prior session. Ten minutes passed before the nephew motioned his hand, and gently stated "enough music". I acknowledged the nephew and Huan while bringing the music to a steady decrescendo. Huan again nodded to me as I prepared to leave. He succumbed to his illness later that day.

Drumming for Release: Case Vignette
The use of drumming to create a meditative space that transcends the physical realm of sensation is supported by centuries of shamanistic and tribal practice in healing.[20] It is of no surprise that drumming as a tangible form of release would have therapeutic implication in the treatment of both physical and emotional pain. The immediate sensory return on the physical investment of playing a drum, offers unique opportunity for an individual to experience release on various levels including emotional, physical, and even visceral.

The thought of creating additional vibration or movement to individuals in the throes of pain crisis can pose a psychological hurdle for such individuals. I have found that in such scenarios, simple psychoeducation about the control that one has in creating the natural release provides invitation to the patient to reclaim a sense of control. The use of small percussion like cabassa, shakers, or the Baoding balls referenced above can provide a seemingly more manageable means by which the fearful patient can move toward effective integration of music therapy toward tension release.

The following case depicts the active use of drumming for release by a 32 year-old flight attendant named Michael. He had been referred to music therapy during his extended hospitalization for posterior spinal fusion required for a debilitating lower lumbar injury sustained over time. Psychosocially, Michael was single and socially active with a large network of friends. He reported an enjoying a good relationship with his parents and an older sister who lived several states away. He also reported enjoying his work in spite of the stress it had placed on him physically, due to the frequent lifting and extended period of time spent on his feet.

At the time of our meeting, Michael had been hospitalized for several weeks following his surgery due to various complications that caused unexpected delays in his ability to transition into the course of physical and occupational therapy necessary for his rehabilitation. Michael's sense of resiliency was severely impacted by the interruptions in his recovery, which resulted in his pronounced state of depression and withdrawal from the care he was receiving. In meeting Michael, I remember being stricken by the incongruous nature of his physical presence with his emotional affect. He appeared to be in very good physical shape, which reflected a lifestyle clearly integrative of self-care and pride. This was a man whose participation in the world was integral to his professional and personal life. By his own report he enjoyed being physically and socially active and felt that his social life was vital to his happiness. His life style, both professionally and personally, while being central to his sense of self and engagement with the world, had also contributed to the injury that had taken its toll on his ability to function effectively. The present circumstances, which were laden with uncertainty, were not only profoundly interrupting his personal and professional life, but were also causing stress and anxiety in regard to mounting hospital expenses and loss of income.

My initial introduction of music therapy services, was met by a polite "thank you, but, I don't think you would do the kind of music I like". I asked him why he would assume that this was true so quickly. My mildly provocative response to Michael's snap judgment caught his attention. He proceeded to tell me that his lifestyle was fast-paced, and that his social life was centralized around nightclubs and dance music. I responded by asking him if he was familiar with several producers (from that genre) by the name of Peter Lutz and Gabriel & Dresden, who had turned out some "cool tracks". Michael had heard of both producers and seemed to immediately shift in attentiveness to what I had to offer him. The dialogue continued about various styles of electronic music that he liked including Drum & Bass and Trance. I asked him questions about how and when he accessed this music in his life. Was it only socially or did it also serve a purpose in his alone time at home?

I've found that in many cases, the initial dialogue regarding music therapy is best served by sensitive query into how the patient has used music in their life, and then connecting it to a dialogue about how they are making sense of their current circumstances. The thread of connection here is that the points of inquiry invite contemplation on how, if at all, they are able to stay connected with those aspects of themselves that remain intact even when their body may not be.

Having established common ground upon which Michael could actually hear and synthesize the possibility that music therapy could function on several levels in his care, I explained the qualities of groove and percussion that could be helpful in creating positive movement in his current state. Michael was receptive to the idea of exploring improvisation on bongos and djembe to an electronic groove that we would select on a synthesizer.

Michael's affect brightened at the prospect of "doing something different", and our first session resulted in a significant personal breakthrough for him as he described in a correspondence months later. Using a Yamaha YPG-225 keyboard/synthesizer, Michael was able to find an electronic groove to his liking, to which we created an improvisation. He selected a set of wood and hide bongos, which he could easily manage in the semi-supine position he held. I provided a synthesized string accompaniment over a cycling progression of chords that offered structure and predictability to create the hypnotic trance-like motion of the music with which Michael most identified. Subtly emphasizing the suspended 4th as a deviation from the modal chord sequence centering on G Mixolydian, the resolution of the interval back to the mode brought a sense of breath with each cycle. Michael created a drumming pattern on the bongos that sophisticatedly fit with the groove he had selected, as we continued through a thirty-minute improvisation that defined our first session. Following several moments of silence, Michael, with his eyes remaining closed, said very simply "yes".

This session was the first of four sessions with Michael over the remaining two weeks prior to his medical clearance for discharge to the acute rehabilitation unit that would serve as the transition back to his life. All of the sessions rendered extended improvisations with Michael immersed in his creations on various combinations of djembes, tubanos, or bongos, underscored by a groove that he would select, and me providing harmonic accompaniment on the keyboard or guitar.

The verbal process that we regularly shared post improvisation was consistently thematic for the reclaimed autonomy and sense of self that he had been challenged to sustain when his losses began to accumulate. There was also a sense of exclusiveness to his use of the music in the particular way that we were working. He would regularly say to me things like, "most people don't get (understand) this type of music (drum & bass, trance), but when you do (like us), there are no limits". I felt this was a form of bonding and testament to the therapeutic alliance we had created, but perhaps more importantly however, was the testament to his reclaimed locus of internal control and identity that this notion supported. The identification of popular genres with personal identity is common, and can extend well past adolescence into adulthood.[22] Creating an exclusive club through the music we had created provided a point of reconnection to the social constructs that had defined his most vital sense-of-self pre-trauma. Pragmatically, the sessions seemed to provide incentive for Michael during the arduous regimen of rehabilitation therapy necessary to his recovery.

Several months after he had been discharged, I received an email to my work address that was on the card I had given him in our first meeting. He notified me of a new release by an artist he thought I would like, and reported that he was "back on the job...back in his life".

Tonal Intervallic Synthesis: Case Vignette
The use of tonal intervallic synthesis in the treatment of pain has found its most profound use in my work with individuals living with head, neck, and throat cancer. For those individuals who have undergone surgical interven-

tion, extreme deficit in functionality in the areas of speech and swallowing, impacting communication and the ability to eat respectively is a reality. The impact on such essential human experiences becomes the criteria by which referrals for psychosocial and spiritual support are made.[23] Music Therapy as a modality may be introduced as not only a forum for emotional process and expression, but as an additional entry point into the reinforcement of the efforts made to assist the individual's retrieval of the physical mechanisms necessary to support speech and swallowing, be it through relearning, reconditioning, or triggering muscle memory.

Mary, a 58 year-old married, woman of Irish-American background, diagnosed with an oropharyngeal squamous cell cancer, found more commonly in men than in women.[24] Mary's diagnosis of a stage 2 cancer required a treatment regimen involving both radiation therapy and surgical intervention. While Mary had an overall favorable prognosis, her treatment required a heroic form of surgery that expectedly resulted in impaired vocal cord function compromising her ability to speak and swallow. In addition, a bone graft from her femur was needed to reconstruct her facial bones. The entire procedure impacted very deeply Mary's self esteem.

I met Mary in follow-up to a referral made by a speech therapist while she was in the intensive care unit. The referral stated that Mary was "teary" and "unmotivated". My experience with individuals moving through this phase of rehabilitation is that self-esteem and traumatic response to the profound losses of these essential human experiences, if even only temporary, can often present as withdrawal and understandable frustration with the tasks ahead. Mary was no exception, and as I sat with her, I wasted no time in establishing the connection of what I had to offer as a music therapist to the reality of the challenges she was immediately facing. I patiently waited as Mary wrote her responses to my questions on a notepad. I learned that Mary's deficits, although explained as possibilities prior to surgery, were more emotionally impacting than she had anticipated. I also learned that the exercises that had been explained by the speech and swallow therapist were uncomfortable for Mary. My initial thought was that the discomfort was physical, but Mary clarified that while she was experiencing numbness and other minor sensations, she was not in significant physical pain. The discomfort, Mary clarified was linked more to feeling "embarrassed" about the sound of her voice and inability to speak. She wrote that she never dreamed that she would have to "sing the ABCs" at her age. My understanding of the exercises that are generally utilized to facilitate functionality allowed me to extrapolate the theory informing speech and swallow interventions to music therapy.

Tonal intervallic synthesis[25] informed my intervention focusing on awakening the vibratory sensations of the tissue around the surgical site. I explained and modeled for Mary how the use of breath and humming could serve as a beginning and additional entry into the work that she was to do. As I initiated a hum on a pitch that seemed appropriate to her range, and invited her to join me. Once immersed in the experience, I would offer challenges to her use of breath and voice by changing the pitch I was singing to a dissonant interval above or below her pitch. Mary followed, and we continued through a sequence of intervals that was manageable. I also modeled for Mary how by changing the vowel, we could proceed through the same sequences but with varying vibratory effect.

This first session was focused on Mary gaining trust in my role and purpose in her care. The beginning of a therapeutic alliance in the work of awakening the tissue developed and while the pragmatism of the work provided the impetus for Mary's receptiveness, I believe it was therapeutic presence that sustained it. I assured Mary that I had the time to wait for her written responses, and to be there with her as she persevered through the challenges of hearing herself attempting to reclaim such a vital part of herself- her voice. We worked together in what I felt to be a dignified manner of exercising vowel shaping and vocal prosody without the use of children's songs.

Additional sessions during Mary's stay focused on expanding the exercise to more complex interval sequences by drawing upon music that was significant to Mary. She identified the late country-pop artist John Denver as one of her "favorites", and so the song "Country Roads" became central to our work leading to discharge. I provided a guitar accompaniment as we sang certain phrases together in unison. I additionally harmonized other phrases to challenge her vocal control in maintaining the melody against my voice. Her attentiveness to forming and vocalizing on the vowels of the words of this song increased with each repetition, and seemed to give her a sense of pride. Additionally, the provision of a tall djembe beside her chair allowed her an additional point of engagement in the music, while also providing the means of tension release.

Mary received six music therapy sessions over the several weeks prior to discharge. As reported by other staff during this time, her affect had gradually shifted from one of flattened and reclusive to animated and positive. Notably, her tolerance of the exercises during her speech and swallow therapy increased, as her context for rehabilitation expanded. I felt that this work was less about physical pain, which was well managed pharmacologically, and more about the physiological and psychoemotional responses to her circumstances. Certainly the outward expression of emotional pain that prompted the referral was validated and dignified by way of the therapeutic relationship that is central to music therapy practiced with a patient and family centered philosophy.

Conclusion

Music therapy holds the unique position of being efficacious across body, mind, and spirit integration in the treatment of pain. A music therapist can focus on any one entity or all three of those presented here, as the needs of the individual present. Notably, practitioners of other disciplines whose scope of clinical focus is narrower often misunderstand such flexibility. The emotional experience of an individual receiving physical intervention is always a consideration in the practice of music therapy even in work that is primarily focused in the physical domain. Needless to say, a referral for pain is understood as broad. Just as the experience of pain itself extends across a range of experiences and layers of functionality, so can the treatment rendered by a music therapist.

The case studies reflect a therapeutic approach that is informed through principal consideration of who the patient is in their own eyes, their family, their workplace, and their community. Such attention to assessment immanently individualizes the care that is rendered by the therapist, and sets criteria by which release strategies are understood and implemented in the context of interdisciplinary pain treatment.

References

1. Valent P. Eight Survival strategies in traumatic stress. Traumatology. 2007; 13: 4-14.
2. Portenoy RK. Contemporary Diagnosis and Management of Pain in Oncologic and AIDS Patients. 3rd ed. Newtown, PA: Handbooks in Health Care Co.; 2001.
3. Beth, Israel, Medical, Center. Our Pledge to Patients. New York, New York: Continuum Health Partners, Inc.
4. Kovacs P, Bellin MH, Fauri D. Family-centered care: A resource for social work in end-of-life and palliative care. Journal of Social Work in end-0f-life and palliative care. 2006;2(1):13-27.
5. Dewees M. Postmodern Social work in interdisciplinary contexts. Social Work Health Care. 2005;39(3):343-360.
6. Family centered care for children in hospitals. 2007.
7. Nicholas E, Walsh M. Rehabilitation of Chronic Pain. Philadelphia, PA: Hanley & Belfus, Inc.; 1991.
8. Macdonald R, Mitchell L, Dillion T, Serpell M, Davies JM, Ashley E. An empirical investigation of the anxiolytic and pain reducing effects of music. Psychology of Music. 2003;3(18).

9. Allred K, Byers JF, Sole M. The effect of music on postoperative pain and anxiety. Pain Management Nursing. 2008;March 11(1):15-25.
10. Huang S, Good M, Zauszniewski J. The effectiveness of music in relieving pain in cancer patients: A randomized controlled trial. International Journal of Nursing Studies. 2010;47:1354-1362.
11. Tan X, Yowler CJ, Super DM, Fratianne RB. The efficacy of music therapy protocols for decreasing pain, anxiety, and muscle tension levels during burn dressing changes: a prospective randomized crossover trial. Journal of burn care & research : official publication of the American Burn Association. Jul-Aug 2010;31(4):590-597.
12. Simcock XC, Yoon RS, Chalmers P, Geller JA, Kiernan HA, Macaulay W. Intraoperative music reduces perceived pain after total knee arthroplasty: a blinded, prospective, randomized, placebo-controlled clinical trial. The journal of knee surgery. Oct 2008;21(4):275-278.
13. Magill L. The use of music to address the suffering in advanced cancer pain. Journal of Palliative Care. 2001;17(3):167-172.
14. Loewy J, Hallan C, Friedman E, Martinez C. Sleep/sedation in children undergoing EEG testing: A comparison of chloral hydrate and music therapy. Journal of PeriAnesthesia Nursing. 2005;20(5):323-331.
15. Siedlecki S, Good M. Effect of music on power, pain, depression, and disability. Journal of advanced nursing. 2006;54(5):553-562.
16. Flauger M. The intervention of music on perceptions of chronic pain, depression, and anxiety in ambulatory individuals with cancer [Doctoral Dissertation]: Music, University of Alabama; 2002.
17. Loewy J. Music psychotherapy assessment. Music Therapy Perspectives. 2000;18(1):47-58.
18. Mitchell L, Macdonald R, Knussen C. A survey investigation of the effects of music listening on chronic pain. Psychology of Music. 2007;35(1):37-57.
19. Dileo C, Bradt J. Entrainment, resonance, and pain-related suffering. In: Dileo C, ed. Music Therapy & Medicine: Theoretical and Clinical Applicatins. Silver Spring, MD: AMTA; 1999:181-188.
20. Friedman RL. The healing power of the drum. Reno, NV: White Ciffs Media; 2000.
21. Loewy J, Azoulay R, Harris B, Rondina E. Clinical improvisation with winds:Enhancing breath in music therapy. In: Azoulay R, Loewy J, eds. Music, the breath and health: Advances in integrative music therapy. New York, NY: Satchnote Press; 2009: pp. 87-102.

22. Whiteley S, ed Sexing the Groove:Popular music and gender. New York, NY: Routledge; 1997.
23. Ramsey DW. Designing Musically Assisted Rehabilitation Systems. Music and Medicine. July, 2011;3(3):141-145.
24. Genden EM, Varvares M. Head and Neck Cancer: An Evidence-Based Team Approach. First ed. New York, NY: Theime; 2008.
25. Loewy J. Tonal intervallic synthesis as integration in medical music therapy In: Baker S, Uhlig S, eds. Voicework in music therapy: Research and practice. London: Jessica Kingsley Publishers; 2011: 252-268).

CHAPTER 10

Analytical Music Therapy for Pain Management and Reinforcement of Self-Directed Neuroplasticity in Patients Recovering from Medical Trauma

Benedikte B. Scheiby, MA, MMEd, DPMT, CMT, AMT, LCAT

"Music may offer the only bridge from inner world to outer reality. It may provide the only means to give expression, in a safe way, to inner feelings. . . . It is important that the music therapist's sphere of interest be the inner life of the patient—that the main concern be with the use of music as a vehicle by which this inner reality can be brought to the surface, to be heard, experienced, and examined in the presence of another."
Florence Tyson

Introduction

Improvisational music therapy used psychotherapeutically is an effective intervention for pain management for patients suffering from pain related medical trauma. I use an integrative perspective in working with the whole person. Working with pain management demands knowledge about music, psychology, brain function, and body function; and about how music, body, mind and spirit can be integrated in the person. It involves helping the person gain insight about how to live in a way that emotions, bodily sensations, physical trauma and spiritual being can work together.

This perspective comes from experiences and insights from a variety of sources: academic and post-academic study in music psychotherapy and body psychotherapy; three years of a formal training in medicine prior to changing to the study of music therapy; clinical work in psychiatry and in a medical rehabilitation context; personal experiences of being a patient in pain at a hospital; and, living a mindful, spiritually connected life. I strongly believe that how I live my life, how I think philosophically and spiritually, and how I receive supervision as a music therapy clinician and researcher deeply influences my ability to be an effective professional.

I work as a clinician with persons with medical trauma as a director of Music Therapy Training and Supervision and Senior Clinician at the

Institute for Music and Neurologic Function (IMNF), located at a facility for short and long term rehabilitation and skilled nursing facility in the Bronx.

As the person in the following case description was suffering from a variety of types of pain: physical pain, psychological pain, spiritual pain and potential psychogenic pain, a short description of the specifics of the four different types of pain follows. See also Figure 1.

Pain Classification
4 different types of Pain:

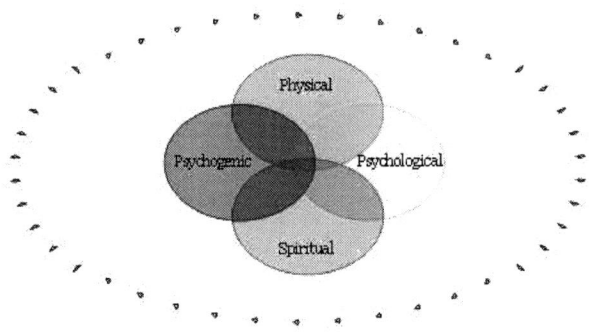

Figure 1

Physical Pain
"Pain is not a concept, but rather a psychical state expressed through localized bodily sensation."[1] Don Ranney[2] defines physical pain as "…a perception, not really a sensation, in the same way that vision and hearing are. It involves sensitivity to chemical changes in the tissues and then interpretation that such changes are harmful. This perception is real, whether or not harm has occurred or is occurring. Cognition is involved in the formulation of this perception. There are emotional consequences, and behavioral responses to the cognitive and emotional aspects of pain."

Psychological Pain
"Sometimes called psychalgia, [psychological pain] is any mental, or mind, or non-physical suffering. Emotional pain is a particular kind of psychological pain, more closely related to emotions. Another kind of psychological pain that is commonly found is spiritual or soul pain. Recent research in neuroscience suggests that physical pain and psychological pain may share some underlying neurological mechanisms."[3]

Spiritual Pain
"Spiritual distress and spiritual crisis" occur when a person is "unable to find sources of meaning, hope, love, peace, comfort, strength, and connection in life or when conflict occurs between their beliefs and what is happening in their life."[4]

Psychogenic Pain
"Also called psychalgia, [psychogenic pain] is physical pain that is caused, increased, or prolonged by mental, emotional, or behavioral factors. Headache, back pain, or stomach pain are some of the most common types of psychogenic pain...sufferers are often stigmatized, because both medical professionals and the general public tend to think that pain from psychological source is not 'real.' However, specialists consider that it is no less real or hurtful than pain from other sources...medicine refers also to psychogenic pain or psychalgia as a form of chronic pain under the name of persistent somatoform pain disorder. Causes may be linked to stress, unexpressed emotional conflicts, psychosocial problems, or various mental disorders. Some specialists believe that psychogenic chronic pain exists as a protective distraction to keep dangerous repressed emotions such as anger or rage unconscious. It remains controversial, however, that chronic pain might arise purely from emotional causes."[5]

The Pain is in the Brain

Music psychotherapy interventions in relation to pain management target areas of the brain where the pain signal is registered. And if the patient's pain is being experienced as lowered in intensity or has disappeared after music psychotherapy treatment we must have created some changes in the parts of the brain, such as the thalamus and the cortex.

"When one takes a look at a representation of pain pathways, stimulation of pain pathways typically begins with the stimulus of a nociceptor, which is a special pain-sensing nerve. That stimulus is propagated along the course of a peripheral nerve toward the spinal cord, but it is not pain yet. Eventually, that signal will reach the spinal cord, where it will be passed from the first order or primary neuron to the second order neuron, but that is still not pain. It is an example of that signal being transmitted from one nerve to another and with that an example of how pain is being transmitted. Eventually, the pain signal will ascend within the spinal cord and reach parts of the brain. First, the thalamus, and then out to the cortex. It is not until that signal reaches the cortex and other areas of the brain that it is interpreted in some emotional context. Only then is it experienced as pain."[6]

Music and Medicine: Integrative Models in the Treatment of Pain

In this context it is important to talk about *neuroplasticity*. This is "the brain's capacity to learn and thus change itself. Usually the results are tiny, incremental alterations in neural structure. Mental activity shapes neural structure."[7] Consequently, music psychotherapy can activate mental activity, create new neural pathways and alter or eliminate perceived pain. It is important here to describe which parts of the brain are activated when a client experiences AMT. The way different parts of the brain activate and work together is similar to how orchestra members work together when they play a symphony. Here I have gathered an overview of the roles of the different areas in the brain:

- Prefrontal cortex (PFC): setting goals, shaping emotions, directing actions,
- creation of expectations, violation of expectations (judgment)
- Anterior (frontal) cingulate cortex (ACC): stabilizes attention, helps integration of thinking and feeling
- Sensory cortex: tactile feedback from playing an instrument
- Motor Cortex: movement, foot tapping, dancing, and playing and instrument
- Auditory cortex: listening to sounds, perception and analysis of tones
- Visual cortex: coordination, looking at one's own and the music therapist's movements
- Insula: senses the internal state of the body including gut feelings, facilitates empathy (for self and others)
- Thalamus: amplification station for sensory information
- Brain stem: sends neuromodulators such as serotonin and dopamine to the rest of the brain when activated
- Corpus Callosum: passes information between two hemispheres of the brain
- Cerebellum: regulates movement such as foot tapping, dancing, and playing an instrument. Involved in emotional reactions to music
- Limbic system: central to emotion and motivation
- Basal ganglia: involved with rewards, stimulation and movement
- Hippocampus: forms new memories, detects threats
- Amygdala: responds particularly to emotionally charged or negative stimuli
- Hypothalamus: regulates primal drives, signals to the adrenal glands to release the "stress hormones" epinephrine (adrenaline) and cortisol

- Pituitary gland: makes endorphins, triggers stress hormones, stores and releases oxytocin which promotes nurturing behaviors associated with blissful closeness and love

For further elucidation on the neurologic functioning of specific regions of the brain, I recommend Daniel J. Levitin's book, *This is Your Brain on Music*, which provides rich detailing and graphics depicting the unique role of music.

Improvisation and Brain Research

In their article in *NeuroImage*,[8] Aaron L. Berkowitz and Daniel Ansari found that improvisation, compared to patterned performance, resulted in increased activity in three areas of the brain: the dorsal premotor cortex (dPMC), the anterior cingulate (ACC), and the inferior frontal gyrus/ventral premotor cortex (IFG/vPMC).

Berkowitz explained it this way[9]: "The dPMC takes information about where the body is in space, makes a motor plan, and sends it to the motor cortex to execute the plan. The fact [that] it's involved in improvisation is not surprising, since it is a motor activity. The ACC is a part of the brain that appears to be involved in conflict monitoring — when you're trying to sort out two conflicting possibilities, like when you to read the word BLUE when it's printed in the color red. It's involved with decision making, which also makes sense — improvisation is decision making, deciding what to play and how to play it." The IFG/vPMC region "is known to be involved when people speak and understand language. It's also active when people hear and understand music. What we've shown is that it's involved when people create music." This research was based upon musicians improvising and not upon music therapists improvising with patients, which might make a difference. Therefore it is important to do research on actual clinical music therapeutic work.

Although not yet implemented, I have designed study that combines Analytical Music Therapy (AMT) with patients with medical trauma, with brain imaging before the treatment, and after the treatment on a portable brain scanner in a natural environment. The hypothesis of this research is that music psychotherapeutic based clinical improvisation facilitates increased activity in a variety of areas in the brain, which means that neuroplasticity is being created.

Music and Medicine: Integrative Models in the Treatment of Pain

How Does the Mind Process Pain?

Melinda Becker asserts that[10] "How you think about pain can have a major impact on how it feels." This is "…the principle behind many mind-body approaches to chronic pain that are proving surprisingly effective in clinical trials." She goes onto quote Josephine Briggs, director of NCCAM, who states, "There is a growing recognition that drugs are only part of the solution and that people who live with chronic pain have to develop a strategy that calls upon some inner resources."

Becker goes onto say that "one technique is attention distraction, simply directing your mind away from the pain…Guided imagery, in which a patient imagines, say, floating on a cloud, also works in part by diverting attention away from the pain. So does mindfulness meditation." In discussing a study that shows how meditation helps ease pain, she quotes Fadel Zeidan the lead investigator of this study who say: "Our subjects really looked at pain differently after meditation. Some said 'I didn't need to say ouch.'"

Becker concludes "experts stress that much still isn't known about pain and the brain, including whom these mind-body therapies are most appropriate for."

It may be possible that improvised music in a music psychotherapy pain management context can facilitate a rewiring of the brain to ease the pain in patients with pain caused by medical trauma. Supporting this possibility, Becker documented that 75 persons who practiced mindfulness meditation while exposed to a heated probe reported a 40 % decrease in pain. Moreover, this article found that there was a 30 % decrease in pain reported by 422 fibromyalgia patients after receiving cognitive behavioral therapy and a 44 % decrease in pain reported by 15 undergraduates when they focused on a loved one's photo while exposed to a heated probe.

This hypothesis is supported by Rick Hanson who speaks about self-directed neuroplasticity. Rick gives lectures and workshops where he demonstrates this phenomenon. I participated in one of these workshops where he showed how psychotherapists can use the mechanisms of experience-dependent neuroplasticity to stimulate and thereby strengthen the neural substrates of positive states of mind through practicing mindfulness meditation and being which is geared towards activation of the neural basis for self compassion and a basic sense of safety.[11] Interested readers can learn further about this practice in Rick Hanson's book *Buddha's Brain*.[7]

Participating in one of Rick Hanson's workshops provided an experience similar to what music therapy practiced in a mindful way can accomplish: psychological and physical pain management and an increased sense of self compassion as documented in the case study in the present chapter.

What is neuroplasticity? Charlotte A. Tomaino defines it as[12] "a physiological ability in the nervous system, referring to its capacity to adapt and change." She discusses how to recognize the red flags that will lead to stressful situations, control the shift from anxious and overwhelmed feelings to calm and collected ones, listen to one's body wisdom and tune into the physical effects of emotions. When new neurons connect, new experiences are created and new skills developed. A physical change occurs in the nervous system accompanies changes in thought, emotion, or behavior. Changes occur on all physical levels from the very small cellular level to the large level of neural networks that interconnect functional locations in the brain. The word *plasticity* is used because your experience shapes the structures of the neurons. Intentional action leads to self-directed neuroplasticity.

In an overview of self-directed neuroplasticity, de Llosa[13] discusses how the breakthrough in imaging techniques, led Dr. Jeffrey Schwartz to question two decades ago, the kind of internal experience that could be better understood by analyzing imaging generated by the neuronal activity captured on a brain scan. The use of knowledge gleaned from scientific discoveries that linked inner experience with brain function, to effect constructive changes in everyday life, was of tremendous intrigue. He reflected on several observations that are interesting here. 1) A student of Buddhist meditation developed a form of therapy to change the faulty chemistry of a well-identified brain circuit- that belonging to patients diagnosed with Obsessive Compulsive Disorder (OCD). The pathological processes of OCD, marked by negative thoughts, could be traced on an MRI. It was suggested that the trademark feelings of doubt experienced by the OCD patient was due to false messaging ensuing from a jammed transmission in the brain; and 2) OCD patients could learn to change the way they thought about their thoughts through regular refocusing, which engaged them in intentional rather than automatic behavior, activating a different brain circuitry. Not only was a new treatment for mental illness introduced, but also hard evidence as to the mind's ability to control the brain's chemistry. He concluded that mindfulness and refocusing has the potential to restore an individual's sense of control and self-empowerment.

How can we use these scientific discoveries linking inner experience with brain function to effect constructive changes in our work as music therapists with patients with medical and psychological pain and trauma? If the mind as shown in the above research can control the brain's chemistry, we can help persons to refocus through practicing AMT that reprograms the brain, and music therapy can give people more control over their lives in relation to physical /psychological pain and trauma.

The context in which AMT is practiced is called music psychotherapy. In 2001 in connection with a lecture given together with Dr. Joanne Loewy we constructed a chart that illustrates the philosophy behind music psychotherapeutic thinking in a medical context.[14] See Figure 2. below.

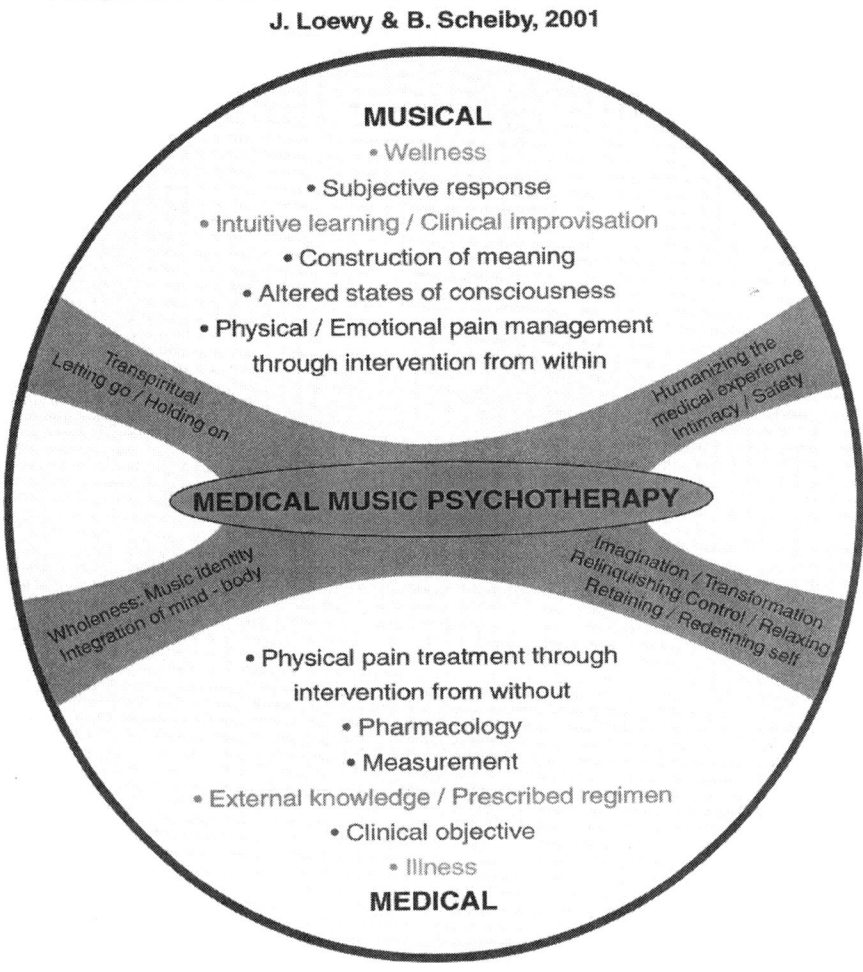

Figure 2

Definition of Medical Music Psychotherapy (Scheiby, 2001):
Medical music psychotherapy is the informed use of improvised or composed music as intervention in order to facilitate therapeutic change in a person's medical and psychological condition. Focused musical interventions, musical experiences and the musical relationship between client and music therapist are the main dynamic factors in the therapeutic process. It is in that context that the following case example should be understood.[14]

At IMNF I have been implementing Analytical Music Therapy (AMT) as a form of integrative music psychotherapeutic treatment method in all areas of the following programs:

Music Therapy Practices at IMNF

- MIDI based Music Therapy (MIDI equipment and recording studio, Use of IPAD 2)
- Community based Music Therapy (Community Drum circles/Wellness, Exercise/Gospel, Concerts, Events, Memorial Services)
- Neurorehabilitation Program (musical cue-based motor and speech rehabilitation)
- Dementia and Alzheimer's Program
- Palliative care Program
- Relaxation and Stress Management Program (Music assisted yoga/meditation, live music to GIM)
- Music assisted Pain Management
- Environmental Music Therapy
- Caring for the Caregivers Program (staff/family members/friends)
- Weight transformation Program
- Smoking Cessation
- I-Pod Program (personalized I-Pod playlists)
- Research (Anxiety, Memory, Dementia, Speech, Depression,)
- Training Program: National and International Internship Programs (BA, MA, Ph.D.), shorter or longer focused specialty training programs, independent studies, professional supervision, consultancy)
- Information dissemination (Publications, conferences, seminars, TV, Radio, Events)
- Outpatient Program for adults and children with neurologic challenges.

What is Analytical Music Therapy?

Its founder, Mary Priestley, developed two Definitions of AMT:

1) "Analytical music therapy is a way of exploring the unconscious with an analytical music therapist by means of sound expression."[15]
2) "So Analytical Music Therapy is the name that has prevailed for the analytically-informed symbolic use of improvised music by the music therapist and client. It is used as a creative tool with which to explore the client's inner life so as to provide the way forward for growth and greater self-knowledge."[16]

In the definition of AMT, the word *analytical* refers to a few different facets:

a) Mary Priestley's theoretical/practical background is in psychoanalysis (Freud, Jung, Klein, Adler, Lowen) and the model involves analyzing clinical musical improvisations from music therapeutic work with patients in psychiatry;
b) Client and music therapist analyze and process the music at a verbal/movement/art level if possible;
c) Music therapist analyzes the audio or videotaped session afterwards and writes a session log.

The process of recovery in this context in general is through musical expression, gaining insight, release of pain, withheld psychic material, etc. For readers interested in reading more about AMT work with persons with medical trauma please read: "Analytical Music Therapy and Integrative Medicine: The impact of Medical Trauma on the Psyche", in: K. Stewart (Ed.), 2010: *Music Therapy and Trauma.* Satchnote Press, New York.

For persons referred to pain management I have developed a practice and a quantitative measurement tool that is used in the beginning and end of each of the sessions. This in order to assess level and intensity of pain before and after treatment and it also serves as empowerment and encouragement for the patient to get to know that the level and intensity of the pain has been lowered or maybe disappeared. See Figure 3. on the following page.

Analytical Music Therapy in Pain from Medical Trauma

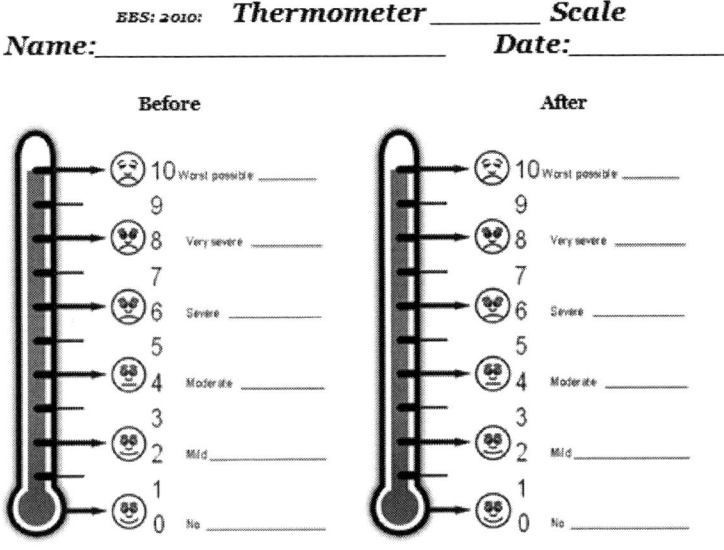

Figure 3

In order to provide the patient with a consistent environment and instrument selection, sessions take place in a Wellness Studio where there are many different instruments available, a warm atmosphere created by special lamps, plants, a photo of a lush nature scene that takes up one whole wall, and a wealth of instruments speaking to any culture available for the patient to use.
- Piano, Keyboard, Accordion
- String instruments: Guitar, Violin, and Auto Harp
- Wind Instruments: North American Flutes, Bird Calls, Whistles, Harmonicas
- Percussion Instruments: Drums, Ocean Drum, Rain Sticks, Rattles, Bells, Gong Bowls, Tibetan Bells, Tambourines, Gongs, Chimes
- MIDI, Sound Beam, iPad 2

Figure 4 illustrates how the sessions proceed in AMT. Sometimes the identification of an issue emerges from starting out in a musical improvisation together, sometimes the theme or issue is identified through verbal processing. Most often it is obvious what the issue is as in the description of this following transcribed session. The patient is extremely angry, yelling and in physical and emotional pain (self reported pain scale: 10)

Procedural Phases in an AMT session: Figure 4

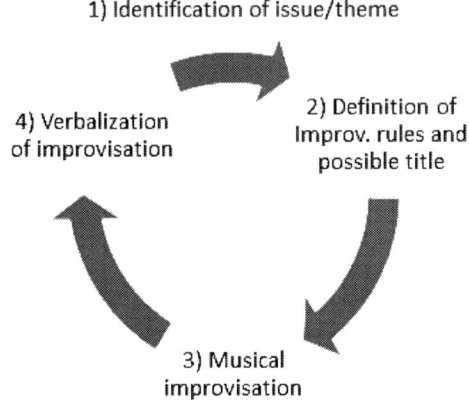

Casework

E. was a 63-year-old male admitted to the facility to receive rehabilitation treatment for post operative care in relation to an operation where a pacemaker was inserted. E. suffered from congestive heart failure, precardial (in front of the heart) chest pains, with a Pain level of 6 on the Wong-Baker faces pain-rating scale at intake. E. was diagnosed as having a mood disorder: bipolar disorder. He had anger management problems, creating conflicts constantly, and he was argumentative, with a strong identification with his past role and status (taxi driver, jewelry seller), along with unsettled relationships. His mood included negative comments, repetitive health complaints, psychological stress, decline in functional abilities, and agitation. Behavioral symptoms: sexual comments to staff and patients that are inappropriate. Former illnesses: motor cycle accident causing hip problems, CVA resulting in paralysis in the left side of body and hemiparesis, one suicide attempt, 5 heart attacks. The interdisciplinary treatment team agreed upon a care plan as follows:

- Encourage independence, improvement of insight/awareness of behavior. Pt. will engage in activities that focus on existing strengths (poetry writing, religion).
- Encourage verbalization of feeling throughout all interaction

- Encourage pt. to explore reasons for feelings
- Reinforce positive coping strategies
- Anger management

E. was referred to music psychotherapy by the medical director with the explicit goals of facilitation of stress management, relaxation, pain management, and anger management skills.

In assessment sessions E. stated that he was not musical and not able to sing or play any instrument. He also stated that he had had several heart attacks before he got the pacemaker inserted. His mental and physical tempo was incredibly fast and he shared that he had not slept well since he arrived to the facility and was extremely exhausted. He was having severe chest pain and mentioned that he had trouble with his roommate and felt like "killing him" sometimes when they had arguments.

He shared that he had been living on the streets before he came to the facility and had lost everything except a book of poems that he had with him. He also shared that he had been physically and emotionally abused as a child by his father, who "made a living as a member of the Jewish mafia" and who "put machine guns" in violin cases. E. shared that he dropped out of college and started being a taxi driver for a living. E. also shared that he had been a platoon leader in the Vietnam War and felt traumatized by what he had to see and do there. This was confirmed by the surfacing of memories and associations when we improvised together in a much later session, and he asked if he could play the instrument called a Chinese bell tree. The sound of this instrument brought him back to a village that he had to lead his group through where bells like that were heard –"chimes ringing when the wind was blowing" and right after his platoon was attacked and he had to kill two men in order to survive.

E. seemed very bright with a fine sense of humor so I connected with him in a light and humorous way, and asked him what his biggest challenge was in the momet. He said that he really needed to get some sleep and relax. I asked if we could make some music together, but he refused to play any instrument or sing and instead "commanded" me to sing and play. Here I became aware of the intersubjective counter transference feeling of "being manipulated" and "forced to" and with that in mind I decided that one major goal besides providing relief and help with self relaxation would be to engage E. in collaborative music-making.

I took note of his several heart attacks and I felt that my heart started racing when I attuned to his tempo. I began thinking about former patients that I had worked with who had histories of heart attacks. I researched a possible connection between heart disease and Post Traumatic Stress Disorder (PTSD), suspecting through my work with him over several sessions, that he might have had a history of trauma. E's psychotherapist also suspected PTSD supporting my impression. An article in *The New York Times*[17] describes that there is a connection between heart attacks, heart problems and PTSD:

- "While it has long been known that a heart attack affects both physical and mental health, most doctors and patients are not aware that the emotional stress of a such a life-threatening trauma can develop into full-blown post-traumatic stress disorder, or P.T.S.D."
- "The disorder, which more typically affects combat veterans and victims of violent crime, can be particularly insidious in heart patients, who live with constant trepidation about their own bodies, frequently paying anxious attention to each heartbeat or twinge of chest discomfort."
- Referring to the Columbia University Medical Center's research: "Their analysis, published online in the journal PLoS One, found not only that P.T.S.D. after a heart attack was far more common than previously believed, but also that the disorder doubled the risk of dying of a second event over the next one to three years, compared with those who did not have post-traumatic stress."
- "Dr. Edmonton said he hoped that future research would focus on ways to minimize the trauma for patients at the time of the heart attack to prevent patients from developing P.T.S.D. symptoms later."
- "'We know where the vast majority of these traumas are going to take place, and that's in emergency departments where heart patients show up,' Dr. Edmonton said. "We are interested now in trying to determine whether there are ways to alter that environment to decrease perceptions of life threat and lack of control so we can reduce the incidence of P.T.S.D in the first place."[17]

Mimi Guarneri confirms what I had suspected[18]: "Research has shown that stress reducers such as visualization, hypnosis, deep breathing, meditation, and yoga have measurable effects on cardiac risk, helping to relax arteries and reduce levels of stress hormones."(p 47)

Based on this idea, I referred E. to group music-assisted yoga and musical meditation as well as individual music therapy sessions. Figure 6 shows patients with medical trauma practicing music-assisted yoga. They move slowly and meditatively and move through the painful places in the body. The improvised music supports the movements that are initiated by the patients. E. enjoyed participating in those sessions tremendously and seemed to start getting a feeling for how one can help oneself with pain management through this activity. Dr. Guarneri's research supports the

Analytical Music Therapy in Pain from Medical Trauma

fact that working with a group doing music-assisted yoga and musical meditation was very helpful for E.:

"Group support is a central part of Dean Ornish's heart disease reversal program, a model for ours. According to Ornish, not only do support groups help participants let down walls, express feelings, and learn to listen compassionately, but group members also motivate one another to sustain lifestyle changes, such as exercise, diet modification, and smoking cessation."[19 (p 82)]

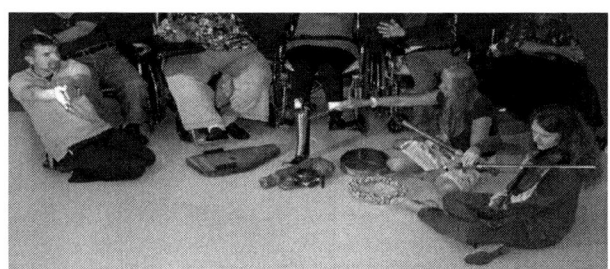

Music assisted group yoga, breathing and musical meditation

Dr. Guarneri goes on to state in her book:

We are all aware of the traditional risk factors for coronary disease that are physically related—obesity, high cholesterol, hypertension, smoking, diabetes, a sedentary lifestyle. But these factors may fail to identify 50 percent of patients with coronary disease. We now know that diseases of the heart can also be caused by other, more subtle factors such as isolation, depression, and hostility that have to do with not only how we live but how we experience our lives.[18(p 63)]

In the transcribed case example one can get an impression of the level of hostility that E. was exhibiting, partly caused by years of abuse as a child, partly caused by the intensity of the pain and not getting enough sleep, partly also caused by depression and isolation having been living his life partly on the streets, and now having no place to go back home to or any family that could take care of him. Additionally, being in an institution awoke images from being in the army, where things are regulated and where certain rules have to be obeyed. I also think the he had internalized a very explosive and angry father as the father had been beating him with a belt every day when he came back from "work" (Jewish mafia).

Guarneri has written about the connection between hostility and coronary disease, something that I believed was relevant in E's case:

Music and Medicine: Integrative Models in the Treatment of Pain

There are recent studies suggesting that hostility, in particular, may be more predictive of coronary disease than more traditional factors such as smoking and high cholesterol. Researchers have found that heart attacks, angina, or other symptoms of coronary disease occurred much more often among men who measured as hostile on a personality test than in those who had more conventional risk factors.[18 (p 63-64)]

I decided to help E. to take an approach to pain management by helping him relax by learning to breathe deeper and slower when necessary. In the initial sessions, I employed music assisted breathing approaches in combination with free association that allowed images, thoughts, feelings and sensations to come and go. E. resisted making music so I started with accompanying his breath and in that way accepting his fear of getting involved in musical actions.

I asked E. to breathe in on the first chord that I played on the piano, then hold his breath, and then release on the second chord. Figure 5 below shows this music. I would start in the tempo in which I could hear him breathe and then gradually slow down the breathing tempo through slowing down the accompaniment on the piano. After the session where I practiced this exercise E. reported that he had been able to take a nap in the afternoon and relax a little bit.

Breath and Voice Chords

Benedikte Scheiby

I took a step in the next session where I introduced him playfully to the harmonica, and shared with him that we could use that for helping him relax also. This time he was willing to play an instrument, and I introduced him to the idea that when he felt like exploding in anger or lost his temper he could play on the harmonica instead of cursing and yelling and screaming. I let him borrow the harmonica for that purpose. See photo: E. on the harmonica.

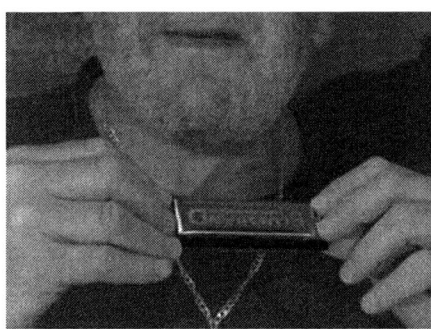

    I also asked him in the same session to breathe in and out on a harmonica in sync with my breathing as I too played a harmonica. Both harmonicas were in the same tonality. I approached this by first encouraging him to breathe in and out in the current breathing tempo that he had. I would then synchronize my breathing and tempo to his on my harmonica. Then I slowly lowered the tempo of the breath, asking him to simultaneously close his eyes and allow himself to connect to his body and his emotions. E. would slowly take over the tempo of breathing that I would manifest, and would quite often fall asleep by the end of the exercise. During sessions where achieving synchrony was more difficult for E., I would add an additional layer of sound. Playing a slow heart beat on the very deep resonator bar, or playing a very long rain stick was effective. The latter sounded like little pebbles coming and going with the ocean waves as they rush to and recede from the beach.
    These interventions helped reduce pain levels 8 or 9 to 5 or 6 degrees during the sessions. I suspected that the pain was not only physical but also emotionally related. We began to think that there might be a connection between the physical pain and emotional pain that he was experiencing. I was very careful not to work directly on the emotional pain initially and I respected his defenses and stayed with working on the physical part of the pain. I suggested that he start writing down every day on his own what came to mind – such as dreams, thoughts, feelings-- as another way to release what was bothering him. I also asked him if it would be permissible to have a student music therapy intern sitting in on his session, and to this he gave permission. Under my direction, the intern, who played the violin, would join the music.

Music and Medicine: Integrative Models in the Treatment of Pain

Dr. Guarneri states:
> suppressed emotions, or ones we are unconscious of, don't just simmer on the back burner indefinitely; they eventually manifest themselves on a physical level and are reflected in our bodies as physical symptoms. And if you lift up the veil of hostility and anger, in my experience, you usually find some kind of emotional pain [18(p65)]

This was illustrated by E.'s experience with emotional pain. In session 5 something seemed to change radically. E. came in to the session very agitated and yelling: (Transcript excerpts from session no. 5. B = music therapist.):

E: Here I am, - taking money and run some errands for some people, wanted to get him a sandwich, another to get a coke, a root beer and some cookies, and some asshole comes along. "Oh! He's taking money from the girls!" So I said: "mind your fucking business!" So the social worker was here, says he caught an attitude. In the meantime I've been trying to get him to see someone that's wanted to see him for two days, and he goes in and sees him and right away I'm upsetting her. She wants a transfer off the floor and she tells me to tell him and this Ms. X, and right away I'm upsetting her. Fucking people are getting me so God damn aggravated! You know... I can't wait to get out of here so I can handle my own shit. Because the harder I work at it, something goes and happens. And I get twice as upset because it all builds up from when I couldn't open my mouth. [Referring to when the patient was not able to speak after a stroke.]
[I am very quiet and listening deeply to the words and the intensity of the anger.]

Guarneri states, "Lynch has spent decades studying how loneliness contributes to a markedly increased risk of developing premature coronary heart disease... people . . . who performed poorly in school and lacked love and were criticized at home, can find communication with others extremely difficult and may avoid it, repeating this pattern throughout their lives. For many depressed and lonely people, communication can be viewed as a threat, triggering the activation of the fight-or-flight response, the secretion of stress hormones that increase blood pressure and makes the heart beat faster."[18(p92)]

[I (Benedikte) am feeling like a very young child being scolded and yelled at and exposed to a tremendous amount of rage (Intersubjective counter-

transference). I take note of this, as this might be important information for making a music therapy intervention later on. The Being in Silence is a very important state of mind here in order to be able to pick up upon the intersubjective counter transference and also in order not to give more fuel to the anger of the patient.]

I wait for quite a while in silence after E. is finished talking and then he says:

E: *"Deeeeeeeeep breath. Yes- I know!!!!"* [This refers to the former sessions where we had been working on using the breath to reach a more relaxed state of consciousness. Here I took the opportunity to as what level the pain was and he answered promptly]: *"It is at a 10".*

I softly suggested that he express and release his frustration and anger on a big table drum in the room. I would support him if he liked. I also encouraged him to free associate and allow images and thoughts and feelings to come and go during the improvisation.

B: *We'll see. Whatever comes to mind.*
E: *I'm just…* [and then he started drumming with all fingers on the drum skin in a furiously fast tempo.]

This is the first time E. expressed his feelings on an instrument, thus moving past his resistance. Then he shortly after stopped the music with a big slap on the drum.
E: *I can put my hand right through this drum, Benny, and that would prove nothing at all.*
B: *Exactly. It's not about sticking the hand through the drum. It's about finding another way of expressing anger than yelling and getting carried away. But it's still your father that you have to face.*

I made a reference to his abusive father, as I thought he might have internalized the angry father on one the one hand. On the other hand, he needed to internalize a good parental figure.
    E.'s experience with his father relates to a study done at Harvard. "According to the Harvard Mastery Study, a forty-two-year follow-up of students at Johns Hopkins University, the parent-child relationship in childhood proved to be a major predictor of major illness, including heart disease and cancer, in midlife."[20(p.93)]

Music and Medicine: Integrative Models in the Treatment of Pain

E: I want respect, love, affection…
B: I tried…[E. interrupts me]
E: Do you want to hear a story? I'll read you a story.

The book E. reads from came about as a result of an assignment I had given him to write down what comes to mind in between sessions. Here I signal to the intern on her violin to accompany the story and express the emotional undertone in the story. I join on the keyboard. E. starts reading with a very loud voice in a very fast tempo.

E: The name of the story is "Little Boy Blue Lost in the Woods." His father was the number one contract killer for the Jewish mafia. He was known by the name of Joe Bullets. He had a long and successful career. And when he asked one of his buddies why they called him by the name of Bullet Joe, his buddy chuckled with a very serious look on his face and then remarked, "because he only needed one shot and then he nevertheless always carried extra ammunition just to be sure." Papa Joe was physically and verbally abusive to his then 5-year-old oldest son, with an IQ that was almost immeasurable compared to his father, who was thrown out of public school with only a 3rd grade education despite a certain natural more cunning as that of a sociopath. For the first five years of his life, the child was called and referred to as "The Little Bastard."

One day the child returned home from kindergarten and threw down in the building's incinerator shaft a leather belt with colored plastic studs that Papa Joe use to brutalize and intimidate and supposedly discipline the child with. When the father returned home to the family apartment that evening, he was told by his wife that the child had thrown away the belt. The father cursed loudly, "that little bastard!" and seemed to be furious. The child heard commotion and backed himself into a far corner of his bedroom, raising clenched tightly his little fists, and waiting the seemingly frightening animal, he was about to be beaten to death. Papa Joe was ons foot's distance with the child. All of a sudden, a certain calm came over the child and he clenched tightly his little fist. Papa Joe raised his large right hand and his fist, and suddenly started to laugh loudly. The child was speechless. Papa Joe remarked: "You know kid, you got more guts than Moxy." Smarts in old time gangster talk. That was the last time the little boy was called "the little bastard".

The music we created reflected the sadness of the child's situation and also the feistiness and guts that the child had shown in throwing out the belt. We also reflected the anger of the father when he talked to the little child. See Figure 6 on the next page.

Excerpt 1: from E's Story
(transcription begins at about 1:15 into the segment)

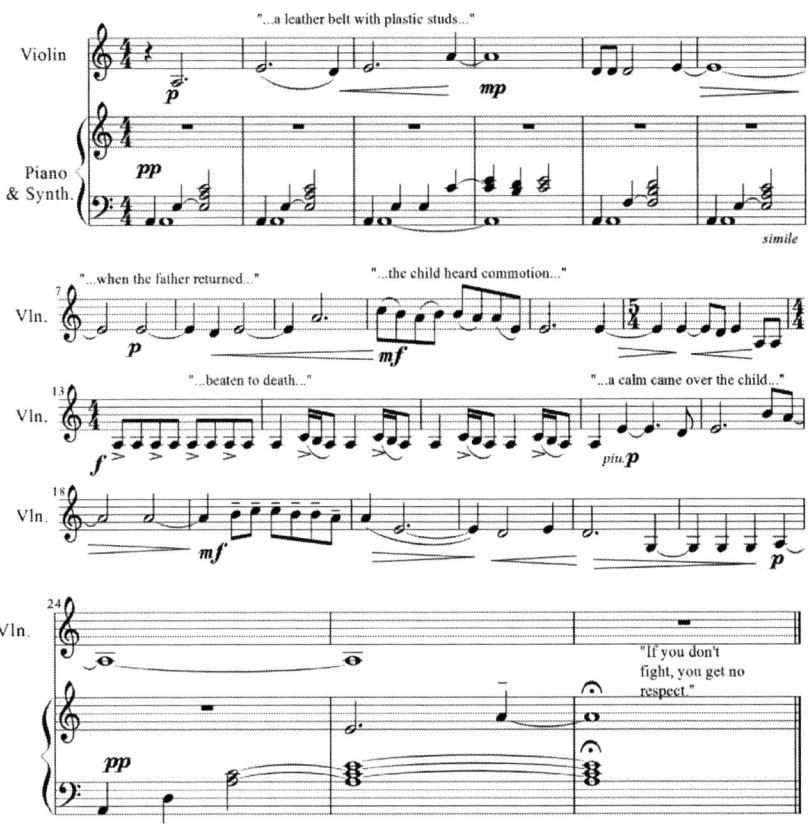

E: *If you don't fight, you get no respect.*
B: *Sad story.*
E: *True story!*
B: *So if you don't fight, you don't get any respect?*
E: *People will take you for a patsy.*
E: *I once got him to take me to the movie. I was reading Sartre. I took him to see Siddhartha. You know what the best part of the picture was to him? When the guy got bitten by the cobra. Sat through three and a half hours worth of a movie and that was the best part. He had this look of death.*

Music and Medicine: Integrative Models in the Treatment of Pain

People have a need to share with others the stories that comprise their lives. Guarneri's research has revealed that within "the act of deep listening and responding, a therapeutic exchange takes place, one that may help heal emotional and psychic wounds."[18]

B: Okay, one little thing more. Come up and sit next to me at this bench.

When I got in touch with an intersubjective countertransference of feeling like the little boy being yelled at by the furious father it led me to make a strong intervention: To musically reflect back in a motherly way how I would have liked to be there for him and protect him. I played extremely slowly in a repeated, harmonic holding pattern supporting my singing voice that sang these words:

B: E., you are good enough as you are. I wish I could have been there to protect you. You deserve somebody to be there for you. You're good enough as you are. You don't have to prove anything. You are special!

I sang this while I looked at E. He started sighing and eventually also crying a little bit. See excerpt from some of the music below Figure 7.

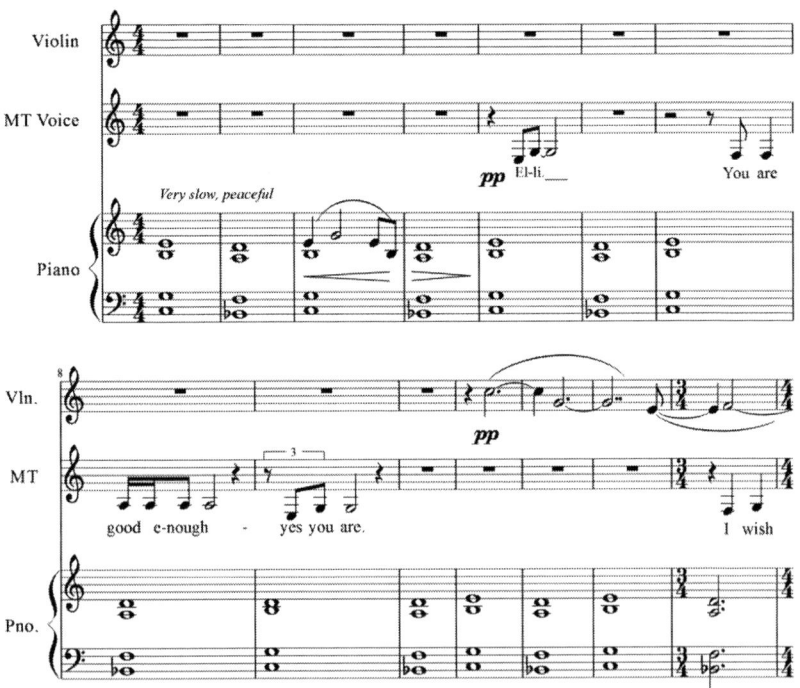

Analytical Music Therapy in Pain from Medical Trauma

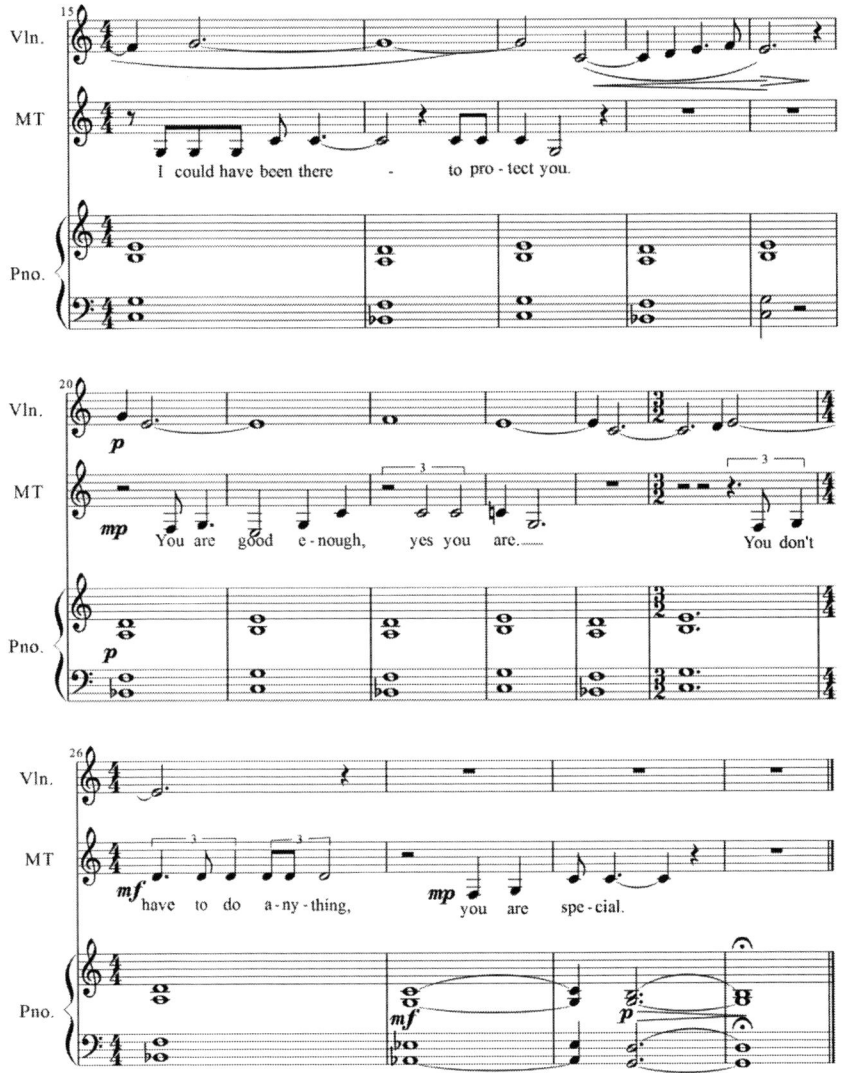

After the end of the music there was a long silence in which tears slowly fell down E.'s cheeks. Then E. started playing the piano in the upper register with both hands. It sounded developmentally like the spontaneous play of a 4 year old. There was a sad and lonely quality in the expression. I accompanied him in the lower register as best as I could, so that it sounded like a whole piece of music with left and right hand is fitting together. The piece was short and intense. Then a long pause again. E., giving me a friendly push on my shoulder indicating that it was a good thing that it happened, broke the pause. I gave E.'s shoulder a friendly push, and he smiled a bit. E. now spoke with a sad and quiet voice:

> *E:* Thanks, Benny.
> *B:* You're welcome.
> *E:* Does it ever go away? Does it ever totally go away?
> *B:* Not totally, it will always be there.
> *E:* It's always going to bother me.
> *B:* You won't be able to let it go.
> *E:* I want to let it go, Benny.
> *B:* How can I help you let it go?
> *E:* This helped. A couple more of these – it will go away. Let's see what happens in church on Sunday.

I asked E. before he left if he could state the level of his pain and he replied:

> *E:* It is gone.

This was a very powerful session in which E was able to open up and allow himself to take in the musical parenting—that the young child in him had needed so desperately. He connected with his inner child. In subsequent sessions, E. was calmer and he did not have any confrontations or angry outbursts at the unit. His physical pain scores were consistently decreased. He also started spending quite some time writing poems, and he became involved in work with the patients' council. Below is an excerpt from a session where the internalization of a good parent seems to have happened. He sings in an improvised lullaby to his "inner child" in a soothing and calming way—just like a parent would sing a lullaby to an upset child. I accompanied him on the accordion, and three interns with whom he had bonded in a variety of ways accompanied him on piano, violin and guitar. The excerpt starts in the beginning of the session where the interns and I are listening to his "theme" of today:

E: And then at my Bar Mitzvah, there were all these hoods with it. And you can see, you know, bulges in their suits – expensive suits. But Mama never let us have anything to do with that side of whatever dad had been involved in. Supposedly he was retired. But what I understood he might have been doing a little freelancing here and there on his business trips. Onetime, we've gone out to a...Borough Park, which was... this part of Borough Park was in the Italian neighborhood, and I was looking in a toy store. And I said to my mother, my...mother, I said "Mommy, Mommy,

Analytical Music Therapy in Pain from Medical Trauma

buy me that toy!" and I made a big stink here – yelling and screaming. He walked over and gave me a whack. I thought my head was gonna come off. I can still feel my ears stinging to this day. He just hauled off and let me have one. I think I was three and a half years old.

<u>B:</u> *Let's sing to that little three and a half year old right now.*
<u>E:</u> *Sing!*

I pick up the accordion and signal to the three interns to improvise on piano, violin and guitar. I decide to challenge E. and ask him to do the work himself, which is important in relation to the internalization process.

<u>B:</u> *You sing to that little E. who got that slap so badly.*
<u>E:</u> *No!*
<u>B:</u> *Yes. Sing to him!!*

E. sings, making up a beautiful song for little E. on the spot.
<u>E:</u> *"Hush little baby, don't you cry. Everything will be all right. Mommy loves you and auntie too. Ain't no reason for you to feel blue. Someday, when you are old enough, you will grow up and be very tough. And nobody will dare slap your face. You are going to be the toughest boy of your race. Hush little baby, don't you cry, mommy is gonna love you…"*
Figure 8 shows the transcription of this music.

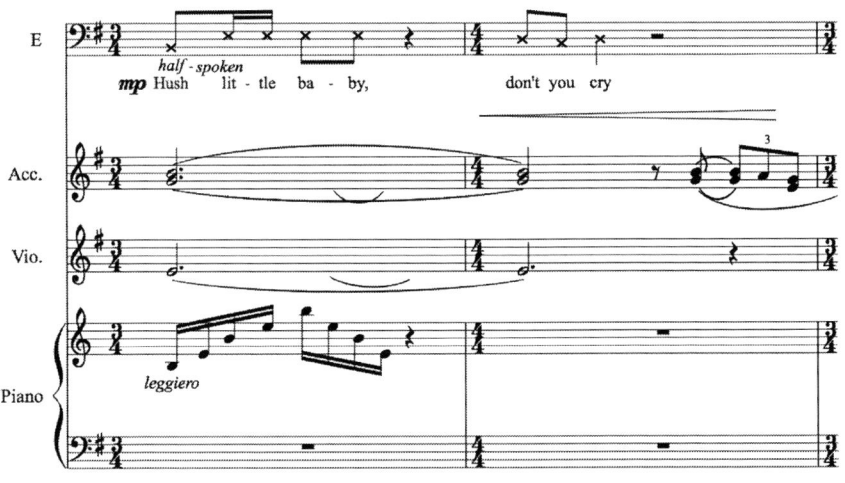

Music and Medicine: Integrative Models in the Treatment of Pain

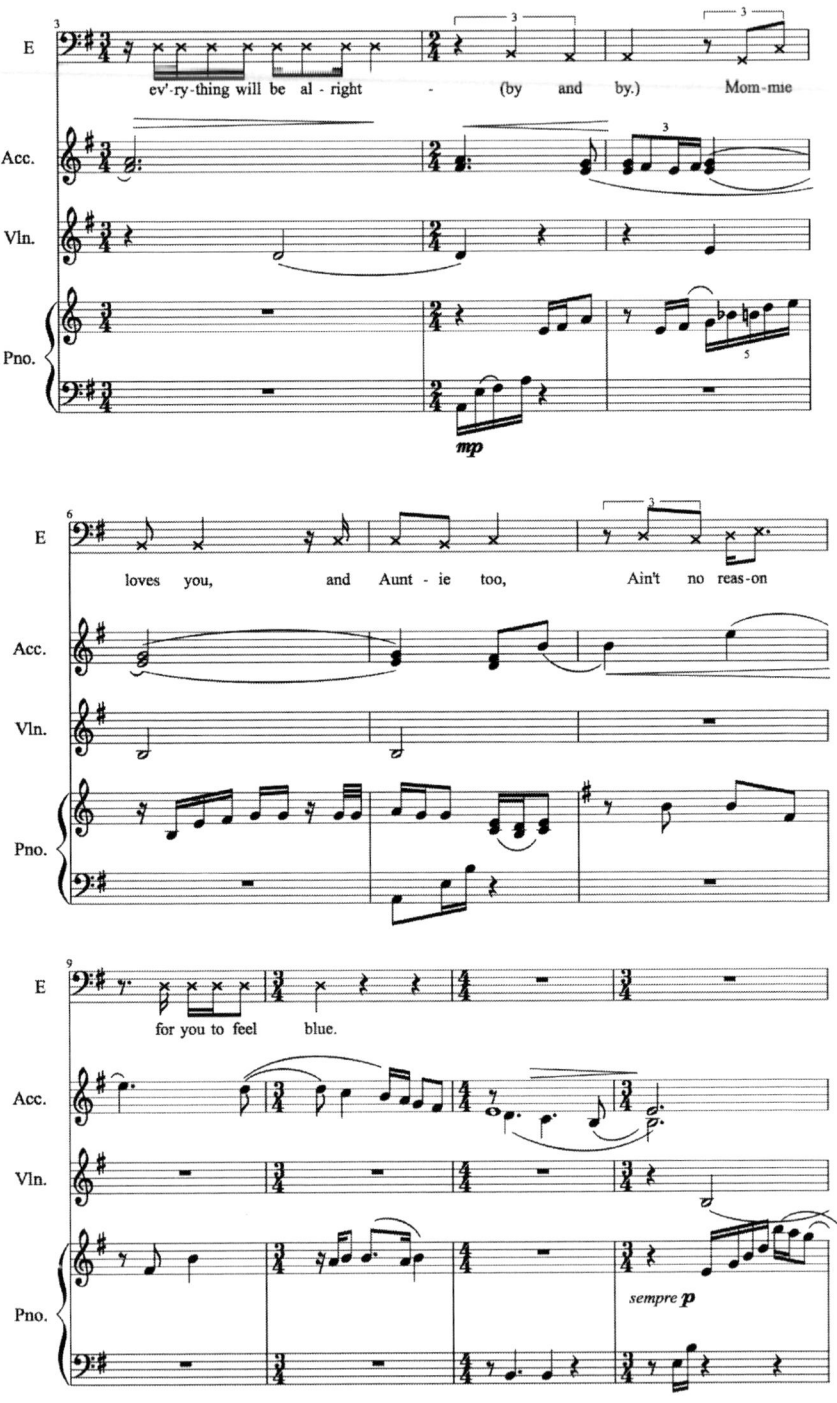

Analytical Music Therapy in Pain from Medical Trauma

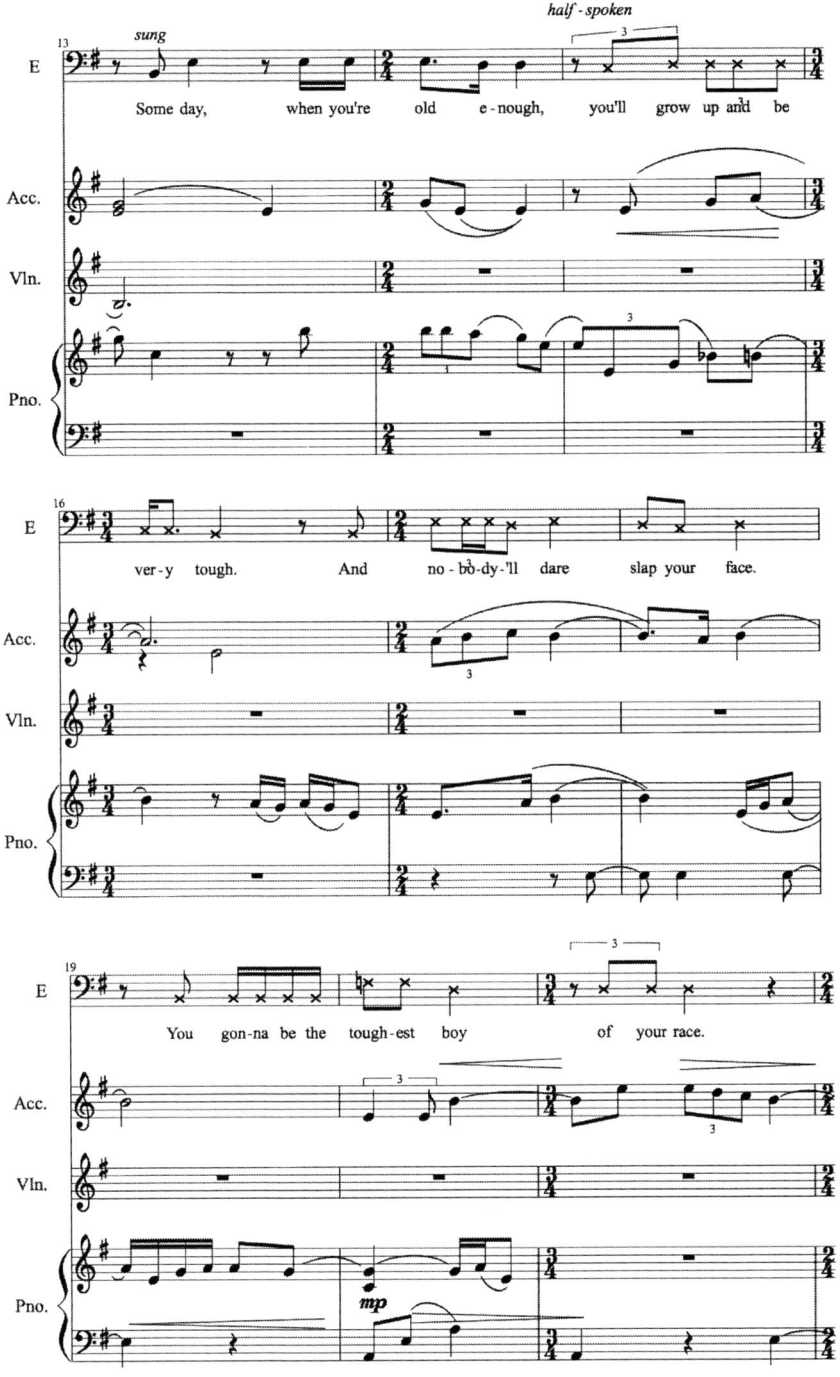

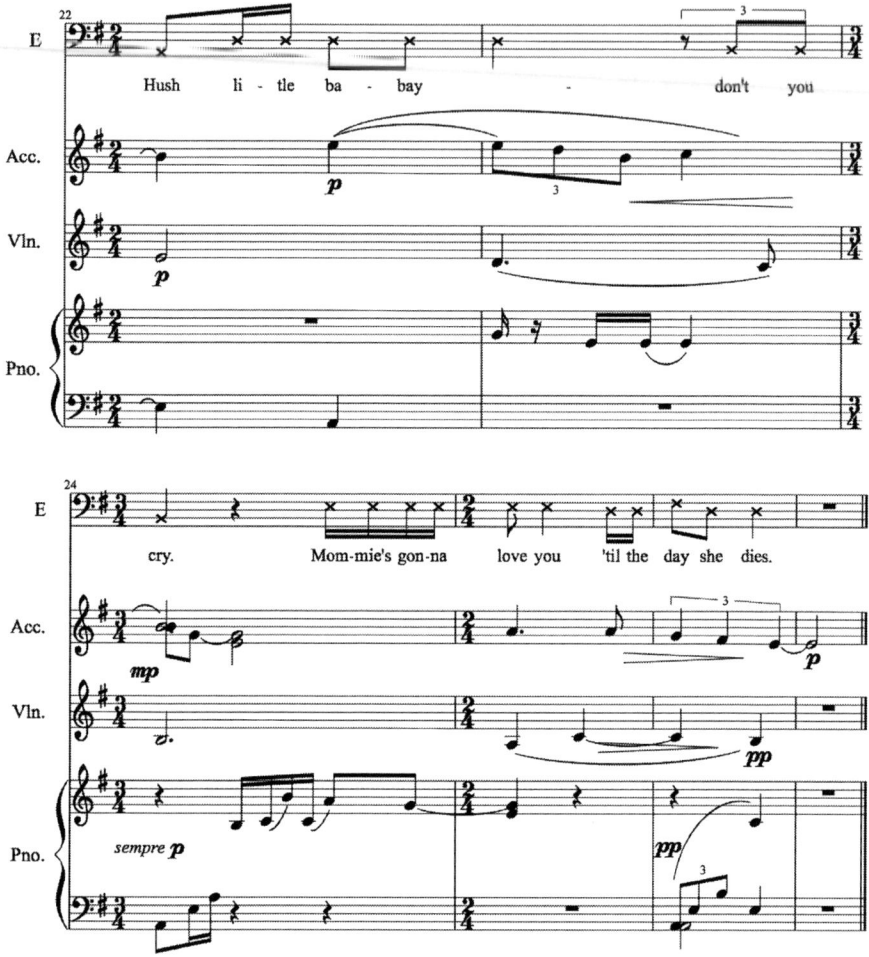

This love and support created through our singing has shown to have a positive influence on coronary artery disease. According to Dr. Guarneri[18]:

> In one study of 149 men and women with angina who were questioned before catheterization about whether they felt loved and supported, those with the greatest perception of love and support displayed the smallest amount of coronary artery disease.(p98)

Moreover, in music therapy research improvised song lullabies have been documented to be very helpful in relation to pain management and stress management with music psychotherapeutic work with premature babies.[21]

Overall, my experience with E. relates to Dr. Guarneri's experience with her patients. She states[18]:

> But I'd changed—my patients had changed me. They had shown me the importance of the heart's biography. They had taught me that coronary disease is physical, spiritual, and emotional. And that there could be a bridge between the conventional world of modern medicine and the type of healing known as alternative medicine."(p85) Yet as the seat of our deepest feelings, the heart is, as we know, all too sensitive, registering through pains, pangs, flutters, and skips the thousand varieties of sufferings that Buddhists claim humans experience—from anger, jealousy, and fear to terror, shame, and, all to often, sadness. (p 85)

Conclusion

The person that suffers from medical trauma can present many challenges for staff and family involved in their care. Not only has the person lost physical function – the person is also suffering emotionally as a secondary result of the medical trauma. Analytical Music Therapy used as a music psychotherapeutic intervention in pain management with persons with medical trauma can provide an integrative entry point into the brain damaged by trauma. The music therapist addresses through improvised music the physical, neural, emotional, cognitive, and spiritual "Pain-Self" to achieve a variety of goals:

- Self-directed neuroplasticity: a global firing of neuronal connections in the cortical and subcortical areas of the brain
- Reconnection to conscious use of breathing to elicit relaxation, ability to self soothe and connecting to deep emotions
- Reconnection to bodily, emotional, cognitive and spiritual flow
- Reconnection to resources and identity before trauma
- Internalization of healthy inner parent
- Reconnection to ability to play, improvise, creativity, "inner child"

This chapter presented clinically derived evidence supporting person centered clinical pain management strategies for persons with medical trauma. As quantitative and qualitative research is needed to further present evidence I am currently developing a research model based upon data being gathered from a mobile brain scanner that can reflect images of the neural connections before and after the patient has received Analytical Music Therapy treatment.

The neural networks you build and continue to reinforce will become the automatic reaction you have and will eventually help to become who you are. Knowing you are a work in progress is the power of the awakened brain. You are the Music! Let me finish with a quote that is important to remember in our work:

> *"Creative work does not usually follow a linear order but builds and destroys itself to find new meaning."*[22]

References

1. International Dictionary of Psychoanalysis online. Psychoanalysis, Pain. Available at: http://www.gale.cengage.com/servlet/ItemDetailServlet?region=9&imprint=000&titleCode=SB33&type=4&id=198545 Accessed July 16, 2012.
2. Anatomy of Pain. Available at: http://jubilation.uwaterloo.ca/~ranney/painanat.html. Accessed July 16, 2012.
3. Wikipedia. Psychological Pain. Available at: http://en.wikipedia.org/wiki/Psychological_pain. Accessed July 16, 2012.
4. Anandarajah G, Hight E. Spirituality and Medical Pratice: Using the HOPE Questions as a Practical Tool for Spiritual Assessment. *American Family Physician*. 2001; 63:81-89.
5. Wikipedia. Psychogenic Pain. Available at: http://en.wikipedia.org/wiki/Psychogenic_pain.Accessed July 16, 2012.
6. Pain is in the brain! YouTube website. http://www.youtube.com/watch?v=n8y04SrkEZU&feature=youtube_gdata_player. Accessed July 18, 2012.
7. Hanson R, Mendius R. *Buddha's Brain: The Practical Neuroscience of Happiness, Love and Wisdom*. Oakland, CA: New Harbinger Publications, Inc; 2009.
8. Berkowitz AL, Ansari D. Generation of novel motor sequences: The neural correlates of musical improvisation. *NeuroImage*.2008;41:535-543. http://www.numericalcognition.org/wpcontent/uploads/2010/08/Berkowitz-Ansari_NeuroImage2008.pdf. Accessed August 29, 2012.
9. Berkowitz AL. Generation of Novel Motor Sequences: The Neural Correlates of Musical Improvisation. Lecture presented

10. at: The 4th Annual Music and the Brain Conference at Stanford University; April 2009; Palo Alto, CA.
10. Becker M. Rewiring the Brain to Ease Pain. *The Wall Street Journal.* November 5, 2011. Available at: http://online.wsj.com/article/SB10001424052970204323904577 038041207168300.html. Accessed July 17, 2012.
11. Hanson R. Buddha's Brain: The Practical Neuroscience of Happiness, Love & Wisdom. PowerPoint presented at: PESI Seminars; April 2012; New York, NY.
12. Tomaino CA. *Awakening the Brain.* New York, NY: Atria Books; 2012.
13. Llosa PD. The Neurobiology of "We". *Parabola Magazine.* 2011. 68-75. Available at: http://drdansiegel.com/uploads/The%20Neurobiology%20of%2 0We%20-%20Patty%20de%20Llosa.pdf. Accessed July 28, 2012.
14. Loewy J, Scheiby B. Developing the culture of music psychotherapy in the medical setting. Paper presented at: the Evening Lecture Series at New York University/Nordoff-Robbins Center for Music Therapy; May 2001; New York, NY.
15. Priestley M. *Music therapy in action.* St Louis, MO: MMB Music; 1975.
16. Priestley M. *Analytical Music Therapy.* Phoenixville, PA: Barcelona Publishers; 1994.
17. Parker-Pope T. Post-Traumatic Stress Rises After Heart Attacks. *The New York Times.* June 21, 2012.
18. Guarneri M. *The Heart Speaks: A Cardiologist Reveals the Secret Language of Healing.* New York, NY: Touchstone of Simon & Schuster, Inc.; 2006.
19. Stewart K. Music therapy, the preterm infant, and the spectrum of traumatic experience. *Music Therapy & Trauma.* New York, NY: Satchnotes Press; 2010.
20. Robbins A. Playing along the porous edge of chaos and discipline: Pathways to the creative analytic process. *Psychoanalytic Inquiry.* 2012:32:225-245.

Music and Medicine: Integrative Models in the Treatment of Pain

CHAPTER 11

Backed into a Corner:
The Use of Guided Imagery and Music in the Care of a Woman with Chronic Pain

Nancy A. Jackson PhD, MT-BC

*"Although the world is full of suffering,
it is full also of the overcoming of it."*
Helen Keller

Introduction

In a 2011 report, the Committee on Advancing Pain Research, Care and Education of the Institute of Medicine indicated that chronic pain affects at least 116 million people in the U.S. with an estimated cost of more than $600 billion dollars each year.[1] One might expect that modern medicine would have developed an effective means of assessment and treatment for an experience that has always been part of the human experience, but it has not. This is largely due to the multidimensional nature of pain, which is a highly complex and individual experience. Bendelow[2] indicates that the experience of pain is both biological and cultural, involving emotional, psychological, social, political and existential aspects. It stands to reason then, that an effective approach to treating pain must move beyond simply responding to the immediate physical/physiological injury or illness, and encompass interventions which recognize the impact of pain on the whole human being.

Studies have shown that psychological difficulties are often comorbid with chronic pain. Tunks, Crook and Weir[3] did a review of published studies and concluded that chronic pain leads to the onset of depression and that depression increases the onset of chronic pain complaints. They note that psychosocial stressors have a direct impact on chronic pain, and must be considered in the prognosis. In exploring the relationship between chronic pain, depression and anxiety, Cui, et al.[4] found that anxiety was even more strongly related to reports of chronic pain than was depression, and that fatigue was an additional mediating factor. Medical interventions often prove to be ineffective for chronic pain sufferers, and these cumulative failures over time along with the impact of pain upon employment and social functioning can lead to a dangerous downward spiral.[5] It is no wonder that those with chronic pain have a lower quality of life than those with other types of medical conditions.[6,7]

As more and more healthcare professionals and researchers ask questions about the nature of pain and its treatment, some interesting ways of conceptualizing chronic pain have been developed. Steihaug and Materud[8] studied group-based pain treatment, and concluded that awareness and understanding of the self is a crucial factor in successful pain treatment. They include bodily, mental, and social processes as the integral parts of a wholistic healing process. Furthermore, they stress that the healthcare provider must be able to perceive more than merely somatic complaints if they are to be successful at assisting those who suffer from chronic pain. Likewise, Smith and Osborn[5] describe chronic pain as an "assault" on the self, noting the impact that pain has on an individual's sense of identity and self-esteem.

Bullington, Nordemar, Nordemar, and Sjöström-Flanagan[9] conceptualize successful treatment of chronic pain as a movement from chaos to a new sense of order and meaning. They discuss the chronic pain patient as an individual with somatic symptoms within the context of a disrupted life experience. Of particular importance in the healing process is the reformation of the person's basic sense of identity and the acceptance of self-responsibility. As the physical pain causes rigidity and decreased movement, it often mirrors rigidity in patterns of thinking, behaving, and feeling that develop in order to protect the individual from cut-off or repressed experiences. Facilitating the flexibility and loosened rigidity of thought, feeling, and behavior through therapy can reintegrate what has been separated or cut-off, allowing an internal reordering that will alleviate the chaos and open the person to new possibilities. This results in a reconnection with one's sense of identity despite the pain, and stimulates renewed interaction with the world.

The use of music in the treatment of chronic pain is an effective way to affect an internal re-ordering and a shift in the perception of pain.[9,10] A recent review of the music and pain literature by Kwan[11] revealed a majority of studies that focused on music used as a form of distraction or as procedural support, similar to an earlier review by Maslar.[12] This included interventions such as music listening, singing and toning, and music-assisted relaxation used largely for treatment of acute pain. A handful of studies have looked specifically at music for non-malignant chronic pain[10,13-16] but they, too, focus mainly on distraction and relaxation training. Three case studies presented by Rider[17] relate the successful use of improvised music to stimulate imagery leading to chronic pain relief. This approach used the concept of entrainment, matching the improvised music to the internal experience of the patient to initiate movement away from pain and stimulate healing. The case presented herein utilized music-evoked imagery to explore a woman's pain and its relationship with thoughts, feelings and behavior patterns to bring about an expression and resolution of buried memories and feelings and an increased sense of empowerment to affect personal change, resulting in an effective shifting of pain perception.

Clinical Work

Background
Colleen (a pseudonym) was a 70 year old woman who had recently had back surgery and was suffering from unresolved, chronic pain. She was divorced and lived alone in her own home with her dear companion, a dog named Paddy. Colleen had been working as a math instructor at the community college, though she expressed strong concern about her ability to continue on with this occupation given her inability to stand for any length of time due to her back pain. She also reported that she was no longer able to do most things that she had previously enjoyed, such as working in her garden or going for walks with Paddy. Her social interactions had greatly decreased because of the pain she experienced while driving, and she seldom attended church or went out with friends as she had in the past. Most troublesome for her, however, was the cognitive impact of the many medications she had been prescribed for pain and depression; indeed, she was taking a cocktail of narcotic pain medication, muscle relaxants, anxiolytics, and antidepressants that was shocking. Colleen was distressed by her inability to do simple tasks such as balancing her check book, and she talked about the "fog" that kept her from being able to accomplish much more than waking mid-day and taking care of only the most basic daily activities.

Colleen was referred to music therapy by one of her physicians with a wholistic orientation (not involved in her pain treatment) who wondered if some form of complimentary treatment might help ease her depression. While Colleen agreed that she was depressed, her perspective on the problem was that the source of difficulty was the chronic pain and how poorly it was being managed. She had repeatedly asked the physicians treating her for her back problems if the medications could be decreased or changed since she was not getting relief. Their response had been to add more, which decreased her cognitive functioning further. Additionally, her complaints about her continued pain and her reluctance to continue taking so many medications led those physicians to begin treating her as a refractory case, a "non-compliant patient."

Music and Medicine: Integrative Models in the Treatment of Pain

During my initial assessment of Colleen, I quickly came to agree with her – that her real problem was very poorly managed, debilitating chronic back and leg pain. I also quickly became aware that Colleen had been, until the onset of her back problems, a highly competent professional woman with a sharp intellect, a keen wit, and a very active lifestyle. But at this time, she was hopeless and wondering why she should want to continue living. I found her to be willing to try anything reasonable that might have an impact on her current state, and she agreed to a trial of four music therapy sessions to determine if this approach might be helpful to her. We identified her goals for treatment as 1) decreasing her perception of her chronic pain, 2) decreasing use of narcotic pain medication and antidepressants, and 3) reconnecting with a sense of meaning and purpose in daily life.

Colleen and I worked together in music therapy for approximately 2 ½ years with sessions scheduled about every four weeks, but more frequently when the pain was at its worst. We engaged in a variety of music experiences including improvisation, music-based relaxation, songwriting, as well as developing recorded compilations of music for inducing and supporting relaxation and sleep. As we worked together, I noticed that she often used descriptive, metaphoric language when she talked about her experience of pain. I also discovered that she had a strong relationship with music, having played clarinet in band through her school years, singing with the Sweet Adelines for many years, and most recently playing in the bell choir at church. For these reasons, the Bonny Method of Guided Imagery and Music seemed to be a good choice of approach for helping Colleen to explore her pain and depression. We had just begun using this approach several sessions prior to the start of this study. The case study described here represents Colleen's work in 10 sessions that occurred over 13 months, beginning about 6 months into her music therapy treatment. Colleen generously gave permission for the use of her session records during this time for analysis and for presentation and publication of the case.

The Treatment Approach
The Bonny Method of Guided Imagery and Music (BMGIM) is a music-centered therapy approach which utilizes specifically programmed music from the masterworks to evoke spontaneous imagery reflecting inner experiences, in order to bring about healing and wholeness. The music initiates movement in the psyche of the individual, which in turn creates opportunity for change and transformation.[18] In a BMGIM session, the therapist (referred to as the "guide") carefully selects a music program that reflects the issues that are the focus of treatment and the patient's physical

and emotional state, helps the patient to enter into a deeply relaxed state, and encourages and supports, in a non-directive, non-suggestive manner, the patient's engagement with the imagery that is evoked by the music. In this approach, the music itself is considered to be the primary "therapist" (and the human therapist, the co-therapist) because of its transformational qualities. After the music and imagery have ended, the therapist assists the client in processing and interpreting the content of the imagery experience.[19]

Those with chronic pain often have imagery that reflects the impact of the pain on the various aspects of their daily lives. Short[20] refers to this as an imagery conglomerate, which usually includes images reflecting physical, emotional, psychological, social and spiritual content. Understanding and integrating the information from these types of images can help the client to internally organize and realign a sense of self and to derive personal meaning.

Backed into a Corner
Colleen was quite guarded about self-disclosure which translated into a lot of avoidant imagery in her early sessions, including images of floating and fog, and having difficulty with describing what she was experiencing. Trust was hard won with Colleen, and as the guide, I felt that I needed to respect her decision about when she was ready to fully engage. This strategy seemed to pay off in a session in which she had spent a good deal of time floating around an area of darkness that she had encountered. She decided that it was "easier" to simply leave the dark alone, but acknowledged that it would continue to be there if she avoided it. I asked where she would go if she was not going to deal with the darkness and in her imagery she found herself in a corner. She described the corner as safe "at least on three sides" (right, left and floor), but then realized that she didn't feel very good about herself for being in the corner and not being willing to leave it.

We continued to explore the corner for a couple of sessions, and Colleen began to describe it as a place in which there was a lot of shame and helplessness. She knew that she chose to be in the corner, and said that it was as a safe place as she could be in given her helplessness. She stated, "At least when you're in the corner you've already been bad. So, now they just leave you alone." During this time, Colleen was using words like "relentless" and "punishing" to describe her physical pain, complaining about how it made her completely useless. Also, when we discussed the content of her imagery, she was beginning to draw parallels between being in the corner and situations in her daily life. In particular she talked about how certain people in her life "backed her into" doing things with or for them. These instances felt subtly abusive to her and brought up feelings of shame and anger. The corner in her imagery was a familiar place, indeed!

Colleen and I talked about her unwillingness to leave the corner, and how this might indicate that there was something that she needed to get from the corner. I felt strongly that she needed to fully acknowledge and own what the corner was for her, and the acquiescence that it seemed to represent in her daily life. She had a "broken backbone." I encouraged her to sit in the corner in her imagery to fully experience and understand it.

Sitting in the Corner
As Colleen continued to explore the corner in her imagery, she began to use words like "stuck," "frozen," and "all-encompassing" to describe her physical pain. She was not fully engaging in her imagery to the extent that I had hoped, and seemed to be as stuck in her progress as she was in her pain. If she was going to be stuck, I wanted her to really experience the feeling and not allow her to sit in one place simply to avoid the issues. At this time I made the decision to move away from the traditional BMGIM programs and to develop a specific program for Colleen's situation. In particular, I wanted to intensify the "stuckness" to the point at which Colleen would have to do something, to change something. I could not make her do this. She needed to make the decision to do something on her own so that she would be empowered to continue to move forward. The music would have to provide the impetus.

I designed a program for Colleen that seemed to reflect her experience of being frozen. It began with a "sinking into the depths" with Bach's *Passacaglia and Fugue in c minor*, a heavy and highly psychodynamic piece that encourages the listener to move inward and which tends to create a bridge to the fringes of the unconscious mind. For Colleen, the movement in this piece moved her focus inward and away from the "noise" of everyday life that typically helped her to ignore her internal experience. Bach's *Komm, süsser Tod* followed with its slow pulse and safe structure, creating a feeling of being "settled" at the bottom of a descent. This piece was important for Colleen to feel safe enough to connect with the feelings and emotions that lived deep inside and to allow those feelings to become a part of the experience in that moment. Then the lengthy, sustained Andante from Goreczki's *3rd Symphony* created the feeling of a barren frozenness. The sustained tones, which at times are held for 10 or 15 seconds without change, have a way of making the listener feel immobilized. The lone woman's voice that floats through the middle of the Andante simultaneously highlights the stark barrenness that the sound creates and conveys a sense of waxing and waning hope and a feeling of longing. This piece truly was a sonic embodiment of the words that Colleen had been using to describe her experience of pain. It produces a strong shift in the perception of time in the listener, an important musical aspect that held Colleen in an active experience of her stuckness so that her own discomfort provided the energy to mobilize and move beyond it. Tchesnekov's *Salvation Is Created* followed as a suggestion of reawakening, encouraging the need to move forward that was built up during the Goreczki. And finally, Vivaldi's *Et in Terra Pax* and Fauré's *In Paradisum* lift and break through into the light. The upward movement of these two pieces propelled Colleen forward so that the momentum begun in the Tchesnekov could come to full resolution in a new experience of hope. Here was the reward for having survived the dark and the pain. This program was used for four successive sessions, re-creating the sense of stuckness not just within each imagery session, but also across sessions over time.

    In these sessions, Colleen struggled with questions about safety and vulnerability. Certainly staying in the corner protected her from vulnerability, but at what cost? She also was increasingly aware of the disappointment she felt in herself for choosing to stay in the corner. In homework between sessions, Colleen began writing about past difficulties in her life. She shared information about her marriage, which was emotionally abusive and debilitating. She began expressing rage towards her ex-husband (now deceased), and grief about the losses that his behavior created for her and her daughter. She also expressed strong anger towards a particular friend who she felt was constantly negative and abusive towards her in very subtle ways. At the same time, Colleen struggled with understanding her physical pain, and came to see that her pain had been with her so long that it had become a part of her. She said, "Every movement seems to make me vulnerable [to more pain]," and asked, "Am I struggling to keep it, or struggling to not have it?"

    Over this time, Colleen had decided on her own to discontinue some of her medications, and at this point had stopped using narcotics and muscle relaxants most of the time and was using only one anxiolytic and two antidepressants. She reported that since the medications were not working anyway, her pain was largely the same as it was before. Her cognitive functioning had improved greatly, however, and this was a great relief to her. I was concerned about her stability as she discontinued anxiolytic and antidepressant medication on her own, but I also understood her frustration with her physicians' unwillingness to work with her to decrease her medications. I developed a safety plan with her because of my concern; secretly, I was pleased that her "backbone" seemed to be healing.

Emerging from the Corner
And finally the change happened. In the second to last session of this series, Colleen had been experiencing tension and frustration in her imagery, and had been moving around in her chair as though she were physically quite uncomfortable. As the Goreczki ended and the Tchesnekov began in the music program, the following exchange occurred between me and Colleen in response to her imagery:

> Me: What do you need right now?
> Colleen: (quiet for a long while, and then laughs) Not going!
> Me: Not going?
> Colleen: Not going. I don't know where they are going, but there are little feet running the other way.
> Me: Whose feet?
> Colleen: Mine.
> Me: Uh-huh! (both of us are silent for some time)
> Colleen: Not running away from myself... as much as running away from what I perceive people want me to do. (silence) Maybe that's what's in the darkness. Anxiety... or expectations. Maybe it's both.

Colleen had emerged from the corner despite the darkness, and was not willing to return. She was now ready to face what the darkness held. In session that followed, Colleen explored the expectations that she and others placed upon her, and questioned which of these were fair and reasonable and which were not. Her imagery contained many forms of taking in light and leaving darkness behind.

The cause of Colleen's back and leg pain had not been resolved. The physician who did her back surgery finally admitted that the surgery had been a failure, and indicated that one of the screws had shifted and was impinging upon a nerve. While she continued to have a high level of pain every day at this point, Colleen was using only an anti-inflammatory medication and one antidepressant. She had discontinued all other medication related to her back and leg pain. She also had begun doing some of the things that she was unable to do previously, like taking walks with Paddy and planting flowers around her house and in her garden. She was consistently using the recorded compilations and relaxation exercises I had developed for her to help herself get to sleep each night. She returned to teaching, carrying a 12 credit hour load.

The Use of GIM in the Care of a Woman with Chronic Pain

Perhaps most remarkable was the empowerment that Colleen began to demonstrate. She "fired" the physicians she had been seeing – two medical doctors and a psychiatrist – and was interviewing new physicians to take over her case. She broke off the relationship with the friend who she realized was abusive and demoralizing, and she began getting involved in new activities at which she was developing new friendships. In a session several months later, she very proudly announced that she was saying "No," to all kinds of things, and she was beaming when she told me this. Clearly, Colleen's backbone had healed, even if her back never would, and this had made all the difference in her daily life and in her perception of her chronic pain.

Conclusion

Colleen was able to access repressed feelings and memories through her music-evoked imagery, and to recognize behavioral patterns that had been hindering her in daily life. The parallels between the content of her imagery and the language with which she described her chronic pain were startling to her when I pointed them out during a session in which we were evaluating her progress in therapy. These parallels demonstrate the powerful nature of internal experience and the impact that it can have on a person's perception of pain. For Colleen, feeling shamed and punished in her relationships with others intensified her perception of her pain as "punishing" and something that made her useless. Feeling stuck in her ability to get past anger and old resentments intensified the perception of being physically stuck in pain, and so on. Working through these feelings and behavior patterns while they were embedded in imagery made them less threatening and overwhelming to Colleen so that she was able to feel competent in creating change for herself, and in integrating and reordering "painful" experiences to make new meaning. The result was not just a shifting of Colleen's perception of pain, but also a demonstrated change in her daily functioning. This is the reconnection with personal identity despite the pain described by Bullington, Nordemar, Nordemar, and Sjöström-Flanagan.[9]

The owning and expressing of anger was an important aspect of Colleen's process. These were feelings that she had repressed, presumably, to keep herself strong enough to get her through difficult situations in her past. It is a reasonable guess that carrying these unresolved emotions played a significant role in "breaking her backbone." As she began to reconnect with these feelings and to grieve over the situations from which they arose, she was also freeing the energy that it took to hold the emotions down so that it could be used in the present to move forward from her stuck place. Owning and working through this type of emotion is a necessity for successfully moving beyond a stuck place mired in emotions of the past.[21] At the beginning of one session, Colleen entered the treatment room, threw a crumpled piece of paper into my lap, and with a scowl on her face said in a belligerent tone of voice, "Here!" On the paper I found expressions of rage replete with expletives scribbled on both sides. I could only imagine the amount of energy it must have taken every day in order to hold such strong emotion at bay.

The therapeutic relationship between me and Colleen was also an important part of her process. Because of her distrust and unwillingness to fully disclose information, I realized that I needed to prove to Colleen not only my trustworthiness, but also my acceptance of who she was and where she was in her process. The therapist's openness to the patient as an individual within a personal context has been noted to be an integral part of a good clinical encounter for pain patients.[9] Colleen responded to this approach more quickly than I expected at the beginning of her therapy with me. On several occasions she recounted incidents from her past to me, stating that she had never told anyone these things. Remaining nonjudgmental and demonstrating that I was capable of withstanding and containing her rage and grief allowed Colleen to feel less fearful of moving into a more vulnerable and open experience of her own life. She was not alone, and she had support.

Ultimately, it was the music that had the most impact on the change that Colleen made happen for herself. The ability of music to connect to emotions and memories from the past and to allow a reworking of the information in order to produce a new experience[22] was at the root of the internal transformation that occurred for Colleen. Only the music could be powerful and persuasive enough to encourage her to sit in and work through such difficult, painful emotion. Only the music could be gentle enough to give her a shove that would mobilize her to move forward. And because the music brought about these things internally for Colleen, it was of her own volition that she reorganized herself and moved forward, not because someone else "made" her or applied an external answer. To look inside and find her own answer was a demonstration that Colleen could find her own sense of wholeness; she could heal her own "backbone".

At the time of this writing, Colleen continues to work as an instructor, carrying 12 credit hours each semester. Most of her hours in the classroom are spent on her feet, walking from student to student. She drives a long distance across the country once or twice a year to visit her daughter. She has created new relationships with people and interacts socially with them on a regular basis. She continues to struggle with ways to decrease her physical pain, but continues to utilize the music recordings for relaxation and assistance with sleep each night. She also utilizes physical therapy and acupuncture to help her maintain her active lifestyle. She has not returned to the use of the medications that she discontinued. If you were to ask her, she would tell you that, "There's just got to be an answer for all this pain," but then she will also tell you that life is "pretty good." And then she will smile.

References

1. Committee on Advancing Pain Research, Care, and Education. *Relieving Pain in America: A Blueprint for Transforming Prevention, Care, Education, and Research.* Washington, D.C.: The National Academies Press; 2011.
2. Bendelow G. *Pain and Gender.* Prentice Hall, London: Prentice Hall; 2000.
3. Tunks ER, Crook J, and Weir R. Epidemiology of chronic pain with psychological comorbidity: prevalence, risk, course, and prognosis. *Canadian Journal of Psychiatry.* 2008; 53:224-234.
4. Cui J, Matsushina E, Aso K, Masuda A, and Makita K. Psychological features and coping styles in patients with chronic pain. *Psychiatry and Clinical Neurosciences.* 2009; 63:147-152.
5. Smith JA and Osborn M. Pain as an assault on the self: an interpretative phenomenological analysis of the psychological impact of chronic benign low back pain. *Psychology and Health.* 2007; 22:517-534.
6. Mitchell LA, MacDonald RAR, Knussen C, and Serpell MG. A survey investigation of the effects of music listening on chronic pain. *Psychology of Music.* 2007; 35:37-57.
7. Silvemark AJ, Källmén H, Portala K, and Molander C. Life satisfaction in patient with long-term non-malignant pain – relation to demographic factors and pain intensity. *Disability and Rehabilitation.* 2008; 30:1929-1937.
8. Steihaug S and Malterud K. Stories about bodies: a narrative on self-understanding and pain. *Scandinavian Journal of Primary Health Care.* 2008; 26:188-192.
9. Bullington J, Nordemar R, Nordemar K and Sjöström-Flanagan C. Meaning out of chaos: a way to understand chronic pain. *Scandinavian Journal of Caring Sciences.* 2003; 17:325-331.
10. Schorr JA. Music and pattern change in chronic pain. *Advances in Nursing Science.* 1993; 15:27-36.

11. Kwan M. Music therapists' experiences with adults in pain: implications for clinical practice. In Hadley, S. ed., *Qualitative Inquiries in Music Therapy, Vol. 5*. Gilsum, NH: Barcelona; 2010:43-85.
12. Maslar PM. The effect of music on the reduction of pain: a review of the literature. *Arts in Psychotherapy*. 1986; 13:215-219.
13. McCaffrey R Using music to interrupt the cycle of chronic pain. *Journal of Pain Management*. 2008; 1:215-221.
14. Kenny DT and Faunce G. The impact of group singing on mood, coping, and perceived pain in chronic pain patients attending multidisciplinary pain clinic. *Journal of Music Therapy*. 2004; 41:241-258.
15. McCaffrey R and Freeman E. Effect of music on chronic osteoarthritis pain in older people. *Journal of Advanced Nursing*. 2003; 44:517-524.
16. Colwell CM. Music as distraction and relaxation to reduce chronic pain and narcotic ingestion: a case. *Music Therapy Perspectives*. 1997; 15:24-31.
17. Rider MS. Treating chronic disease and pain with music-mediated imagery. *Arts in Psychotherapy*. 1987; 12:113-120.
18. Clark M. Evolution of the Bonny method of guided imagery and music (BMGIM). In: Bruscia KE, Groke DE, eds. *Guided Imagery and Music: The Bonny Method and Beyond*. Gilsum, NH:Barcelona, 2002:5-28.
19. Ventre M. The individual form og the Bonny method of guided imagery and music (BMGIM). In: Bruscia KE, Groke DE, eds. *Guided Imagery and Music: The Bonny Method and Beyond*. Gilsum, NH:Barcelona, 2002:30-35.
20. Short A. Guided imagery and music (GIM) in medical care. In: Bruscia KE, Groke DE, eds. *Guided Imagery and Music: The Bonny Method and Beyond*. Gilsum, NH:Barcelona, 2002:151-170.
21. Jackson NA. Models of response to client anger in music therapy. *Arts in Psychotherapy*. 2010; 37:46-55.
22. Bonny H, Savary L. *Music and your mind*. NY: Collins Associates;1973.

CHAPTER 12

The Listening Room

Trisha Ready PhD

To Music
Music. The breathing of statues. Perhaps:
The quiet of images. You, language where
languages end. You, time
standing straight from the direction
of transpiring hearts.
Rainer Maria Rilke

Introduction

"Can you download 'Spirit in the Sky'?"[1] Andrew asked. He considered it "appropriate" to share with other patients at the acute psychiatric hospital. The song, written in 1969 by Norman Greenbaum,[1] includes the lines: "When I die and they lay me to rest, gonna go to the place that's the best."

The appropriateness of the song was dubious given Andrew's serious suicide attempt with pills one week prior to his hospital admission. Several other patients on the unit had made equally serious attempts.

"I wonder what the song means to you?" I asked.

Andrew replied, "It just keeps going through my mind."

Andrew arrived at the hospital, locked inside a tenacious state of despair. He had foreclosed on the possibility of a future. Looking ahead would have required inventing another life: one that began after his upcoming divorce from his wife of twenty years. In therapeutic groups, he stared out the window.

Fetching and listening to "Spirit in the Sky"[1] with Andrew was a slow process of therapeutic attunement. The song reminded him of hopeful times; it also referred to his urge to depart life. In the process of exploring the song, we discovered that "Spirit in the Sky"[1] was written in fifteen minutes by Norman Greenbaum, a young rock composer, who modeled the song on a traditional Christian hymn, inspired by watching country, gospel singer Porter Wagoner on television.

Fetching the song for Andrew, in terms of both finding the song as object, and exploring the song and its meanings (i.e., despair, suffering, hope, redemption), was akin to bridge building. Along the way, Andrew and I discussed his lethal urges, his withdrawal from life, and his youthful memories. After seven days of listening to and discussing other songs Andrew selected, I downloaded "Spirit in the Sky." In the process of slowly arriving at the song, Andrew's suicidal urges diminished, and his openness to connection increased by establishing a method for breaking down difficult emotions together.

Methods and Modalities

This chapter is an inquiry into how a patient's emotional pain might be briefly, incrementally lifted, and digested, by listening to preferred music with a professional. Thus, attuning to patient's preferred music and establishing a musical connection with a patient, facilitates and motivates rapport.

This work centers on music-based research at an acute psychiatric hospital focused on crisis stabilization and milieu therapy. Only brief slices of time are available for one-to-one therapeutic sessions. Patients' diagnoses range from schizophrenia and other psychoses, to mood disorders, personality disorders, co-occurring disorders and substance related issues. Besides hospital vignettes, this essay features the results of mixed method research, including examining one of eight case studies conducted with patients diagnosed with early stage psychosis. I met with each research participant for ten- 30-minute listening sessions based on participant selected music played on a portable IPod stereo system.

Each case study participant was given a Rorschach assessment at the beginning and end of the ten sessions. The Rorschach is a psychodynamic instrument that measures such indices as affect, containment, expression, and projections. Participants responses to the ten ink blot images were especially considered according to the following categories: control or delay of affect (pure F); appropriate use of form (X-%, XA%, WDA%); reality testing (FC:CF +C, X-%); affect modulation (Afr.); emotional distress (Sum Shading: FM +m); openness to new experiences (human content and movement: H, Hd, Hx, and M); and the capacity to respond to external sensory stimuli input (special scores: DV, DR, INCOM, FABCOM, ALOG, MORB).

This inquiry is predominantly based on attachment, neurobiological theorists, psychoanalytic theorists, and other empirically supported explorations of the calming and soothing effects of music and the music of the human voice. Panksepp and Trevarthen refer to the brain as an "organ of intersubjective collaboration with systems of emotional regulation that are fundamentally musical."[2] My hope is to illustrate that the same dynamics, which animate and compel emotional regulation and attunement in the mother-infant dyad are present and equally essential when working with adult patients in states of intense and ineffable emotional distress.

The Listening Room

Soundtracks

In establishing therapeutic rapport with patients, it was helpful to acknowledge patients' existing relationships to music. I have been inspired by the work of Joanne Loewy [3] who developed the technique of song sensitation to work elaboratively with patient's familiar music. Dileo and Parker [4,5] have used familiar songs in working with hospice patients. Overall, stronger effects seem to be achieved when participant selected music is used. [6,7] In general, there is a growing trend in music research to focus on participant selected pieces. [8-11] Listening to preferred music has been associated with positive change in affect with purgative, or cathartic effect for adolescent/young adults in distress. [12-14]

One challenge for clinicians using preferred music is that some songs, such as music by Eminem or Lil Wayne include disturbing content or provocative language. Michigan based Music Therapist Jennifer Wyatt [15] stressed the importance of limiting glamorous references to drugs, violence, cutting, suicide, sex, or other sex explicit lyrics, or songs with heavy religious or political content. She also advised limits on the use of love songs, and music that might cause emotional dysregulation. Wyatt preferred hopeful lyrics. [15]

I endeavored to download "clean" versions of songs; however, I first used music that patients found familiar and comforting, then gradually shifted with the patient from there. Particularly for patients with psychosis, musical choice is communication.

Tarrant, North and Hargreaves noted in 2000 --years before the advent of the mp3 player-- that young adults in the United Kingdom and the United States listened to from 2.5 to 4 hours of music each day. [16] We are what we listen to: living in an era where a personal mp3 player filled with one's own musical soundtrack is an accepted, culturally relevant container of self or identity. [17] Portable music devices reflect cultures and sub-cultures and are, thereby, self-defining. [18-21]

People of all ages in modern societies use music to regulate enhance and change qualities and levels of emotion. [22] Acute psychiatric patients walk through hospital hallways listening to music, albeit unconsciously, for emotional regulation, containment and expression.

Personal music players also serve as transformers of self. Music has the power to change our psychological space and to allow the listener to be– within the container of the musical piece– another kind of person than the everyday self. [22] Thus, music can also help construct (vs. express) a sense of identity. [22-24]

This is especially important for patients trying to reconstruct a sense of self after an experience of profound disorganization, complex grief, or traumatic crisis. Music can engage core brain mechanisms that regulate well-being in the body and guide the formation of self confident association and memories in affectionate relationships.[25-27]

Urge to Connect

Since music can foster human connection, how can we use music to inspire people suffering from severe mental health issues and isolation to reconnect with others? An abundance of research exists on positive physiological changes resulting from listening to music. That music promotes relaxation, and reduces stress can be gauged by heart rate, cardiac output, skin temperature, and glucose count.[28-33]

According to scholar and musician, Ellen Dissanayake[34] beginning 1.8 million years ago humans discovered that coping together through musical expression was better than being solitary. She noted that our primal urge to connect and attach in relationships is interwoven in the invention of music. Panksepp[35] suggested that the appeal of music for humans might relate to the activation of social emotional processes, some of which, like mother infant bonding are addictive. These addictive aspects of music may be beneficial to fostering a socially bonded life.

Sharing music may help cope with the chemistry of stress and uncertainty. Music helps mitigate release of cortisol, which might otherwise negatively impact immunity, mental performance, growth, tissue repair, and reproduction.[36-40] Music can induce the release and action of oxytocin, thus helping to re-enforce strong positive emotional memories, and supplant negative emotions.[41] Another positive impact of music, verified by pharmacological and brain imaging studies, relates to its affect on the brain dopamine system,[42,43] which integrates the search for appreciation and reward. Alcaro, Huber, & Panksepp[44] also noted changes in human's norepinehprine attention systems.

Communicative Musicality

In the psychiatric hospital music helps to allay the anxieties of patients who are often facing the unknown in terms of housing, jobs, benefits, relationships, or even next treatment steps. Caroline arrived at the hospital after having been diagnosed with stage 4 cancer and after having refused chemotherapy. Her paranoia and anger were understandable given the combination of schizophrenia and the internal siege of a terminal illness. Caroline initially attacked any linking with staff and peers. Her gestures illustrated how isolating grief and loss can be for a person experiencing the overarching sense of loss of control over environment and mind that accompany schizophrenia. Complex and dense emotions may become ineffable but patients with schizophrenia still have the urge and the longing to express them. Thus, the act of choosing and sharing familiar, emotional music with a therapeutic professional can be reparative: providing tangible opportunities for meaningful connection and reconciliation. After ten days, Caroline began participating in music appreciation groups. Gradually, her participation increased to requesting songs and responding at the end of each song with weeping or nodding, followed by giving me boxes of breakfast cereal. "You look so hungry, honey," she would say. Caroline's offer of nourishment in exchange for nourishing music caused me to first wonder about listening to music as a bidirectional process requiring the embodied presence of both people listening together. Caroline's gestures echoed the back and forth dynamics of the infant/mother dyad.

According to Langer[45] the inner life has similar properties to music. There are similar patterns of motion and rest, tension and release, agreement and disagreement, as well as preparation, fulfillment, excitation, and sudden changes. Many people who arrive at the hospital have a lost connection to an inner life.

Trevarthen and Aiken[46] noted that infants are biologically prone to seek mutual coordination of dynamic mental states with their caregivers. Trevarthen[47] refers to the incremental and melodic rhythmic co-creativity between mother and child as "communicative musicality." According to Trevarthen,[47] there is a coordinated and often playful non-verbal, exchange of gestures: facial expression, coos, squawks and other musical sounds between baby and caregiver. The dynamics of communicative musicality are based on pulse, quality, and narrative. Pulse refers to the regular succession of discrete behavioral events (gestures and sounds) through time in the process of conversation.[48] Malloch and Trevarthen[49] noted that babies were born with a musical readiness that allowed them to respond to rhythmically presented facial and body movements.

Much like Trevarthen, Medical Psychologist, Beatrice Beebe[50] emphasized bi-directional communication and emotional regulation between mother and child. Beebe[50] noted young babies' profound sensitivity to the contingency and authenticity of a communication partner's rhythm of expression and to the sympathy of feelings expressed by gesture and tone of voice. This same bi-directional modality operates when a clinical therapist listens to music with an adult or teenager in distress or in emotional pain. The act of "listening with" includes an intersubjective dialogue.[51,52] We listen, and there is an "us" who listens; the existence of an "us" helps keep a sense of safety in the experience.

The connection between therapist and patient, like mother and infant, does not need to be perfect. Trust and safety are built upon moments of mis-attunement and repair. There can be differences in terms of taste, or a therapist can get a song meaning wrong. Repair is a flexible "interactive" process involving matching, mismatching, and re-matching.[51-53] Moving back and forth between similarity and difference constructs and fine-tunes rapport.[51,54,55] What is ideal for an infant are caregiver responses that assist self-regulation and facilitate down regulation of arousal.[51]

Here we circle back to applying these concepts to therapeutic settings. Music could help us learn with patients what qualities and rhythm of voice might be most essential in creating a "good enough fit" or listening rooms between patient and therapist? Music could fill the spaces where language has failed; it could allow access to what Beebe[51] termed "implicit and pre-linguistic forms of communicative competency and intersubjectivity."

The musical space of the listening room, relates to Winnicott's[56] potential space or that intermediate space between therapist and patient, which mirrors what once existed between mother and child. It is a play space between fantasy and reality.[56] Panksepp[57] referred to musical space as a place where therapist and patient could explore projective identifications and promote pro-social interactions. Hug and Lohne[58] name this same space the "Third Area."[59] Noting the importance of an auxiliary object in the room, such as therapist or an iPod to avoid intense direct focus on the patient.

Music of Therapy

Let's transition now toward the mechanics of what happens in the listening room. It's a place where the unconscious or our implicit memories have a safe frame in which to express themselves.[59,60] The power of bringing unconscious material into the therapeutic room has been explored by music therapists who use Guided Imagery.[61]

Wilhelm Reich[62,63] posited that the unconscious was expressed in physical gestures, postures, facial expressions, and somatic symptoms. He advocated that a therapist pay precise attention to the patient's body, and to the therapist's own body. Presence and attentiveness would allow a therapist to note the transference, or unconscious, archaic images the patient imposed on the therapist. Likewise, a therapist could also discern countertransference, or his own unconscious reactions to patients, and significant people in the patient's life, in addition to his own ideation and transference. McDougall[64] stated, "some people use actions and somatic symptoms as forms of communication. Music seems to have the potential to reach through to deeper layers of unconscious silence where language may be too complex or threatening.

Tustin offered guidance to therapists in saying, "The interpretation of primitive bodily states requires the capacity to enter into someone's else's physical states without losing one's head."[65] The question arises: How do we safely and therapeutically enter into physical states of patients in acute settings? The therapist's function may be to help digest, distressing emotions through words, symbols or actions. This could happen on two levels with self-selected music. First, the music could express a level of articulated emotion. Secondly, the therapist could attend to what is transferred through the patient's response to the music while noting her own embodied countertransference. Samuels[66] referred to embodied countertransference as the "physical, actual, material, sensual expression in the analyst of something in the patient's inner world. Possible therapist responses are falling asleep, anger, or fantasy responses such as the sensory rich image of a bird in flight. Attending to embodied countertransference is especially helpful with patients who have suffered preverbal trauma, which they cannot communicate verbally. Stone[67] described the therapist's body as a tuning fork to a patient's unconscious material.

One research participant danced facing hospital surveillance cameras in response to hip-hop music. She danced as if she were in a nightclub: talking loudly and engaging in disputes. Through her performances she revealed present tense feelings about hospital confinement, and memories of a traumatic past, in which she was watched and controlled.

Musical dialogue occurs constantly between patient and therapist. Knoblauch[68] noted "subtle state shifts—in tone, and patterned rhythms of speech, plus changes in breathing and awareness of subjectivity—which impact the therapeutic process. Knoblauch,[55,68] referred to these contours of therapy that emerge in dialogues (volume, tone, tempo, rhythm and turn taking) as the "musical edge." He advised attunement to all levels of communication—"intimate, primitive, poetic or musical edges"---for a "broader and richer range of meaning and affect" to construct and inhabit.[55]

Metabolizing Emotions

After establishing a theoretical basis for musical attunement, potential space and embodied countertransference, we turn toward particular challenges people experiencing psychosis face when sitting with a therapist. Likewise, the therapists are equally challenged to contain a psychotic patient's emotional states such as horror, despair, emptiness, aggression, deadness, or lack of contact with an emotional inner life.

For many people suffering with psychosis, no mechanism was established for breaking down experience into digestible pieces or for putting words around those experiences. Psychopathology in general may be caused by a serious developmental or environmental trauma particularly impactful to people highly sensitive to environmental stimuli.[69-72] Without sufficient caregiver mediation in breaking down experiences, sensations, and emotions, and digesting them through the help of imagination, fantasy, illusion, and symbolization, infants can become overwhelmed beyond their nervous system threshold capacity.[73-75]

Grotstein[76] noted that if a psychotic person synthesized words into thoughts he would be exposed to dreaded, preferably avoided, aspects of the self. Rather than letting sensory impressions or memories enter the mind, the person with psychosis attacks building blocks of thought. Thus, music with its already chosen lyrics can express anger, for example, which merely fantasizes about destroying the world such as in Lil Wayne's song, "Drop the World."[77]

The neurobiology of a defense against feeling might be experienced by, people with psychosis as increased right hemispheric activity.[78] Dominance of this hemisphere relates to a tendency for more primary process thinking[59] not subject to the rules of logic or oriented to reality (i.e., dreams, hallucinations), more intrusion of implicit, unconscious memories, and more intense unbounded emotions.[78] In psychosis there can also be a strong sense of isolation and lack of ability to feel safe and join with others.[79] It can be a terrifying and disorienting state. Music may be better suited than language to address unbounded implicit and unconscious memories until a therapist learns to meet and match the patient's music.

Wilfred Bion,[69,80] who worked extensively with psychotic patients, described the attunement and emotional regulation processes as a kind of metabolization, which he called the alpha function. Bion's alpha function described a mother converting raw sensations, impressions and emotions (known as beta) by receiving them as projections into her own mind and transforming them, by digesting these projections, into bearable small pieces.[69,80] The mother, breaking beta pieces down into semiotic elements such as language, helps a child experience containment and the ability to organize and think about his affective experience.[80-82] Bion saw the alpha function as being as essential to the therapeutic process as to the mother infant dyad.[69]

Researchers have observed that music has a relaxing and organizing effect on schizophrenic patients.[83,84] Music based interventions diminish negative symptoms and improve interpersonal contact for patients with psychosis which might facilitate reintegratation into the community.[85] Listening to preferred music with a facilitator may help persons with psychosis develop a safe container in a relational setting where language is broken down into the beta elements of rhythm and tone.

The Listening Room

One example of a shared metabolization process can be illustrated in listening to the live version of, "Folsom Prison Blues" by Johnny Cash,[86] a song popular among hospital patients I have encountered. Cash played at Folsom Prison to join with inmates[86]; he was enthusiastically received. Thus, patients can be contained simultaneously by the prosody of Cash's steady rhythms, while sitting with a therapist metabolizing the emotional experience of being locked-in and longing for freedom.[86]

Clinical Work

Within Silence
The case study that follows applies theories regarding attachment, embodiment, and the pro-social and soothing effects of music to the case of a young man in an early stage of psychosis. According to the stage model, the early stages of schizophrenia are more responsive to treatment.[87] Treating schizophrenia in its earliest stages with medication management, structured activity, family therapy and case management may have more positive future outcomes.[87]

Seneca, an 18-year old Caucasian male, was diagnosed with Schizophrenia, Paranoid type and Poly-substance Dependency. He had maternal relatives with schizophrenia and his father had been an addict. Seneca described what brought him to the hospital: "I have taken too many psychotic drugs and I don't have someone to love."

Seneca had been in the hospital twice previously. After each stay, he subsequently fell off medication compliance. Originally, Seneca had played guitar and composed songs, noting music helped distract from hallucinations.

Seneca was attracted to participating in the research study after listening to another participant singing karaoke. In his first session, Seneca stated his musical preferences: "I like rock, rap, most everything really. I know classic rock from my father, and my mother liked '90s music. I like what I like. What do you like?" In the first session, he switched from song to song eventually settling on Evanescence's, "Together Again."[88] "It's opera for you," he said.

Seneca seemed to connect through a process similar to communicative musicality. He communicated through physical expression, songs, and somatic symptoms. When listening to Death Cab For Cutie's[89] "I Will Follow You into the Dark," he averted his eyes; he rubbed his head, then rubbed his hands on the table. When the song finished, he said: "This one is like my soul." Seneca seemed to convey the fear of the cost of being uncontained and alive[90] as well as his devotion and longing for the ideal woman. He also expressed a longing to return to rave culture. Early raves were spontaneous parties held in warehouse and other spaces in urban areas. Raves were remarkable for their itinerant sense of community and connection.

In the second session, Seneca chose Lil Wayne's "Drop The World"[77] and three Alice in Chains songs. He also selected Daft Punk's rave theme "Around the World."[91] Seneca stared at the wall, throughout the session. In the next few sessions, Seneca avoided forming symbols, connecting, or articulating emotions.[69] The closer we would get to words, the stronger Seneca's somatic responses became. He literally itched with affects. This phenomenon seemed akin to Bion's[69,80] concept of evacuating unprocessed proto-emotions into muscular action as a feature of psychosis. Seneca's anger became more pronounced in "Cleaning Out My Closet."[92] left during Led Zeppelin, "Going To California,"[93] then returned. He was restless and anxious.

Session seven and eight focused on Beatles songs from the White Album including, "Mother Nature's Son".[94] He scrolled through other songs without making a selection. His Mother, who planned to testify in court the next morning for Seneca's further detainment, came to visit. She brought him clothes; he left her standing in the hallway. Seneca chose "Together Again"[88] "There's nowhere for me to go from here," he said. Next, he chose Tool's "The Grudge,"[95] and two Eminem songs. He asked if he could leave early because he felt sick, and didn't want to make me sick also, as if to stop the splitting and projection of destructive parts outward. The next day Seneca was notified of his upcoming transfer to the state hospital.

In the 9th session Seneca and I attuned. Seneca asked at the beginning of the session: "How are you today? You seem sad?" He selected five songs from Tool's, *Lateralus*[95-97] I dreaded listening to Tool; however, by the fourth song I could hear more subtle levels of emotion in the music. "Do you get it now?" Seneca asked; he had been otherwise intently staring at the table. Searles[98] wrote about "silence between persons" as "not necessarily a gulf, a void," but as something which "may be tangibly richer communion than any words could constitute." I was drawn through Seneca's music to a glimpse into his inner world.

Before the final session I searched the hallways for Seneca, then turned to find him standing beside me. Seneca chose, "Cleaning Out my Closet" [92] and an angry ranting song about a cheating girlfriend. Then he chose several Tool songs including "Schism"[97] "Do you still like Tool?" he asked. I nodded. For his last song: he chose Led Zeppelin's "Ramble On,"[99] which seemed appropriate for its double entendre and expression of longing for love.

The Listening Room

Seneca was like a vigilant and stealth feral cat. He drew close. Then pulled away. There was an ebb and flow to the angles of Seneca's intimacy. The link between us became thinner once the sessions were completed as he prepared for relocating to the state hospital. Bion's theory of Minus K came to mind in thinking about Seneca, reconstructing the world out of the emptiness he felt.[69,80,81]

With Seneca, the silences carried significant amounts of transference and countertransference. I had anxiety whenever I couldn't find Seneca, combined with vigilant caution about not abandoning him. On the other hand, it was difficult to find Seneca psychologically. In terms of verbal communication and activity, much less occurred during Seneca's sessions, as compared to the other case studies; yet, Seneca's sessions were the hardest to metabolize and put into words.

One aspect of emotionally digesting sessions with Seneca and other patients, involved exploring musical choices as communications. Tool's music, which was popular among younger hospital patients, typified a depth experience.[100] The music had a ritual quality: marked by pounding, repeating rhythms and trance-like effects.[101] Tool was focused on the philosophy of Jung with a particular interest in the collective unconscious and archetypes.[100,101] In Tools' music, there was a perpetual tension that waited for release: resembling the internal experience of psychosis. Tool's music had been described as, bleak and idiosyncratic" and "probing of the most desperate emotions." Common Tool themes were "wrath and pain, desire and self-loathing, and ferocity and meditation."[101] The album *Lateralus* was described as a search for a way out of the apocalypse, the path leading away from "negativity, blindness and cynicism."[101]

Another of Seneca's favorite bands, Evanescence, was originally a Christian metal band. Their song, "Together Again,"[88] articulated the affective resonance of Seneca's losses: romance, family, loss of connection with others, and loss of his own coherent self. Music journalists described Evanescence's lead singer, Amy Lee, as a "sweet Southern girl with a freaky Goth side," and as "the voice of her generation,"[102] Together Again,"[88] was originally written for *The Lion, The Witch and the Wardrobe*.[103,104] Lee, as an expression of pain, and of longing for home donated the song to a United Nations fundraising site for Haiti earthquake relief. She wanted the song to bring people relief from suffering.[105]

Eminem was another of Seneca's interesting choices. We noted earlier that schizophrenia and other psychoses, involve disturbances in verbal language and abnormalties in processing auditory and visual sensory stimuli,[106-108] Eminem models a kind of alpha function in which he takes raw elements of language and spins them into rhymes.[111] Eminem's manager compared him to John Nash, the Nobel Prize–winning economist, who struggled with schizophrenia.[109,110] Eminem organizes and synthesize a panoply of echoing voices from the past, with the word salad of ongoing impressions, into musical form. He has been described as having a "vexatious obsession with violence and social dysfunction."[111] By self-description Eminem is a kind of monstrosity, a disturbing mirror for social distortion who traces his rage back to early childhood experiences of abuse and neglect.[111] Seneca was lost in an inner chamber of psychosis where he could not verbally express the range and intensity of emotions Eminem could metabolize and express safely for him.

Rorschach Results
Another method of analyzing Seneca's progress from the first to the final session was through Rorschach results.[112-114] Initially, Seneca had strong unfulfilled needs for closeness due to emotional losses from the past exacerbated by the present. He experienced feelings of deprivation (eb, 3:4) and torment (Shading Blends). He was irritated by his own longing and loneliness (Sum T, 2). Seneca ruminated about himself (FD, 5; Sum V, 0) and was critical and over-focused on his body (An +Xy, 2). Initially, he had a hard time with attention and with holding images in short term memory (DQ sequencing). He perceived himself as monstrous and primitive (i.e., a dog or a monkey), as a frozen statue, as a dragon with tears coming out, and as a demon, with green intestines, possessed with a virus that others could catch. Seneca believed that something essential was escaping out of him (blood from head) and that all parts of him, except one, were dead (Minus Form, MORB 4). Seneca conveyed through his Rorschach responses that he was like a monkey, exploring love and curious about the prospect of a heart His own emotions were strange to him (FM, 2 and m,1).[114-116]

After the ten music sessions, Seneca's answers were more within normal limits (DQ Distribution and Sequencing), although he was still coping with strong intellectual defenses (Intellect Index, 5). Responses were more subdued and less bizarre (Critical Special Scores) and he tended to hide his distortions (decreased Minus Distortions). His scores indicated that he would do better in an uncomplicated, structured environment where feelings were prized (EB, O:4; Lambda, 1.0). He internalized feelings that he longed to externalize; some emotions were translated into somatic responses (eb, 1:2). He experienced unusually high distress and discomfort but the magnitude of his emotions were not in proportion to his circumstances (FC: CF +C, 1:3). His negative ruminations and self-inspection decreased in the post test (FD,1, Sum V,O) with less concern for his body (An + Xy, 0). He also paused quietly to look at his sadness with less combativeness (MORB, 1). Seneca indicated that something primitive he needed for protection was escaping him (Minus Scores). He had less longing for closeness and a wish for more space than in the previous test (Sum T, 0). His sense of isolation also increased due to painful interactions with others (M, 0, Fm, 1). He described two people in love with inherent dangers in their coming together.[114-116]

Conclusion

Seneca and Andrew re-enforced the importance of communicating and attuning through preferred music. As therapists we ask patients to sit with and tolerate avoided emotions, or emotions they might prefer to project back into the environment. Likewise, a therapist may need to tolerate music that initially seems alien, or inappropriate. In the process of developing a kind of communicative musicality and attunement with adult patients in acute crisis settings, connections are more easily fostered when the focus is on a third, such as an iPod filled with various musical choices. Music can move between the therapist and patient establishing rhythm, resonance, and potential space within which some semblance of safety and inquiry can occur. With Andrew, who was struggling with complex grief and bipolar depression, we embarked upon an inquiry into understanding a song with multiple meanings. With Seneca I paid close attention to his somatic responses, and countertransference. Yet it was actually listening to Seneca's beloved music with him that helped show me the importance of what exists in the suspended silences of "negative capability"[69,80,115] wherein meanings emerge without grabbing or trying to control them. Outside of the listening sessions I attempted to metabolize Seneca's (and Andrew's) non-verbal emotional material. It was particularly complicated to work with Seneca on building a trusting and consistent frame, while he was navigating the emotional and legal complexities of the court system.

With patients in an acute hospital setting, there are sometimes only small windows of time and opportunity within which to connect with people who are suffering emotional pain. If a therapist can listen to music with a patient who is in a state of chronic isolation, emotional overwhelm, dread, or disorganization, she can also be listening for that patient. She can listen for the moments of dyadic openness, where a sense of "us," fills the room even in the rhythmic silences between beloved songs.

References

1. Greenbaum N. Spirit in the sky. [Recorded by Norman Greenbaum]. On Spirit in the Sky. [Digital download] London, UK: Reprise Records;1969.
2. Panksepp J, Trevarthen C. The neuroscience of emotion in music. In Trevarthen C, Malloch S, eds. Communicative musicality: Exploring the basis of human companionship. Oxford, UK: Oxford University Press;2009:105-146.
3. Loewy J. Song sensitization: How fragile we are. Caringor the caregiver: The use of music and music therapy in grief and trauma. Silver Spring, MD US: American Music Therapy Association; 2002:33-43. Available from: PsycINFO, Ipswich, MA. Accessed March 12, 2011.
4. Dileo C, Parker C. Final moments: The use of song in relationship completion. Music therapy at the end of life. Cherry Hill, NJ New York, NY US: Jeffrey Books; 2005:43-56. Available from: PsycINFO, Ipswich, MA. Accessed March 12, 2011.
5. Dileo C. Songs for living: The use of songs in the treatment of oncology patients. In C. Dileo ed., Music therapy and medicine: Theoretical and clinical applications. Silver Spring, MD: American Music Therapy Association; 1999: 151-66.
6. Carter FA, Wilson JS, Lawson RH, Bulick CM. Mood induction procedure. Importance of individualizing music. Behav Change. 1995;12:159-161.
7. Thaut MH, Davis WB. The Influence of Subject-selected versus experimenter-chosen music on affect, anxiety and relaxation. J Music Ther. 1993;30;4:210-223.
8. Guhn M, Hamm A, Zentner M. Phsyiological and musico-acoustico correlates of the chill response. Music Percep. 2007;24:170-180.
9. Iwaki T, Tanka H, Hori T. The effects of preferred familiar music on falling asleep. J Music Ther. 2003;40;1:15-26.
10. Mitchell LA, MacDonald RA. An Experimental Investigation of the Effects of Preferred and Relaxing Music Listening on Pain Perception. J Music Ther. 2006;43;4:295-316.
11. Rickard NS. Intense emotions responses to music: a test of the physiological arousal hypothesis. Psychology of music. Psych Music. 2004;32;4:371-388.
12. Baker F, Bor W. Can music preference indicate mental health status in young people? Australasian Psy. 2008;16;4:284-288.

13. Lacourse E, Claes, M, Villeneuve, M. Heavy metal music and adolescent suicide. J Youth Adolesc. 2001;30;3:321. Available from EBSCOhost, Ipswich, MA. Accessed January 15, 2011.
14. Martin G, Clarke, M, Pearce, C. Adolescent suicide: Music preference as an indicator of vulnerability. J Am Acad Child Adolesc Psy. 1993;32;3: 530-535. Available from EBSCOhost, Ipswich, MA. Accessed May 7, 2011.
15. Wyatt JG. From the field: Clinical resources for music therapy with juvenile offenders. Music Ther Persp. 2002;20;2:80-88. Available from EBSCOhost, Ipswich, MA. Accessed July 7, 2012.
16. Tarrant M, North AC, Hargreaves D J. English and American adolescents' reasons for listening to music. Psy Music.2002:28;2:166-173. .
17. Bohlman P. Music as representation. J Music Resrch. 2005;24;3/4:205-226. Available from EBSCOhost, Ipswich, MA. Accessed February 20, 2011.
18. Hargreaves DJ, North A. The functions of music in everyday life: Redefining the social in music psychology. Psy Music. 1999 27;1:71-83.
19. Mickel E, Mickel C. Family therapy in transition: Choice theory and music. Intl J Real Ther. 2002;21;2:37-40. Available from EBSCOhost, Ipswich, MA. Accessed February 20, 2011.
20. Schulkind, MD, Hennis L, Rubin DC. Music, emotion, and autobiographical memory: They're playing your song. Mem Cog. 1999;27;6:948-955.
21. Tekman HG, Hortacsu N. Music and social identity: Stylistic identification as a response to musical style. Intl J Psych. 2002;37;5:277-285.
22. DeNora T. Aesthetic agency and musical practice: New directions in the sociology of music and emotion. In Jusline PN, Sloboda JA, eds. Music and emotion: Theory and research. Oxford, UK: Oxford University Press; 2001:161-180.
23. Becker J. Anthropological perspectives on music and emotion. In Jusline PN, Sloboda JA, eds. Music and emotion: Theory and research. Oxford, UK: Oxford University Press; 2001:135-160.
24. Seeger A. Why Suya sing: A musical anthropology of an Amazonian People. Cambridge, UK: Cambridge University Press;1987.
25. Peretz I, Zatorre R. The cognitive neuroscience of music. NY: Oxford University Press; 2003.
26. Klockars M, Peltoman M. Music Meets Medicine. Helsinki: Oy Nord; 2007.

27. Osborne N. Music for children in zones of conflict and post-conflict: A psychobiological approach. In Malloch S, Trevarthen C, eds. Communicative Musicality. NY, NY: Oxford University Press; 2009:331-356
28. Boudewyns PA. A comparison of the effects of stress vs. relaxation instruction on the finger temperature response. Behav Ther.1976;7;1:54-67.
29. Burns J, Labbé E, Williams K, McCall J. Perceived and physiological indicators of relaxation: As different as Mozart and Alice in Chains. Appld Psychophys Biofdbk.1999;24;3:197-202. Available from EBSCOhost, Ipswich, MA. Accessed January 12, 2011.
30. Kibler V, Rider M. Effects of progressive muscle relaxation and music on stress as measured by finger temperature response. J Clin Psych.1983;39;2:213-215. Available from EBSCOhost, Ipswich, MA. Accessed January 12, 2011.
31. Landreth J E, Landreth HF. Effects of music on physiological response. J Resrch Music Ed. 1974;22;1:4-12.
32. Maranto C. Music therapy and stress management. In Lehrer P, Woolfolk R., eds. Principles and practice in stress management. 2nd ed, New York, NY: Guilford Press; 1993:407-442.
33. Peretti PO, Swenson K. Effects of music on anxiety as determined by physiological skin responses. Journal of Research in Music Education. 1974 22;4: 278-283. Available from EBSCOhost, Ipswich, MA. Accessed January 12, 2011.
34. Dissanayake E. Root, leaf, blossom, or bole: Concerning the origin and adaptive function of music. In Trevarthen C, Malloch S, eds. Communicative musicality: Exploring the basis of human companionship. Oxford, UK: Oxford University Press; 2009:17-30.
35. Panksepp J. The neuroevolutionary and neuroaffective psychobiology of the prosocial brain. Oxford handbook of evolutionary psychology. Chap 12. Oxford, UK: Oxford Library of Psychology; 2007:17-30.
36. Dissanayake, E. Art and intimacy: How the arts began. University of Washington Press, Seattle,WA: University of Washington Press; 2000.
37. Mithen S. The singing Neanderthals: The origins of music, language, mind and body. London, UK: Weidenfeld and Nicolson; 2005.
38. Nakata T, Trehub SE. Infants' responsiveness to maternal speech and singing. Infant Behav Dev. 2004;27;4:455-464.
39. Trehub S. Human processing predispositions and musical universals. In Wallin NL, Merker B, Brown, S. eds, The origins of music.

40. E. Cambridge, MA: Massachusetts Institute of Technology;2000:427-448.
40. Trehub S. The developmental origins of musicality. Nat Neurosci. 2003;6;7: 669. Available from EBSCOhost, Ipswich, MA. Accessed January 11, 2011.
41. Freeman W J. Societies of brains. A study in the neurobiology of love and hate. Mahwah, NJ: Erlbaum;1995.
42. Blood AJ, Zatorre RJ. Intensely pleasurable responses to music correlate with activity in brain regions implicated in reward and emotion. Proceedings Natl Acad Sci USA. 2001;98;20; 11818. Available from EBSCOhost, Ipswich, MA. Accessed January 12, 2011.
43. Menon V, Levitin DJ. The rewards of music listening: Response and physiological connective of the mesolimbic system. Neuroimage. 2005;28;1:175-184.
44. Alcaro A, Huber R, Panksepp J. Behavioral functions of the mesolimbic dopamanergic system. An affective neuroethological perspective. Brain Resrch Rev. 2007;56;2:283-321.
45. Langer SK. Philosophy in a new key. Cambridge,MA: Harbard University Press; 1942.
46. Trevarthen C, Aitken, KJ. Brain development, infant communication and empathy disorders. Intrinsic factors in child mental health. Dev Psychopathol. 1995;6:597-633.
47. Trevarthen C. Action and emotion in development of the human self, its sociability and cultural intelligence. Why infants have feelings like ours. In J. Nadel J, Muir D, eds. Emotional development, Oxford, UK: Oxford Unversity Press; 2005:61-91.
48. Malloch, S. Mother and infant and communicative musicality. Musicae Scientae, Special Issue 1999-2000;1999: 29-57.
49. Malloch S, Trevarthen C. Musicality: Communicating the vitality interests of life. In Trevarthen C, Malloch S, eds. Communicative musicality: Exploring the basis of human companionship. Oxford, UK: Oxford University Press; 2009:1-15.
50. Beebe B. Brief mother-infant treatment: psychoanalytically informed video feedback. Inft Mentl Hlth J. 2003;24;1:24-52.
51. Beebe B. Co-constructing mother-infant distress in face-to-face interactions: Contribution of microanalysis. Infnt Observ. 2006;9;2:151-164.
52. Beebe B, & Lachman F. Representation and internalization in infancy: Three principles of silence. Psychanal Psych.1994;11:127-165.

53. Tronick E, Cohn J. Infant-mother face-to-face interaction: Age and gender differences in coordination and the occurrence of miscoordination. Chld Dev.1989,60:85-92
54. Benjamin J. Like subjects, love objects, essays on recognition and sexual difference. New Haven, CT: Yale University Press;1995.
55. Knoblauch SH. The musical edge of therapeutic dialogue. Hillsdale, NJ: The Analytic Press; 2000.
56. Winnicott DW. Playing: Its theoretical status in the clinical situation. Intl J Psychanal.1968;49:591-599.
57. Panksepp J. The neuroevolutionary and neuroaffective psychobiology of the prosocial brain. Oxford handbook of evolutionary psychology. Oxford: Oxford Library of Psychology;2007:Chap. 12.
58. Hug E, Lohne P, (2009, February 1). A case study of the treatment of a patient with psychosis and drug dependence: Towards an integration of psychoanalytic and neuorscientific perspective. Psychosis. February 2009;1:82-92.
59. Freud S. Instincts and their vicissitudes. In Strachey J. ed. trans. The standard edition of the complete psychological works of Sigmund Freud. Vol.14. London, UK: Hogarth Press:1957/1915:109-140.
60. Jung CG. Symbols of transformation. In Read H, Fordham M, Adler G, W. McGuire, W. eds. Hull, RFC. Trans. The collected works of C. G. Jun,g 2nd ed, Vol. 5. Princeton, NJ: Princeton University Press;1977/1956:394-446.
61. Wärja M. Sounds of music through the spiraling path of individuation: A Jungian approach to music psychotherapy. Music Ther Persp.1994;12;2:75-83. Available from: EBSCOhost, Ipswich, MA. Accessed January 7, 2011.
62. Reich W. Character analysis. 3rd ed. Garfagno, VR, Trans. New York, NY: Farrar, Strauss & Giroux. 1972/1945.
63. Reich W. Selected writings: An introduction to orgonomy. New York, NY: Farrar, Strauss & Giroux; 1973/1951.
64. McDougall J. Primitive communication and the use of countertransference—reflections on early psychic trauma and its transference effects. Contemp Psychanal.1978;14:173-209.
65. Tustin, F. Autism and childhood psychosis. London, UK: Karnac Books;1972.
66. Samuels A. Countertransference, The "Mundus Imaginalis" and a research project. J Analytic Psych. 1985;30;1:47-71.
67. Stone M, The analyst's body as tuning fork: Embodied resonance in countertransference. J Analyt Psych. 2006;51;1:109-124.
68. Knoblauch SH. Body rhythms and the unconscious: Toward an expanding of clinical attention. Psychan Dialogues. 2005;15;6:807-

827. Available from: EBSCOhost, Ipswich, MA. Accessed January 7, 2011.
69. Bion WR. Second thoughts: Selected papers on psychoanalysis. New York, NY: Karnac; 1984.
70. Schore AN. Implications of a psychoneurological model. In Alhanti S, ed. Primitive mental states, Vol 2: Psychobiological and psychoanalytic perspectives on early trauma and personality development. New York, NY: Karnac; 2002:1-64.
71. Schore AN. Affect regulation and the origins of the self. Mahwah, NJ: Lawrence Erlbaum;1994.
72. van der Kolk B, Roth S, Pelcovitz D, Sunday S, Spinazzola J. Disorders of extreme stress: The empirical foundation of a complex adaptation to trauma J Traum Stress. 2005;18;5:389-399.
73. McEwen BS. Early life influences on life-long patterns of behavior and health. Mental Retardation & Developmental Disabilities Research Reviews.2003;9;3: 149-154. Available from: EBSCOhost, Ipswich, MA. Accessed January 2, 2011.
74. Mulvihill D. The health impact of childhood trauma: An interdisciplinary review, 1997-2003. Issues Comp Ped Nurs. 2005;28;2:115-136. Available from: EBSCOhost, Ipswich, MA. Accessed January 2, 2011.
75. Nijenhuis ES. Somatoform dissociation: Phenomena, measurement, & theoretical issues. New York, NY: WW Norton; 2004.
76. Grotstein J. "Orphans of the "Real": II. The future of object relations theory in the treatment of the. Bull Menninger Clin. 1995;59;3:312-332.
77. Carter DM. Drop The world. [Recorded by Lil Wayne]. On Rebirth [Digital download]. New York, NY: Cash Money Records; 2009.
78. Cozolino L. The neuroscience of psychotherapy: Building and rebuilding the human brain. New York, NY: W. W. Norton; 2002.
79. Rosenbaum, B. Psychosis and the structure of homosexuality: Understanding the pathogenesis of schizophrenic states of mind. Scand Psychanal Rvw. 2005;28;2:82-89.
80. Bion WR. Learning from experience. London,UK: Karnac; 1984.
81. Bion WR. Cogitations. London, UK: Karnac; 1992/1957.
82. Bleandonu G. Wilfred Bion: His life and works 1897-1979. New York, NY: Other Press;1994.
83. Glickson J, Cohen Y. Can music alleviate cognitive dysfunction in schizophrenia? Psychopath. 2000;33:43-47.
84. Neilzén S, Cesarec, Z. On the perception of emotional meaning in music. Psych Music.1981;9;2:17-31.

85. Ulrich G, Houtmans T, Gold C. The additional therapeutic effect of group music therapy for schizophrenic patients:a randomized study. Acta Psych 2007,116;5: 362-370
86. Cash J, Jenkins G. Folsom prison blues. [Recorded by J. Cash]. On Live at Folsom Prison [Digital download]. Folsom, CA: Columbia;1968.
87. McGorry PD, Killackey E, Elkins K, Lambert M, Lambert T. Summary Australian and New Zealand clinical practice guideline for the treatment of schizophrenia. Australasian Psy. 2003;11;2:136-147. Available from EBSCOhost, Ipswich, MA. Accessed November 2, 2010.
88. Lee A. Together again. [Recorded by Evanescence]. On United Nations: Haiti earthquake relief [Digital download]. New York, NY: Wind-Up Records;2010.
89. Gibbard B. I will follow you into the dark. [Recorded by Death Cab for Cutie]. On Plans [Digital download]. North Brookfield, MA: Atlantic;2006.
90. Grotstein JS. A beam of intense darkness. London, UK: Karnac;2007.
91. Bangalter T, de Homen-Christo GM. Around the world. [Recorded by Daft Punk]. On Homework [Digital download]. Paris, FR: Virgin Records;1997.
92. Eminem, Bass J. Cleanin' out my closet. [Recorded by Eminem]. On The Eminem show [CD]. Los Angeles, CA: Shady Records;2002.
93. Page J, Plant R. Going to California. [Recorded by Led Zeppelin]. On Led Zeppelin IV [Digital Download]. Los Angeles, CA: Atlantic; 1971.
94. Lennon J, McCartney P. Mother Nature's Son. [Recorded by The Beatles]. On The White Album [CD]. London, UK: G. Martin;1968.
95. Tool. The grudge. On Lateralus [Digital download]. Hollywood, CA: Volcanoe Entertainment;2001.
96. Tool. The patient. On Lateralus [Digital download]. Hollywood, CA: Volcanoe Entertainment;2001.
97. Tool. Schism. On Lateralus [Digital download]. Hollywood, CA: Volcanoe Entertainment;2001.
98. Searles, HF. Countertransference and related subjects. New York, NY: International Universities Press, Inc;1979.
99. Page J, Plant R. Ramble on. [Recorded by Led Zeppelin]. On Led Zeppelin II. London [Digital download]. London, UK: Atlantic;1969.

100. Loder K. Maynard James Keenan: Not yet a legend, not yet dead. Available from MTV.com http://www.mtv.com, Retrieved on November 26, 2010; 2001.
101. Pareles J. Pop review: Flailing wildly to escape the darkness. The New York Times. October 6, 2001:21.
102. Dolan J. Music review: The open door. Entertainment Weekly. Available from http://www.ew.com/ew/article; October 9, 2006.
103. Peacock A, Adamson, A. The Lion, the Witch and the Wardrobe [Motion Picture]; 2005.
104. Staff. Wardrobe closed to Evanescence singer. New Zealand Herald. November 27, 2004. Accessed from http://www.newzealandherald.com.
105. Fuoco, C. Evanescence Biography. Accessed from www.Allmusic.com. Retrieved on December 18, 2011
106. Kestenbaum CJ. Thoughts on the precursors of affective and cognitive disturbance in schizophrenia. In Feinsilver DB ed, Towards a comprehensive model for Schizophrenic Disorders. Psychoanalytic essays in memory of Ping-Nie-Pao. Hillsdale, NJ: Analytic Press;1986:211-236.
107. Feinsilver DB. Pao's telescopic overview of treatment. In Feinsilver DB. ed, Towards a comprehensive model for Schizophrenic Disorders. Psychoanalytic essays in memory of Ping-Nie-Pao. Hillsdale, NJ: Analytic Press;1986.
108. Peccecia M, Benedetti G. The integration of sensorial chanels through progressive mirror drawing in the psychotherapy of schizophrenic patients with disturbances in verbal language. J Am Acad Psychoanal.1998; 26;1:109-122.
109. Caramanica J. Eminem resurfaces in a new role, memoirist. The New York Times. October 2, 2008. Accessed from http://nytimes.com. Retrieved on December 12, 2011.
110. Caramanica J. Eminem. The New York Times. June 22, 2011. Accessed from http://topics.nytimes.com. Retrieved on December 12, 2011.
111. Sanneh K. The new season/pop music: Eminem vs. Eminem vs. Eminem. The New York Times. September 12, 2004. Accessed from EBSCOhost. Retrieved on Decembe 14, 2011: 67.
112. Exner JE. The Rorschach: A comprehensive system. Volume 1:Basic foundations. 3rd ed. New York, NY: Wiley; 1993.
113. Exner JE. A primer for Rorschach interpretation. Asheville, NC: Rorschach Workshops; 2000.
114. Exner JE. A Rorschach workbook for the comprehensive sytem, 5th ed. Asheville: Rorschach Workshops; 2001.

115. Keats J. Letter, dated Sunday, 21 December. In Rollins HE. ed, Letters of John Keats. Vol I & II. Cambridge, MA: Havard University Press; 1817.

CHAPTER 13

Improvisational Singing: A Nordoff-Robbins Based Vocal Music Therapy Intervention in the Treatment of Pain

Melanie May Po Acosta MA, LCAT, MT-BC, NRMT

"The inner nature of man is the province of music."
Confucius

Introduction

Music therapists have, at their disposal, a powerful, unique and invaluable instrument. Often overlooked and underutilized, this instrument has intricacies, nuances and characteristics that, when used clinically and combined with knowledge of the vast components and elements of music can facilitate, enhance, and deepen connections that are essential for therapeutic growth and change. This instrument, stated simply, is the voice.
Understanding the musical aspects and elements that make up a vocal music therapy intervention is crucial to the process of implementing *music as medicine* and using the voice as an effective clinical instrument. The subtle intricacies of the voice, the vocal quality and the musical elements applied to the use of the voice during a vocal music therapy intervention can exponentially increase the opportunities for achieving therapeutic goals in a clinical setting. By carefully analyzing and dissecting these elements the therapist can begin to understand the efficacy of the interventions and use the voice with intention and purpose in order to reach his or her clinical goals. The purpose of this chapter is to provide an in depth analysis of the use of the voice as a clinical instrument in the treatment of acute pain from the perspective of a Nordoff-Robbins based music therapist. The chapter will focus primarily on the use of improvisational singing as a vocally led relaxation intervention designed to promote overall full body relaxation and flow of breath in the treatment of pain in a hospital setting.

A Nordoff Robbins Approach to Vocal Music Therapy Work

As a music therapist, my philosophies of music and therapy resonate with the music-centered work of music therapy pioneers, Paul Nordoff and Clive Robbins and their concept of the *music child*.

Music and Medicine: Integrative Models in the Treatment of Pain

Nordoff and Robbins define the music child as "the individualized musicality inborn in every child: the term has reference to the universality of human musical sensitivity-the heritage of complex and subtle sensitivity to the ordering and relationship of tonal and rhythmic movement-and to the uniquely personal significance of each child's musical responsiveness".[1(p3)] The efficacy of music therapy relies on the ability of the therapist to facilitate and then maintain a connection to the music child, or in inborn musicality, within each patient. The universality of music makes it an accessible medium with which to establish connections on many levels, whether physical, emotional or spiritual.

This universal musicality of the human condition is an important element to understand when studying the efficacy of a music therapy intervention. Whether it is because of the evolutionary origins of the development of language in the human species or due to the rhythmic and vibratory make-up of the human's bodily systems (heart rate, respiratory rate, pulse etc.) the human condition predisposes us to an innate understanding of music and musical communication. Further, there is an innate human propensity to respond to vocal communication. Singing reconnects us with our most primitive selves through the stimulation of musical faculties that have evolved over time.

Dissecting and analyzing the musical elements involved in a music therapy session in order to study and understand the effects of the music and musical interaction with a client is a crucial component of the Nordoff-Robbins approach to Music Therapy. Similarly, dissecting and analyzing the elements (musical and physiological) involved in vocal music therapy is crucial to understanding ways that the voice and singing can be used with clinical intention and to discover effective ways to replicate the results as effective treatments. A thorough understanding of all of the involving elements provides the therapist the information necessary to implement treatments and achieve a variety of clinical goals.

The Intervention: Improvisational Singing to Induce Full Body Relaxation and Flow of Breath in the Treatment of pain

Background

Pain is now viewed by the medical community as a multidimensional, complex experience influenced by psychological[2] and emotional factors,[3] stress levels, and the cyclical processing of neurological pain impulses.[4] Music has been shown to facilitate relaxation and reduce fear and anxiety in pre-operative[5] and post-operative situations.[6] In work with children, music therapy has been shown to be an effective intervention to lower anxiety and reduce pain sensations during painful procedures.[7] Recent studies on music and pain have demonstrated the effects of individual musical elements, such as mood or tempo on the sensation of pain.

Live music therapy has been shown to be an effective intervention in the treatment of pain. In studies with patients of all ages, with a variety of diagnoses and diseases, such as areas of critical care,[8-10] or trauma units,[11-13] music has been shown to alter the perception of pain and decrease anxiety.[14-16]

In the following music therapy intervention, pain is addressed utilizing vocal improvisation and two key principles: the iso-principle and the principle of entrainment.

The Iso-Principle is defined as a concept in which a "patient's musical mood can be matched to assist him or her in becoming aware of thoughts and recapture memories."[17] According to Dileo, the iso-principle can be used to consciously impact the patient's mood by matching the music to the patient's emotional state.[18] In the case of a patient experiencing pain, matching the patient's mood may include matching the sounds and rhythms of the physiological and somatic responses, such as rapid breathing, physical movements or vocalizations as well as matching the perceived emotional state and stress levels. With improvisational singing, the iso-principle can be implemented by isolating specific responses of the patient and matching them by clinically applying different musical and vocal elements to the therapist's vocalizations.

In addressing issues of pain, it is important to note the significance of rhythm and vibration within the human body. Invasive procedures, such as surgery, physical illness, or injury cause sensory and neurological stimulations that result in the perception of pain. However, emotional responses can also result from these sensory stimulations as well as from the reactions to the situations themselves, causing anxiety, fear or sadness, for example. Together, this contributes to an overall disruption of the body's natural rhythms.

Guiding the patient towards more stable and regulated bodily rhythms is often the first physiological goal in dealing with pain issues. Fortunately for a music therapist, music can be a powerful way to achieve that goal through the phenomenon known as entrainment. Gaynor states:

> "Scientists have also determined that there is a tendency in the universe toward harmony, a phenomenon known as 'entrainment'...The reason that entrainment occurs is that the more powerful rhythmic vibrations of one object, when projected upon a second object with a similar frequency, will

cause that object to begin to vibrate in resonance with the first object. We human beings also react in resonance with the vibrations and fluctuations in our surroundings, so it follows that our physiological functioning may be altered by the impact of sound waves, whether produced by our own voices or by objects or instruments in our environment.[19(p49)]"

By embracing the musical elements of rhythm, tempo and vibration, the music therapist can utilize the phenomenon of entrainment. Adding a harmonic instrument to support the voice when utilizing improvisational singing as an intervention can add further emphasis to the rhythm and tempo of the intervention. As the patient enters into a relaxed state, the attention to the rhythm and tempo will occur for him or her on an unconscious level as the phenomenon of entrainment takes place.

Why the Voice?

The voice is the closest and most intimate of instruments, as it resonates, literally, within the body. The natural sounds emitted by the voice when made spontaneously, are always truthful expressions and often have their own melodic elements, such as melody, pitch, or rhythm. Studies have been done on nonverbal vocalizations, such as spontaneous expressions of emotions or pain (whimper, groan, whine etc.) and results indicate that such vocalizations are cross culturally recognized[20] and universally understood. The cultural universality of these natural sounds suggest that they are biologically adaptive,[21] stimulating discussions over the origin of music and language[22,23] and giving credence to the belief in the predisposition of humans to respond to vocal communication.

In very young children, vocalizations tend to emerge from these natural sounds as they first begin to discover their voices. These early singing sounds are the first introduction to the natural singing voice. The natural singing voice refers to the individual's vocalizations before, beyond or extracted from the constraints and rules of speech development. Cook refers to the singing sound as it first emerges from the very young as "another wordless communication linked directly to the feeling state".[24(p27)] Often, with the development of speech, these natural sounds are altered, as the individual finds himself conforming to various rules of society and culture. As a result, the instinctive impulse is stifled, and the instinctive sounds are no longer allowed to be released freely. Austin states, "Just as we restrain our breathing in order to control our feelings, many of us consciously or unconsciously learn to control and repress our instinctive impulses and the sounds that accompany them out of fear of judgment, rejection or harm."[25(p27)] Harrison states, "Speech...having deranged the throat's original natural vocal activity, is in no position to instruct the voice how to sing. On the contrary, speech has taught the voice how not to sing.[26(p14)]

A therapist must understand the difference between the natural and the affected voice and be able to freely model the use of the voice as a tool for communication. By analyzing and understanding the various elemental components involved in these natural nonverbal vocalizations (musical, physiological and emotional) the therapist can gain deeper understanding of his or her patient's expression, facilitating the building of a deeper therapeutic relationship. However, by additionally rediscovering his or her own natural singing voice and thoroughly studying and dissecting the elements involved in his or her own natural nonverbal vocalizations, a therapist can intentionally use the voice as an instrument to enhance his or her own authentic emotions and intentions, facilitating the pathway to a wider variety of important therapeutic connections, including the use of the voice to implement music as medicine.

Research and publications documenting effective voice work and vocal music therapy techniques have increased over the past few years bringing heightened recognition to the voice as an important instrument in therapy work.[27] Many of these techniques used by music therapists encourage expression and facilitate engagement from the client, whether vocal or through other musical expressions, and demonstrate the efficacy of the voice as a medium of communication and as a tool for therapeutic change.

However, in this chapter, the intervention discussed utilizes vocal improvisation performed by the therapist as a type of musical *medicine* in the treatment of pain from a music-centered music psychotherapy perspective. The intervention requires only active listening by the patient. The focus of the work involves the therapist's own careful and intentional use of the clinical voice, including a keen awareness of the workings of his or her own vocal instrument, a vast knowledge of the musical elements and musical components as they affect the voice and the vocal quality of his or her sound in conjunction with the music, and the ability to vocally improvise. Finally, the intervention requires that the therapist have a thorough understanding of the iso-principle and entrainment in the context of vibration, resonance and pain management. Most importantly, it requires that the therapist have a thorough understanding of his or her own voice, and how to use it effectively to communicate his or her feelings through nonverbal vocally improvised sound. As Uhlig states:

> "the impact and effect of the sound of the voice is determined by the quality, the color and nuances, the ranges and its limits, tone stability, breathing techtechniques...vibration and resonation...positive and negative attributes of intonation, rhythm, emotional signals...acoustic symbols and sensitivity and perception about what is being communicated verbally and nonverbally."[28(p3)]

This particular intervention also requires that the therapist conduct a thorough assessment of the patient, gathering as much information as possible regarding the intensity, location and quality of the pain being experienced.

Improvisational Singing as an Intervention

The ability to improvise vocally is essential to a music therapist because it conveys a sense of freedom and relaxation and allows for true musical expressivity. Subsequently it is understood that true vocal improvisation requires relaxation, both physically and mentally, as well as an open awareness of the communication occurring between the participants.

Vocal improvisation allows the therapist to add truthful parts of him or herself to the musical conversation because the vocalizations come directly from, and are part of the therapist's actual being. Because of the intimacy of the vocal instrument, vocal improvisation can also emphasize the authenticity of the therapeutic communication, as it requires the natural, fluid, primitive, and expressive freedom of the therapist's natural singing voice. Just as the ability to freely improvise on a harmonic instrument facilitates the therapist's ability to musically meet a patient, vocal improvisation can be used to melodically impact the consonance or dissonance of harmonic structure, to dramatically change the dynamics, rhythmic or tonal elements of the music for example, or even greatly change the mood or emotions thereby adding to the overall scope of musical communication.

Each individual person has a unique timbre to his or her voice. The timbre of a person's voice refers to the tone quality or color of the sound. To a certain degree, the timbre of a person's voice is not in the person's control as it relies heavily on the physical structure of the person's actual physical body and shape of the resonance cavities. However, there are many ways to consciously affect the timbre of the voice. When used clinically, these affects can potentially enhance or impede the efficacy of the intervention. The position of the head and neck as well as posture can greatly affect the openness of the vocal tract. Changes to physical positioning of the head and neck, as well as tongue base (forward or back) and position of the palate affects the diameter of the vocal openings, resonance cavity and amplification of the sound produced.[29] For example, Dr. Heman-Acka further explains that "elevation of the palate helps to open the vocal tract in the back of the mouth and seals the nasal cavity to minimize a nasal-sounding voice"[29(p32)]. Intentionally producing or manipulating the timbre of the voice during singing interventions requires understanding of the physiology of how the sound is produced. Physical manipulation of the sound, particularly when done from a manipulation of the physical body or within the oral cavity (tongue, palate positioning) or the head and neck can cause dangerous strain on the vocal folds or may lead to unhealthy singing habits when done without understanding of the vocal production and knowledge of safe and healthy singing techniques.

People who have a natural 'breathy' quality to their speaking or singing voice may also present with voice disorders including vocal nodules, vocal fold cysts or polyps, among other symptoms.[30(p40)] However with proper understanding and sufficient knowledge the timbre of the sound can be affected intentionally in a safe way, resulting in a different vocal quality and color that can enhance a vocal therapy intervention. This type of vocal versatility expands the therapist's repertoire of possible vocal interventions and ways to form connections with patients. Uhlig's descriptions of qualitative and quantitative vocal techniques involve this type of awareness of vocal timbre.[28] Similarly, Uhlig goes on to describe ways to use the voice to achieve "corporeal attunement" on a physical level.[28(p94)] This type of voicework, requires sustained tones and vibratory resonance as part of the treatment. These different tones, depending on the phonation and use of breath and physical body control used in the production of sound, can take on vastly different timbres. Many music therapists use toning clinically with a variety of populations to address different issues.[25,31,28] In the intervention described in this chapter, the use of toning refers to the therapist's use of different tones, which the client receives in an active listening experience. The timbre of the therapist's voice can play an important factor in the efficacy and flow of the intervention.

The following section describes several key elements of improvisational singing, which greatly impact the timbre of the vocal sound. While these elements could be labeled as stylistic affects, isolating these elements and understanding how these affects are produced as well as the effect on the resulting sound is important for any professional who uses the voice as an instrument.

Respiratory Elements of Improvisational Singing

The following elements of vocal sounds are important for a therapist to consider when using improvisational singing because of the immediate effect on the timbre of the voice:

The Breath
The breath is one of the most important elements involved in singing. When using improvisational singing as a music therapy intervention, focus on the breath is imperative as it can be used as an assessment tool for the client while simultaneously affecting the intentionality of the therapist.

Awareness of the Patient's Breath and Breathing Pattern
Nonverbal expression of emotions, the patient's breath and breathing pattern during a vocal interaction, whether speaking, singing or nonverbally vocalizing (whimper, whine, sigh etc) can provide a great deal of information for the therapist. Awareness and understanding of the emotions communicated nonverbally is extremely important for the therapist. The perceived pain level often is reflected through the client's breath, even if only revealed in a subtle sound such as a sigh or one word response. The quality of a patient's breath and breathing pattern can also provide a nonverbal indication of the patient's needs in the moment.

Intentionality of the Use of the Breath
By focusing on the specific quality and amount of breath involved in each tone that he or she sings, the therapist can intentionally increase or decrease the intimacy of the therapeutic space and respond appropriately to the needs of his or her patient. For example, if during an assessment the therapist determines that a patient needs to feel more warmth and openness from the therapist before reciprocally engaging, the therapist can warm the quality of his or her voice by adding breath to each note sung. By lowering the pitch to a conversational level and combining the pitch with a soft breathiness, the quality of the therapist's voice can convey a warmer, more inviting tone. Similarly, if a patient responds negatively to a therapist's initial tones and the therapist determines that the patient needs more time and space, the therapist can decrease the intimacy of the therapeutic environment by decreasing the amount of breath of each note, thus reducing the breathy quality of the tone and removing some of the perceived warmth. For the therapist, the ability to translate his or her own emotions and intensions in an authentic and knowledgeable way through this type of vocal and breath manipulation can greatly enhance his or her practice.

Vowel Choice during Vocalizations

The choice of vowel or vocal sound produced when toning can greatly affect the timbre and resonance of a note. For the therapist, the difference vowels toned or sung affects the physical resonance of the oral cavity, the head, throat, chest and abdominal area. This in turn affects the frequency vibration and resonance of the tone produced. Clinically, this information can be useful in the treatment of pain as the application of different musical tones will produce sound waves and frequencies that resonate in different areas of the patient's body during the intervention.

For example, in the intervention described below, the phonation and actual physical pronunciation of the vowel E ("ee") placed on a particular high pitch in the therapist's voice will resonate in the therapist's head region, and will produce a specific tone. During such intervention, the therapist when applying the iso-principle may choose the vibration and resonance of the tone while attempting to meet the patient at their cognitive, physiological and emotional starting point during an intervention. If the therapist's intention is to initiate a progressive relaxation, working the vowels slowly through the different regions of the body with clinical intention and purpose will facilitate the relaxation process.

My choice of vowel sounds for the intervention described in this chapter, was influenced by Loewy's "Corresponding Vowel Sounds for Chakras"[31(p268)] and based on the theory that the vibration and resonance produced by the toning of certain vowels ("A" pronounced "Ay", "E" pronounced "ee", "I" pronounced "Ah" "O" pronounced "oh", "U", pronounced "oo") can be clinically applied in order to bring relief and harmony to particular body regions. Loewy substantiates the theory of vowel sound production and body regions in her work using tonal vocal holding[31,32] and tonal intervallic synthesis.[31] The theory behind toning, resonance, frequency vibration and body work is also substantiated by many of the other music therapists practicing voicework in the field.[33,28,25]

Musical Elements of Improvisational Singing

Pitch
In choosing how high or low to sing a note the therapist must consider the goal of the immediate intervention. Higher pitches resonate in the head cavity (head voice) and can have a bright sound, depending on placement of the pitch (whether placed with emphasis in the nasal cavity or lower in the throat area). A pitch sung in the head cavity with a bright sound may be stimulating to a patient. If the goal of that pitch is to match a patient who is clearly engaged in thought, a head tone with a bright sound may be appro-

priate at that moment. Conversely, a low pitch sung near the very bottom of a therapist's register will have more air, thus taking on a more breathy tone. It also may resonate so that the therapist can feel the tone in his or her lower abdomen area. If the goal of the progressive relaxation is to unconsciously move the focus of flow and breath into the lower region of the body and the patient has entered into the state of relaxation, a low breathy pitch may be the most appropriate reflection of the patient's physical and emotional state. Understanding how pitch changes the timbre of the voice is important when conducting an intervention.

Intervals
The choice of intervals used in improvisational nonverbal singing can facilitate the creation of a particular mood and effect the environment that the therapist wishes to create. For example, a minor 2nd sung in a repetitive pattern creates a much different mood than a major 5th. When intentionally combined with the harmonic support (guitar, piano or other harmonic instrument) the therapist can use the intentional singing of specific intervals to convey different moods, based on the needs or desires of the moment.

Melodic and Rhythmic Phrasing
When using improvisational singing, the melodic and rhythmic phrasing, (i.e. the use of melody and choice of musical phrasing), can enhance and emphasize the therapist's intentions. The intentional use of melodic and rhythmic phrasing can mimic speech prosody and convey intention even without the use of words or lyrics.

Tempo
The simple use of tempo regarding improvisational singing is simply to focus on how fast or slow one sings during an intervention. The speed with which one sings can greatly affect the stimulating or sedating effect of one's voice. However, there are many ways to intentionally use tempo in a vocal improvisational singing intervention that effectively juxtaposes the voice against the harmonic supporting instrument, utilizing two opposing sources of tempo to reach a particular single clinical goal. For example, during a progressive relaxation intervention, such as the one described in the session below, the tempo and rhythm of the voice and the guitar are juxtaposed during the introduction section in order to vocally reflect and match the patient's early emotional and physiological state while simultaneously creating a safe, steady rhythm on the guitar. The voice and the guitar, at this particular starting moment, are musically part of the same harmonic and rhythmic musical composition, yet within the composition the two instruments are focused on different elements of the patient's overall state.

A Nordoff-Robbins Based Vocal Music Therapy Intervention

Meter
The meter of an improvised piece of music plays an important part in the efficacy of the intervention. In an intervention intended to promote relaxation or possibly aid in sedation, such as the intervention described in this chapter, the meter is designed to lull the person into a slower physiological and emotional state, thus emulating a lullaby. For this reason, the music is set in ¾ time, with a possible shift here and there to compound 6/8 time.

Dynamics
Like tempo, how loud and soft one sings during an intervention greatly affects the quality of the therapist's voice and thus plays a significant part in the clinical and intentional use. Dynamics in relation to the voice, also, however, can be juxtaposed against various other musical elements to increase or decrease the efficacy of the intervention. For example, the soft singing of a minor 2nd interval against a loud rhythmic chord played on either piano or guitar can effectively create an ominous or scary mood, each instrument reinforcing the effects of the other.

Melody
In vocal music therapy work, melody is an extremely important element. Whether combined with lyrics or used in nonverbal vocalization, melody is often the most accessible element for the patient, creating a bridge toward client participation. The use of familiar melody, contemporary or popular songs often provides an immediate connection with a patient in that he or she can instantly share an experience with the therapist. Using familiar melody can facilitate intimacy with a patient by increasing motivation for participation allowing the therapist to share an experience with a patient that is normally experienced in his or her outside, home life. Composing based on favorite melody is also an effective intervention as it provides a safe and familiar point of connection by offering a place for immediate participation (the familiar melody) and a platform for improvisation (composition). Such intervention can render multiple entry points to the processing of more intimate and deeper issues.

Conversely, the use of unfamiliar, improvised melody can be an effective way to engage a patient's interest without stimulating melodic memories or invoking emotional thoughts.

The Use of Modes and Idioms

When using free improvisation the use of modes and idioms can greatly increase the opportunities for connection on many levels. As with other types of improvisational music therapy interventions, playing in modal

music can free the therapist from the "habitual, excessive use of the dominant-tonic progression"[1(p462)] and provide a wider musical platform to begin an intervention. Popular Western music or conventional familiar lullabies generally follow the dominant-tonic progression. In simple form a lullaby is meant to gently lull an individual, usually a child or infant, to sleep. Lullabies used in a music therapy session, in many instances, will promote sedation and encourage sleep and can be effective interventions for promoting relaxation. However, one of the main challenges to the therapist in a relaxation intervention intended to address pain is to establish an open musical sound environment that will follow the ebb and flow of breath, and any ensuing changes in the patient's breathing pattern.
This work can thoroughly support the patient's stream of consciousness while encouraging the cognitive freedom necessary to promote complete and total body relaxation.

In my experience with improvisational music therapy interventions, providing musical motifs that avoid the dominant-tonic progression, such as modal music (Dorian, Phrygian, Lydian, Mixolydian, Aolian, Locrian), whole tone, pentatonic scales etc, can effectively promote relaxation by reducing the triggering of melodic memory. For example, a patient may hear an improvised melody following a dominant-tonic progression and associate the melody with a familiar song following the same musical progression. They may then find that the song evokes certain feelings or memories associated with that particular song. In certain instances that association may result in increasing the feelings of relaxation, which ultimately will aid in the overall goal for the therapist. However, in other instances the patient's associations with the familiar melody may evoke thoughts or feelings that become counterproductive to the relaxation process by stimulating the mind and then the other body systems, (respiratory, heart rate, etc). They also may find the stop and start thought processes associated with the triggering of memories or evoking of emotions too abrupt or jarring, resulting in subtle physical movements or changes in body systems, and exacerbation of the physiological pain. Improvised modal music can provide an open forum that supports the stream of consciousness while following the spontaneous physiological changes as the person passes through different phases of relaxation and release.

Although subjective and at the discretion of the therapist, improvised modal music also has the potential to influence different moods, thereby establishing different sound environments. Combining the use of modes and idioms with the clinical voice provides the therapist an even wider platform to seek levels of connection, whether to match a perceived emotional state, a physiological state, or to meet a patient's musical preferences or desires. The intimacy of the voice, the intentional use of the

A Nordoff-Robbins Based Vocal Music Therapy Intervention

various elements discussed above, and the use of various musical motifs exponentially increases the opportunities for the therapist to clinically meet the patient and form important therapeutic connections.

Style

The ability to sing effectively in different styles provides the therapist with a wider platform for meeting a client's tastes or musical preferences. Even when using improvisational singing, rather than popular or familiar music, the addition of a stylistic affect can increase the opportunities for connection with a patient, particularly when a thorough assessment is performed before a session, including an intake of the patient's history with music. Analyzing particular styles of song from a vocal perspective is crucial for a therapist to learn to emulate that particular style. For example, in comparing and contrasting the vocal styles of country music and opera music, what vocal qualities differ in the presentation of particular notes? What characterizes the vocal quality or phrasing, whether melodic or rhythmic, of the singer in a reggae song? Often the emphasis is placed on the harmonic chord structure and patterns in the analysis of song style. The vocal qualities of different styles also play a marked part of characterizing the song style.

    A good exercise in learning to sing in different styles is to take the same song and change the style while singing accapella. This practice forces the singer to pay attention to all of the elements (breath, breathing pattern, rhythmic phrasing, melodic phrasing, vocal quality, pronunciation of lyrics, etc.) involved in a particular style of music.

Examples of Different Styles
Blues
Gospel
Pop
Classical
Operatic
Rhythm and Blues
Soul
Musical Theater

Clinical Work

Vignette: Jamie
Jamie was a 14 year old female patient in the Pediatric Intensive Care Unit (PICU). She had just undergone spinal fusion surgery, to treat scoliosis and was experiencing high levels of pain. Idiopathic (of an unknown cause)

scoliosis is an abnormal condition characterized by a lateral curvature of the spine.[34] Although scoliosis can occur at any age, Jamie's type of scoliosis, adolescent idiopathic scoliosis, presents during the preadolescent or adolescent years. Surgical intervention, such as in Jamie's case, involves fusing of the involved vertebrae in order to prevent further deformity. Postsurgical pain management is often an issue for patients undergoing spinal fusion surgery. Jamie was referred to Music Therapy to aid in her pain management.

The Assessment
When I first met Jamie, she was sitting up in bed as her mother attempted to brush her hair. Her whining and complaints appeared to be exasperating her mother who seemed anxious and frustrated as she attempted to accommodate Jamie's many demands. I explained that I could attempt to use music therapy to address some of her pain issues. Jamie very quietly agreed to try a session. Jamie's self-reported pain rating was high at 10 out of 10. She responded with facial grimaces and high pitched vocal sounds in response to the offer for her to actively participate in musical play and made clear vocal nonverbal protests when I led the discussion toward the idea of her participating through imagery and visualization. Her voice was high pitched with a constricted, tight timbre, characteristic of a much younger child. Her breathing was shallow. Her nonverbal vocalizations and overall physical and emotional presentation suggested that she was anxious, angry and clearly frustrated in addition to appearing uncomfortable and possibly experiencing a high degree of pain. She did not want to have to do anything. She displayed clearly regressive behavior, observed during the interaction with her mother as well as in her vocal and physical responses to my questions. I quickly determined that Jamie was in need of a receptive music therapy intervention only; one which required only active listening, with a goal of facilitating overall full body relaxation and possibly assisting her in falling asleep. I decided to utilize improvisational singing.

The Intervention
Phase I: The Introduction-Vowel-"E" (pronounced "ee")
I began by plucking open chords on the guitar (Dm, Am and Em) in a ¾ meter and singing an improvised melody in a D Dorian scale. The chord progression in the introduction phase was simple, open chords, chosen to support free flow of the vocal improvisation in the D Dorian mode. The meter of the intervention (3/4) established by the guitar plucking pattern provided a stable, steady lullaby rhythm which became the grounding force behind the intervention. It established a holding pattern that I would use to eventually introduce entrainment. I chose the Dorian mode to begin the

intervention for several reasons. In this particular pain intervention, my intention as the therapist was not only to promote relaxation and possibly encourage entrance to a sleep state, but to encourage the flow of the client's breath throughout the body.

In order to utilize the Iso-principle and match Jamie's starting point both physiologically and emotionally I needed to support her stream of consciousness without stimulating the thought process by triggering familiar sound or melody associations. In this particular Dorian improvisation, the musical motif provided was an improvised melody, unfamiliar to the patient and not following the dominant-tonic progression. The movement of the melody was guided solely by Jamie's breathing rate and pattern and did not follow a predictable or measurable melody. The Dorian mode and the melodic pattern established in the early part of the introduction phase provided the musical environment to support the movement of Jamie's thoughts and cognitive state. Because Jamie's mind and thought process was moving and changing sporadically and unpredictably at the start of the intervention, my clinical goal was to match her state musically by creating an open sound environment that moved and changed with her, supporting her "journey" with an ambient, non-judgmental soundtrack. To me, the Dorian mode provided an effective mood to meet that goal.

Jamie's face was grimacing slightly as she fidgeted in her bed, making small adjustments in her body and limbs, followed by small vocal whimpers. Her body appeared tense. Picking a relatively high pitch and making sure that I could feel the resonance vibrating in my own head I sang the "E" vowel, allowing the improvised melody to travel up and down the D Dorian scale. The melodic pattern moved up and down the scale as I vocalized nonverbally on an improvised melody using the vowel "E" (pronounced with a long "ee"). The vowel choice and pitch (E vowel in a high head tone resonance) were chosen because Jamie's thought process was very much engaged and flitting from moment to moment; clearly "in her head". A head tone resonance vibrates at a higher pitch. The E vowel can be manipulated to take on a slightly nasal quality, which also places emphasis on the forehead and sinus region, matching the focus of the intervention to the head region. Singing in this place allowed me to empathize and meet Jamie where she was at that particular moment.

Watching Jamie's face for reactions I began to slow the movement of the melodic pattern, sustaining the tones and adding more audible breath sounds as well as glissandi. The movement of the melody and the melodic pattern, traveling up and down the Dorian scale reflected both the movements of Jamie's thoughts, the rapid changing of emotions and the small physical movements of her body as she struggled to settle into a safe, comfortable place.

With each passing phrase I began to slow the melodic movement while simultaneously lowering the pitches of the improvisation, until the melody only involved three to four different changing notes. Harmonically I continued to use the three open Dm Am and Em chords on the guitar, maintaining a relatively constant tempo through an improvised plucking pattern, which I based loosely on Jamie's breathing rate. I began to slow the movement of the melodic pattern on the vowel "E" with each phrase containing only between three and four different notes and ending each phrase with a sustained and breathy "ay" sound on the descending glissando indicating a transition to the next phase. With each "A" vowel, I lowered the pitch and concentrated on feeling the resonance of the tone move from my head to my throat. In this new vocal register, I continued the improvisation slowing the melodic pattern, phasing out the "E" vowel and replacing it slowly with the A vowel until I was improvising solely with one sound.

Phase II: Descension-Vowel "A" (pronounced "Ay")
Jamie's facial grimaces had stopped and her face seemed at rest as she appeared to be concentrating on her breathing, with her eyes closed. I lowered the pitch and manipulated the resonance of the sound until I felt the buzzing in my neck and throat area, vocally and physically reflecting the movements in Jamie as I observed her motion decrease, particularly in her forehead and face indicating her initial steps toward relaxation. The change in vowel as well as the lowering of the pitch changed the shape of my vocal cavity (head, mouth, and neck region) to a more open space, in turn changing the tone frequency, vibration and overall timbre of the vocal sound. Throughout this second phase I continued the "A" vowel improvisation, lessening the melodic movement until it involved only two to three changing sustained notes, and lowering the pitches of the improvised melody, musically encouraging Jamie to descend further into the relaxation. The slowing of the tempo, the decreasing of the melodic and rhythmic movement, and the decrease in the number of notes sung all reflected Jamie's descension into the relaxation. I continued to use only descending two-tone intervals, slowly decreasing the dynamic and sustaining the last note of each phrase, signally a transition to Phase III.

Phase III: Entrainment-Vowel "I"
(pronounced without the "Y" as in "ah")
I continued to emphasize the breath by increasing the breathy quality of my own voice as I sang each "Ah". The continual descension of the body relaxation into the chest region began the actual focus on entrainment. Throughout this second phase I dropped to two chords, Am and Em as I transitioned into the A Aolian mode. Changing the mode from D Dorian to

A Nordoff-Robbins Based Vocal Music Therapy Intervention

A Aolian was a subjective decision on my part to reflect the process changing from an open journey to a floating suspension, as if the body has fallen into an open vacuous space and was now suspended in the air. The shift to two chords and two tones sung on the descending intervals with the emphasis on the glissandi reflected the floating and then descension deeper and deeper into the relaxation.

Watching Jamie's chest rise and fall and using Jamie's breathing pattern as a guide, I began to slow the tempo of the improvisation, initiating the phenomenon of *entrainment*. I supported this process by slowly decreasing the number of vocal tones until I was singing only two notes. I further supported the process by singing the first tone with the inhalation and the second tone with the exhalation. The matching of Jamie's inhalation and exhalation to the movement of the tones and chords emphasized and encouraged the entrainment process.

Each initial note was followed by a glissandi down to the subsequent note, reflecting the descension into deeper relaxation. Throughout this phase of the intervention Jamie's body movements gradually ceased, with the exception of a few hand twitches, indicating to me her descent into a light sleep state. Her breathing appeared rhythmic, light and steady and her face was calm.

Phase IV: Deepening-Vowel "O" (pronounced "oh")
Once I felt entrainment had been solidly established, I continued the gradual descension into the lower body by transitioning to the vowel "O" (pronounced long "Oh") manipulating the resonance until the sound was fully open and resonating in my lower chest and abdomen region, a vocal reflection of the movement of the relaxation into Jamie's lower region. The pitch was quite low in my own register. Lower pitches vibrate at a slower frequency. In order to create the low sound on an "O" vowel I focused on keeping the air flowing while simultaneously creating an open sound deep within my own chest and abdomen. I continued with the Am and Em chords on the guitar and using two low tones on the vowel "O", and carefully watched Jamie's breathing pattern as I slowed the tempo, decreased the dynamic and lowered the pitches even more. I observed a few more hand twitches as Jamie appeared to fall deeper into sleep. Once again, as with each previous transition, I gradually changed the vowel from "O" to the vowel "U" (pronounced "ooh") on the second note by adding it to the end of the phrase and then eventually phasing out the "O". The pitches were very low in my register.

Phase V: Holding-Vowel "U" (pronounced "Ooh")
At this point in the improvisation, Jamie appeared to be sleeping so my goal was to maintain and support this sleeping state by creating a holding pattern, possibly allowing her to fall into an even deeper sleep state. My guitar pattern was still switching between Am and Em at this phase. I began to repeat only the playing of the Em chord and sustaining the vocal "U", using long breathy, very low tones at the bottom of my register, feeling the buzzing at the very base of my chest cavity and lower abdomen.

I then played a sustained Em chord followed by a G major chord, softly, strumming once in the same pattern, one long slow strum allowing the time for the strings to vibrate softly. I slowly and softly sang the same low pitched sustained "U" over the G chord. The transition to the U (ooh) vowel, sustained in a very low tone, along with the shift to just one G chord reflected the shift from descension into a stable, steady place of ultimate relaxation and sleep. The musical movements at this time were subtle, slow and careful so as to support a seamless transition. Jamie's breathing was light, her face was calm and her mouth was slightly open. In order to continue the final transition to the holding pattern that would hold and continue to "rock" Jamie as she slept, I added a C chord, re-introducing a ¾ lullaby rhythm once again in a very slow tempo.

The musical reflection of Jamie's being held and rocked as she slept was produced by the transition to the G major I-V chord pattern and the vocal reflection of a sustained unmoving stable "ooh" vowel. I held this "place" of rest and sleep for Jamie for several minutes. Often when I am conducting a progressive relaxation, the client will awaken slightly after several moments of sleeping, guiding me to transition from a relaxation to a gradual re-awakening and re-energizing process, which I carry out by reversing my process, working backwards through the different body regions and vowels, adding movement, tempo, dynamic and ascending intervals and elevating pitches. However, after several minutes of observing Jamie sleep, I determined that the intervention was over, as Jamie was in the state she needed to attain, a deep restful sleep. Eventually I faded out the vocals, followed by the guitar and then waited in the silence. Jamie was soundly sleeping. As quietly as possible, I nodded goodbye to Jamie's father, and left the room.

Conclusion

The intervention described above is a common vocal intervention that I use in the treatment of pain. While the musical choices and vocal improvisation were spontaneous and subjective on my part, they were based on clinical experience working with the voice in the treatment of patients experiencing pain in a hospital setting. I have found that the conscious, intentional use of the elements described in this chapter make this intervention effective in inducing relaxation and increasing breath flow in the clients thus reducing the sensation and experience of pain.

From a music centered music psychotherapy perspective, the efficacy of the intervention was determined by the music created, including the production of the sound, the quality of the tones, resonance of the vibration, and all of the musical elements involved, including the pitch, melody, rhythm, dynamic, intervals, meter, etc. The clinical application of each musical element relied on my ability, as the therapist, to respond to Jamie's spontaneous physiological, emotional and cognitive movements using knowledge of the voice, vocal cavity, sound production and vocal musical improvisation. Because the voice is my primary instrument for both musical creation and clinical communication, a thorough understanding of ways to use the voice to adapt and change with Jamie's spontaneous and subtle physiological and emotional states was imperative to the success of the treatment.

References

1. Nordoff P, Robbins C. *Creative Music Therapy: A Guide to Fostering Clinical Musicianship.* 2nd ed. Gilsum, NH: Barcelona; 2007.
2. Zhao H, Chen A. Both happy and sad melodies modulate tonic human heat pain. *J Pain.* 2009; 10 (9): 953-960.
3. Loewy J. The use of music psychotherapy in the treatment of pediatric pain. In: Dileo C. ed. *Music Therapy and Medicine: Theoretical and Clinical Applications.* Silver Spring, MD; American Music Therapy Association; 1999: 189-206.
4. Sand-Jecklin D, Emerson H. The impact of a live therapeutic music intervention on patients' experience of pain, anxiety, and muscle tension. *Holist Nurs Pract.* 2010; 24(1): 7-15.
5. Robb S, Nichols R, Rutan R, Bishop B, Parker J. The effects of music assisted relaxation on preoperative anxiety. *J Music Ther.* 1995; 32(1):2-22.
6. Good M, Anderson G, Ahn S, Cong X, Stanton-Hicks M. Relaxation and music reduce pain following intestinal surgery. *Res Nurs Health.* 2005; 28(3)240-251.
7. Klassen JA, Liang Y, Tjosvold L, Klassen TP, Hartling L. Music for pain and anxiety in children undergoing medical procedures: a systemized review of randomized clinical trials. *Ambul Pediatr.* 2008; 8(2):117-128.

8. Austin D. The psychophysiological effects of music therapy in intensive care units: music therapy is inexpensive with significant physiological and psychological benefits says donna austin. *Ped Nurs.* 22:14-20.
9. Henry L. Music therapy: a nursing intervention for the control of pain and anxiety in the icu: a review of recent literature. *Dimens Crit Care Nurs.* 1995; 14(6):295-304.
10. Hunter BC, Oliva R, Sahler OJ, Gaisser D, Salipante DM, Arezina CH. Music therapy as an adjunctive treatment in the management of stress for patients being weaned from mechanical ventilation. *J Music Ther.* 2010. XLVII (3): 198-219.
11. Mazer S. Music noise and the environment of care: history, theory and practice. *Music Med* 2010; 2(3):182-191.
12. Schneider A, Biebuyck J. Music in the operating room. *Lance.* 1990; 335 (8702): 1407.
13. Short A, Ahern N, Holdgate A, Morris J, Sidhu B. Using music to reduce noise stress for patients in the emergency department: a pilot study. *Music Med.* 2010; 2(4):201-207.
14. Muller BJ. Working with children in pain: the music therapist's perspective. In Loewy JV, ed. *Music Therapy and Pediatric Pain.* Cherry Hill, NJ: Jeffrey Books; 1997: 69-80.
15. Standley J. Meta-analysis of research in music and medical treatment: effect size as a basis for comparisons across multiple dependent and independent variables. In: Spintge R, Droh R, ed. *Music medicine;* St. Louis, MO: Barcelona; 1992; 364-378.
16. Standley J. Music research in medical treatment. In: *Effectiveness of music therapy procedures: documentation of research and clinical practice.* Silver Spring, MD: American Music Therapy Association; 2000.
17. Jonas: Mosby's Dictionary of Complementary and Alternative Medicine. Iso-principle. The Free Dictionary by Farlex. http://medical-dictionary.thefreedictionary.com/iso+principle. Published 2005. Accessed June 29, 2012.
18. Dileo C. ed. *Music therapy and medicine: theoretical and clinical applications.* Silver Spring, MD: American Music Therapy Association; 1999.
19. Gaynor M. *The healing power of sound: recovery from life threatening illness using sound, voice and music.* Boston, MA and London, England, Shambhala: 2002.
20. Sauter D, Eisner F, Ekman P, Scott S. Cross-cultural recognition of basic emotions through nonverbal emotional vocalizations. *PNAS.* 2010; 107 (6): 2408-2412.

21. Scherer K. Expression of emotion in voice and music. *J Voice*.1995; 9 (3): 235-248.
22. Mithin S. *The Singing Neanderthals: The Origins of Music, Language, Mind and Body*. Cambridge, MA: Harvard University Press; 2006.
23. Levman B. The genesis of music and language. *Ethnomusicology*. 1992; 36: 147-170.
24. Cook, O. *Singing with your own voice*. London, England: Nick Hern Books; 2004.
25. Austin, D. *The Theory and Practice of Vocal Psychotherapy: Songs of the Self*. London, England and Philadelphia, PA; Jessica Kingsley Publishers; 2008.
26. Harrison P. *The Human Nature of the Singing Voice: Exploring a Holistic Basis for Sound Teaching and Learning*. Edinburgh, Scotland: Dunedin Academic Press; 2005.
27. Uhlig S, Baker F. ed. *Voicework in Music Therapy*. London, England and Philadelphia, PA; Jessica Kingsley; 2011.
28. Uhlig S. *Authentic Voices, Authentic Singing: A Multicultural Approach to Vocal Music Therapy*. Gilsum, NH: Barcelona; 2006.
29. Heman-Acka YD. The science of breath and the voice. In: Boston J, Cook R, ed. *Breath in Action: The Art of Breath in Vocal and Holistic Practice*. London, England and Philadelphia, PA; Jessica Kingsley; 2009:21-32.
30. Martin S. A short history of breath from womb to tomb. In: Boston J, Cook R, ed. *Breath in Action: The Art of Breath in Vocal and Holistic Practice*. London, England and Philadelphia, PA; Jessica Kingsley; 2009: 33-42.
31. Loewy J. Tonal intervallic synthesis as integration in medical music therapy. In: Baker F, Uhlig S, ed. *Voicework in Music Therapy*. London, England and Philadelphia, PA; Jessica Kingsley Publishers; 2011:252-268.
32. Loewy J. The musical stages of speech: a developmental model of pre-verbal sound making. *Music Ther*. 1995; 13 (1):47-73.
33. Thane E. A vocal-led relaxation for children with autism spectrum disorders. In: Baker F, Uhlig S, ed. *Voicework in Music Therapy*. London, England and Philadelphia, PA; Jessica Kingsley Publishers; 2011: 41-62.
34. Idiopathic scoliosis. Mosby's Medical Dictionary, 8th edition. http://medicaldictioary.thefreedictionary.com/idiopathic+scoliosis. Published 2009. Accessed June 1, 2012.

Music and Medicine: Integrative Models in the Treatment of Pain

CHAPTER 14

A Symphony of Life: Harvesting Emotions by Preserving Legacy and Honoring Pain

Brian H. Schreck MA, MT-BC

"So I think there is again this word love. It's capable of so many transformations that can be then something quite practical. And it all comes down to—It's all celebration. Adventure and celebration. Music is the one way in which you can imagine that world—Music that speaks to the human soul, but originates somewhere else, that tells the music, the human soul, that you originate somewhere else. This is the voice of home."
Clive Robbins, 2005

Introduction
Movement 1: Introductory Motif

The first movements in a symphony are commonly fast, weighty in content and feeling—striving towards beauty. It is my intention that this overture structures this composition of life to illuminate innovative practices of medical music therapy to combat pain. Pain, in musical terms, acts as the "accidental", which as we know is a sign that raises or lowers a given diatonic pitch, deviating from its key signature. It is easy to think that we are the writers of our symphonies, but as strong as the mind is, the body is often holding the pencil and eraser. When pain puts an accidental in our patient's melody it is the job of the music therapist to make that note resolve, resound, and more importantly, sound and feel right.

The word "symphony" means sounding together.[1] Creating musical life during all stages of illness is an adventure, and with any adventure it is not known exactly how it will end; there must be the hope that we will get somewhere together, even if it is not exactly where we expected. In this act of creation, as music therapists we can shape what the end of the symphony could sound like while the composition is still being written. This unknown unfolds the wondrous capability that music can facilitate at every critical, vulnerable, and fragile part of life. In this crucial time constraint music can provide a synergistic symphony of life in an environment that may be actively moving towards the opposite, for not only the patient, but for their families, friends, and attending medical staff as well.

Music and Medicine: Integrative Models in the Treatment of Pain

For the chronically ill patient and their families, illness and the progression of treatments may be the prominent melody of their symphonic life. At times the patient's disease and emotional state modulates without audible support of the symphonic body. My fellow music therapists and I can aid by serving as beckoning horn in the recapitulation, bringing back tonality and harmony to life at the time of the unknown progression. It is an honor to be with someone's pain. It is an honor to be with people in their worse day thus far. To know that there may be more terrible days ahead is a dark, looming realization. Despite this, it is a music therapist's privilege to reintroduce joy through this practical love with music to structure each patient and family's symphony of life through their amazing adventure and struggle with moving in and out of the hospital.

For the past eight years I have served hundreds of patients and their families from the introduction of palliative care through the end of the life. I have harvested 1,840 recordings with the patients and families I have served. These recordings immortalize our experiences in music therapy and in their lives. The legacy created is timeless and accessible. These gifts of time—to quote a very special physician in our palliative care service—are "Priceless. The ability of a parent or adolescent to leave an audio/musical memory…the ability to play a siblings words and songs while their brother/sister is dying and they can't be present…priceless!".[2]

In my current practice at our pediatric hospice we offer bereavement service for two years with the bereaved. I am grateful for this possibility and time to have been a part of their loved one's past, their present and, with clinical rationale, their future. Music therapy can successfully engage with ease throughout these milestones and realities of life and continue to flourish, grow and celebrate the pain and suffering that make up our stories of existence and of living.

Is it possible for acute and chronic illness to have beauty in sterility, hope in terrible crisis, and meaning throughout the entire experience of living with disease? Dr. Joanne Loewy writes:

> What would it mean to rejoice in all that occurred in one's lifetime with a finale? A finale is defined as "the last and often climactic event or item in a sequence".[3(p469)] A finale of a symphonic work often has shadows or remembrances of themes that occurred throughout the entire piece. Although the circumstances of one's death may be complex and replete with pain and illness, how wondrous it could be if we were able to plan the way we die with more dignity, intention and focus.[4(p xvi)]

As a clinical-creative music therapist, I do everything in my imagination to accompany and structure my patient's emotional and physical pain. Through harvesting their stories and emotions, recordings can be created together. Once this is made available, it can then be a functional source of reflection and remembrance. This can then be accessed at the listener's will, throughout the beginning, middle and end of illness. It is also this writer's hope that these recordings will remain functional throughout the listener's life.

Stories make up our lives and when told, paint pictures of every emotion we are capable of experiencing. Despair, hope, terror, joy, anger, laughter, nausea, needles, tubes, air, breath, blood, sweat and tears are often present during the act of birth and the act of death. Finding comfort in this discomfort takes practice.

And like our patients and their families, we too will one day be in a similar situation. Using the philosophy of today, instead of yesterday or tomorrow, we as music therapists, being a strong component of the multi-disciplinary medical team, can promote, advocate, and transform the transition that each of us will all go through one day. We can help create a bridge between mind, body, and heart throughout the medical experience. This will be achieved by using the day as a sacred gift of time to pioneer the implementation of music therapy in meeting, assessing and treating emotional and physical pain.

Movement 2: Making Every Moment Count

The second movement in a symphony may be slow and solemn. In this movement I will describe my work in perinatal hospice and the interventions that transformed emotional and physical pain by making every moment count. The ability to be with patients and families in their homes has been such a gift. Through this continuum of care, a deeper relationship can be formed outside of the sterile hospital facilitates allowing for an ease in the delivery of music therapy interventions both in and out of the home.

To daily affirm and practice before entering a patient's room, to: First, look at the (dying) person in front of you and think of that person as just like you, with the same needs, the same fundamental desire to be happy and avoid suffering, the same loneliness, the same fear of the unknown, the same secret areas of sadness, the same half-acknowledged feelings of helplessness.[5]

Our perinatal hospice program is for women (and their families) who learn during pregnancy that the baby they are carrying has a terminal health condition. We help these families through pregnancy and delivery, and after. The following story describes these events and the clinical outcomes that were possible through the use of music therapy in peri-natal hospice and bereavement.

From the Hippocratic Oath: In every house where I come I will enter only for the good of my patients.[6]

Amy's Song of Kin
My first perinatal visit was co-treated with the bereavement coordinator. We met the couple at the extended-stay hotel they lived in until they could save enough money for an apartment. I try to picture myself as them; answering the door and letting me come in. What would I expect a music therapist to do for me, my significant other, and our unborn child, who after delivery may live for a minute, for a week, or for months? This uncertainty is enough to cause a forecast of dissonance that has the potential to make the symphony sound like a scene in a horror movie.

I was told that Adam (dad) works nights and has been asleep for the past two visits. Adam sat up and joined us at the table near the window. They had a young black cat who instinctually knew that I was allergic to it, and from that moment of shared realization, did not leave me alone throughout the session. I asked Amy if she liked to sing. She shyly smiled and nodded yes. I followed up with, "Is there a song that you connect with your unborn child or feelings that you have been feeling lately?" She replied, "Alicia Keys' "If I Ain't Got You"." The chorus of this song reads: "Some people want it all/ But I don't want nothing at all/ If it ain't you baby/ If I ain't got you baby".[7] Using GarageBand on a Macintosh laptop, Amy recorded her vocals alongside Alicia Keys. At first she was embarrassed to sing in front of us, so the bereavement coordinator and I went outside and sat in my car.

Adam was smiling as he motioned us back in the hotel room. To give her a break I asked him similar questions. He spoke about his other three children (from a previous relationship) and the music they like. Since the news of the complications surrounding her pregnancy, Amy stated that it was very difficult for her to be around other kids. Adam respected Amy's wishes. It had been a few weeks since they had seen Adam's other three children. He reported calling the three at their mother's house every day. I invited the couple to video record a message that could be sent to their current address. Adam liked this idea. The bereavement coordinator and I stepped out again. The couple recorded a five-minute message telling the kids how much they loved them and how they couldn't wait to have a space that was comfortable for all of them to be together, once they were back on their feet. The DVD was mailed to where Adam's children lived.

I then asked Amy about a Song of Kin. She replied, "I wrote this down in a notebook once I found out I was pregnant." By this point in the

Harvesting Emotions by Preserving Legacy & Honoring Pain

session, she felt comfortable enough to sing it in front of us. She began to sing: "Please put your hands down on me/ Show the world what you can do/ Thanks for giving me this baby/ I beg to see his life through/ I know I'm not perfect, but I give my life to you/ Please shine your light on me/ Show the world what you can do!" Using the guitar, I played a simple chord progression in the key she was singing. She sang it over and over. I pressed record on GarageBand. Adam looked proud as he watched Amy sing while holding her belly.

The CD with her Song of Kin was brought to the hospital when Amy was in active labor. Many of the alarms had been turned off. I had my guitar and asked her if I could play to help her relax. She agreed and was smiling with her eyes closed. After the session was finished, I showed Adam where the CD player was and we put her CD in the player. He pressed play as myself, the bereavement coordinator and the chaplain exited. The bereavement coordinator and the chaplain went over the birthing plan with the nurse.

What could be one of the happiest days in this couple's lives now is shadowed by sadness. Amy's stance was focused on the baby living and even if for just a short while. She had two wishes of things she wanted to do while her baby lived: to feel the baby's breath and dress her in an outfit she had chosen for this occasion. I cannot express to the reader how intense this feeling of love and hope for their unborn child was while sharing time with this couple. In the end her labor lasted for over 24 hours during which she lost a lot of blood. The baby girl was rushed from Amy after delivery. The baby girl was returned to her, dead and fully clothed. Amy reported how excruciating it was to have this experience of dressing her baby taken away from her.

The three of us (bereavement coordinator, chaplain) arrived the next morning on the maternity unit. Amy was sobbing audibly from the hall. She was exhausted and in a state of emotional panic. No family was present other than Adam. Amy had a phobia of blood and was desperately trying to get the nurse to turn off the transfusion she was receiving due to the loss of blood during delivery. Amy was terrified she was going to get AIDS from the blood and screamed, "All I want to do is get the fuck out of here and go home!" Adam was on the couch with the covers pulled over his head. As a team we worked together to first assist in decreasing Amy's anxiety of the blood transfusion. Live music was created using the acoustic guitar. I sat next to Adam on the couch. He emerged from his covers and nodded. The gentle music appeared to initiate a structure to contain Amy and Adam's emotional pain, allowing both to calm down and begin to talk. Amy's nurse made eye contact with me as she hung another bag of blood and mouthed "Thank you," as the chaplain and bereavement coordinator openly listened and supported Amy's processing of the previous night. Adam engaged in active conversation with me as the live-music-assisted-relaxation was implemented.

It was at the end of our initial assessment session in the hotel room that Amy discovered the song "Beautiful" by the hip-hop artist Eminem. She found the song to be "justifying" in regards to her pregnancy experience as it compared to that of others. The chorus reads:

> *In my shoes, just to see / What it's like to be me I'll be you, let's trade shoes/ Just to see what it'd be like To feel your pain, you feel mine/ Go inside each other's minds /Just to see what we'd find / Look at '*stuff' through each other's eyes.*[8]

A brief a capella version was facilitated during this bereavement visit to present a prepared prerecorded CD mix of songs that were important to Amy and Adam as well as songs that were appropriate for this time in the hospital, including the aforementioned Eminem song. The CD was placed in the DVD player. Adam was invited by us to sit on Amy's bed. The couples' emotional pain appeared to be significantly diminished and manageable upon our exit. Medical staff was appreciative as we left the unit.

In a follow up visit, Amy reported that she was glad to have the recordings, but was not yet ready to listen to them. Amy and Adam continued to utilize our bereavement services. During a recent bereavement visit Amy reported listening to the song she wrote, "when I need to cry." On another visit near mother's day the bereavement coordinator shared with the team that Adam had written Amy a letter. He wrote, "You are a mother, and you always will be." Amy and Adam can't wait to try to have more children together.

With a limited number of visits before Amy's baby died, we used the philosophy of making every moment count to decrease this young couple's emotional and physical pain. In our last bereavement visit Amy and Adam requested the bereavement coordinator and I meet them at a park to release balloons to celebrate/honor their lost child's first birthday. Amy requested for the song "So Hard To Say Goodbye To Yesterday" by Boyz II Men to be played during the release. Amy brought enough balloons for each of us to write a message on. The song was played while we let go of the balloons. Adam held Amy as she cried. The couple opened their arms to embrace the bereavement coordinator and I. Amy and Adam said, "We don't know if we could've gotten through all of this without you guys." Amy and Adam are expecting their second baby.

Harvesting Emotions by Preserving Legacy & Honoring Pain

Movement 3: Scherzo, "What We Play Is Life!"
(Louis Armstrong[9])

The third movement in a symphony may be fast-moving and humorous. Being in a hospital can feel very much the same. Days last forever and there is a quiet heaviness of uncertainty that weighs over everyone. When a family member makes eye contact as you pass one another in the hall, there is an unspoken transmission of emotions beyond the conjured smile. All of the agonizing days, months, and years inside the confines of the hospital that patients and their families endure can obscure the positive feelings patients experience when home.

This movement will describe a patient that was both fast-moving and humorous throughout his countless hospitalizations. This patient was nicknamed by his little sister who could not pronounce "Christopher." She crowned him with the nickname "Critter", that fit him so exquisitely it stuck forever. I met Critter when he was nine and worked with him through his thirteenth birthday. In one of our first sessions, I introduced the electric guitar to him. Much like his name, it fit him so exactly, it stayed by his side in and out of the hospital much like a warrior's sword supplies strength and power. Critter once said, "When I pick up the guitar and start playing, it clears my mind...when I play I think I'm famous...it just erases everything, and helps me get through it."[10]

Critter was a horror movie aficionado and a lover of the rock band KISS. He had pure rock n' roll running through his veins. When the electric guitar was placed in his arms for the first time he began taking a tremelo solo like Neil Young with such intention and love it made everyone present laugh with joy! The first riff Critter learned was Metallica's "Entersandman." It was his go-to melody to play whenever first picking up his axe. We played this riff together one time through the halls with battery-powered amplifiers all the way into his surgery. Surgeons and nursing staff looked at us both with initial puzzlement that morphed into curious smiling as we rolled passed them.

It was discovered in one of these exploratory scopes that Critter had developed a fungal infection in one of his lungs that required resection. This surgery was complicated due to his current health and there was a chance he would not make it out of the surgery. Critter did. This was one of many medical hardships Critter endured often with the odds stacked up against him. We recorded our time together before this major surgery to regain focus and redirect anxiety for everyone present in his room.

After the surgery we began to record everything he learned on the guitar from Deep Purple to Kiss to more Metallica, to Blue Oyster Cult, to Pearl Jam to Blind Melon to Lynyrd Skynyrd. As his sixth grade talent show approached, Critter in his second relapse of leukemia asked me if I would play a song with him for this important show. I suggested we write a song instead of playing someone else's. He agreed and in a few sessions had written the following song in one of his school notebooks.

"The Battlefield"

My Cancer's like a battlefield
That I just keep on rockin' through
Every day and night I fight
And I just keep on rockin' through
Fartin' and makin' it right
Hoagies, fries and sprite
I just keep rockin' through

My Cancer Is A Battlefield

Cancer is a battlefield
IV pumps and hospital beds
That I just keep on rockin' through
Doctors and nurses all around
That I just keep on rockin' through
Pepsi, steak, & corn
That I just keep on rockin' through

Battlefield, battlefield
My cancer is a battlefield!"

Upholding his stylistic preferences as well as supporting his abilities on the guitar, I helped by offering chords that he could play to accompany his phenomenal lyrics. After listening to the finished recording together, a look of accomplishment and satisfaction washed over his face.

In speaking directly to Critter about his disease he stated:
"When I sat down to ask God to help me with cancer, I wasn't specific enough…cancer is going good, but they found another spot on my lung, a few spots on my brain."

Through struggling with emotional and physical pain, Critter began to want more and more pain medicine to get through his hospitalizations as well as just to feel good. Critter was hospitalized once from saving a few of these strong medications and taking them all at once to get "drunk" and feel good. Weaning him off of these powerful drugs was difficult for the young man. During this hospitalization we used vocal improvisation and free association to work through the emotional layers of the episode. Critter began singing about wanting to go back to school and to be normal: "I'm finally at school! Guess who I'm talking to now...all of those girls, all of my friends, my mama in the office, giving candies, giving me drinks, giving me everything I want...Thank you, thank you, thank you, I appreciate it so very much, later!"

Both of us had no idea this would be our last recording together. He requested to sing "Free bird" by Lynyrd Skynyrd. The intervention involved reading which stimulated cognition and focus. Critter read and sang as I played the chords.

During his next and last hospitalization, Critter was depressed. For the first time ever, he did not want to play or listen to music. Our last discussion was about his talent show and he did not say much other than nodding in agreement with playing "The Battlefield." Critter went into septic shock and was in the ICU for a number of days sedated and intubated.

CDs were made and pictures were printed off of our experiences together. Music medicine was created of all of his favorite music and played in the room. I engaged his family in singing songs around his bed. One of Critter's cousins was given a guitar to borrow so that he could continue to play for him.

Upon walking into the hospital a few days later, Critter's mother, father, and family greeted me crying. His mother hugged me and said, "My baby's dying." His father said, "I just want to trade places with him...he is too young." His mother then asked me, "What about his talent show? Will you still play it?" I responded, "Of course."

Critter's family wished to have him transported to the hematology and onconlogy floor where he had spent all of his time as an inpatient. There he would be with all of his favorite nurses and medical staff. The palliative care room was the closest place to home we could find --jam-packed with forty of Critter's closest family, friends and medical staff.

A nurse present that day writes: "On the day it became evident that Critter would lose his battle, Brian stayed with him and his family in the ICU, playing the songs that Critter loved, singing with the family and providing them with CD copies of the recordings. As we walked Critter back to A5 South in his bed, still on the ventilator, Brian was there, playing the music that meant so much to Critter. When the family gathered around Critter's bedside to say a final goodbye, his father requested that Brian come and be close to the family. He was an essential part of Critter's care team, and his presence and music at the end of the journey provided such a comfort to the family."

When approaching the bedside with his immediate family, Critter's attending physician in the Intensive Care Unit explained with such compassion, calmness and beauty what was about to happen when Critter was extubated. He invited everyone to say what they wanted to before this occurred. I began playing "Release" by Pearl Jam, which was one of the family's favorite bands. Lyrics include: "I hold the pain, release me."[11] His father gave me a nod in acknowledgement of this choice. Within seconds of extubation Critter left his body. His father looked around with a sad exclamation of laughter and said, "Look at that smile! He's smiling!"

At the funeral I sat next to Critter's open casket. I used prerecorded music to accompany my live electric and acoustic guitar. The Vitamin String Quartet's renditions of "Entersandman," "Back In Black," "Jeremy," "I Don't Wanna Miss A Thing," "Sweet Child O' Mine," and "Carry On" were played with live electric guitar during the processional. As more people arrived I played and sang Pearl Jam's "Just Breathe," The Pretenders' "I'll Stand By You," The Offspring's "Gone Away." Every song was important to different family members and it was a live review of their life shared with this young man. The same nurse present throughout Critter's experience wrote: "Critter's best friend is a current patient, and at the funeral, he wanted to sing a song he had written. Brian assisted him in playing, and I believe that in the difficult months ahead for this child, Brian will also bring comfort through the love of music that all three share."

As the family said their last goodbyes a prerecording of Kiss's "Shout It Outloud," "Detroit Rock City," and "Rock n' Roll All Nite" was played in the parlor.

A few months later it was time for the talent show. Our last recording of Critter's vocal improvisation was used to introduce us. Using our previous recordings, my laptop was plugged into the P.A. Through the harvesting of Critter's stories, time and music, his classmates and teachers were able to hear his own voice singing praise once again and give a final goodbye: "Thank you, thank you, thank you, I appreciate it very much…later!" This was such a gift! I accompanied with live guitar Critter's Battlefield, sung by Critter just like we would've done it if he were there.

For four years Critter and his family lived with uncertainty and tumultuous emotional and physical pain. When we were together and "Shouting Outloud" his symphony of life, our shared time was fast-moving and humorous. Critter's mother recounts:

> "Well I know for me music was like an outlet to help forget about all the pain Critter was in and all the worry of the possibility of maybe one day having to let him go. It's like when you came into the room his smile did as well. He'd grab that guitar and all of us would sing and put

everything else to the side. I was listening to his CD's, it's funny you can hear beneath all the music and singing the pump beeping. But it was almost like we weren't even in the hospital when you were around. Not one of us mentioned it though. It reminded me of being at home with my family, doing what we did best, singing and playing the guitar. I don't think my life will ever be the same. I know that was the worst time of my life but yet the best as well. I spent so much time with my Critter, more than most parents, because we had a lot of one on one time. I miss so much laying on that bed with him, snuggling him, sleeping with him, and listening to "our music!" I'm so grateful for all the good times we had because of you Brian. You made all of us forget, even though it was for a little while each visit. I guess music therapy helps more people than the patients alone, so thank you."

Movement 4: The Voice of Home

It is our job to be grounded in the present. We as clinicians have to be aware of all of the information we are blessed to gain in our constant reevaluation of our projected outcome goals. It is of great importance that we use this information that is given to us to create meaningful interventions.

A twenty-four-year-old I spent five sessions with in our pediatric hospice program makes me think of this quote from my favorite movie, Ferris Bueler's Day Off, "Yep, I said it before and I'll say it again, Life moves pretty fast, you don't stop and look around once in a while, you could miss it!".[12] Chris lived his life with Duchenne muscular dystrophy. His favorite song was the "King of Wishful Thinking" by Go West. To learn from each patient and family we work with is what this is all about. Chris's optimism and happy-go-lucky attitude was contagious when spending time with him. These gifts of time have stayed with me when I think that I am having a bad day.

In all of our sessions at Chris's home, he was waiting in his room sitting up in his wheelchair. Chris's musical interests were in electronic music and due to his limited physical abilities his computer and the Internet were his window to the outside world. We used midi-controllers to create original electronic music. In one session we used NPR's "StoryCorps" questions to record stories that would've been otherwise unknown if not asked in this facilitated fashion.

Music and Medicine: Integrative Models in the Treatment of Pain

In what was not known at the time to be our second-to-last session, Chris presented for the first time lying in his bed. I did not have a session plan. Upon arrival Chris's mom stopped me in the hall before entering his room and commented that she noticed that he was much more weak and she felt uncertain how much time they had left with him. I asked her, "What would you like me to do today?" She responded, "I have heard from other bereaved DMD mom's that one thing they miss is the sound of the electric wheelchair." This was my starting point for the session.

Chris showed me and the child life specialist a YouTube video of Diego Stocco's, Music from a Tree.[13] In this clip Diego uses a multi-track to record with many different microphones rhythms and creativity to create music from a tree.

Since Chris had spent much of the last part of his life in his room, we agreed that we would record the music of his room. Chris's suction machine was turned on and with intention he maneuvered his mouth to make an interesting sound. We turned on his electric wheelchair and got every sound we could out of it. I used drum sticks on the railings and mattress of his bed. He had many re-used grocery store plastic bags to discard medical supplies in that I shook around and hit in the air. We discovered in this session that Chris had been collecting key rings from all over the world. This was kept in his closet in a plastic storage container. Hundreds of key rings were shook around to add to this symphony that had become his life. All that was left was to create a rhythm to hold all of this together. The microphone was placed close to Chris's mouth and he beat-boxed a rhythm much like a club beat: "Mmm cha Mmm cha, Mmm cha Mmm cha." This was looped as the foundation of this creative creation. This piece was in need of a title and Chris quickly retorted, "Music from an 8x8 room." This was recorded, distorted, and placed strategically throughout this electronic masterpiece. These were the sounds of his life. I added a synthesizer to pull it all together.

Before leaving Chris stated, "You know my favorite band's new album is coming out in a few months."

Upon returning to the hospital, I e-mailed the manager of this band. I expressed that one of their number one fans will most likely not be alive to hear their new album, and we would be grateful if Chris could hear one song as soon as possible. Their manager quickly responded and said he had spoken with the band and they were willing to share the entire album with Chris.

Sometimes in life miracles do happen. The manager e-mailed me and described that the singer of the band was coming to Cincinnati in the upcoming weekend, and asked if it was ok for him to hand-deliver the CD to Chris. Amazing right? As the Saturday approached I was phoned by one of our hospice team's nurses who said, "I think if it is possible, we should make this happen sooner than later." Chris's mom recounts:

> "Chris was more shocked, delighted, and excited than I had seen him in recent memory. The night before Brian came was a very hard one physically for Chris. Chris kept calling to me because he was in so much pain. Between IV medications, I was working on a cookie bouquet for him to give to the band, and at one point I said to him, "Do you want me to work on the cookies or take care of you?" His answer was, "Make the cookies, forget all about me." Can you imagine?"

The singer was available to change his plans to drop off the CD first thing upon arriving in Cincinnati. Chris was very tired but still up for this visit. I waited for the singer outside of the house and prepped him for what he was about to walk into. I also asked permission to record this experience. He agreed. Inside Chris's room were his immediate family and best friend.

He came in with the first pressing of their new CD as well as everything they had ever done including wristbands and t-shirts. We immediately turned on the record. Chris was able to talk and said, "This is the most awaited album of the year!" I told the singer that Chris and I had been working on a piece of music and invited him (if it was ok with Chris) to sing whatever he wanted on it. Chris's favorite band's singer recorded a fun and outrageous finale to this symphony of his life. Chris was smiling under his bi-pap and his eyes were alert and focused as this was occurring.

Chris's mom baked ornate cookies with the band's logo on them as a measure of gratitude for making such a special visit. The singer was overwhelmed with appreciation.

After the generous musician left I came back into Chris's room, put one of their wristbands on his wrist and asked, "How cool was that?" Chris responded, "Soooo coool!" I put the CD back on and said, "I love you buddy, everything is going to be fine!" He responded in his sweet and complete understanding, "I know," and closed his eyes. Chris died one hour later. A DVD and CD recording of these experiences were given to his family at his funeral. How wondrous it was by making every moment count, to be able to plan (as best as possible) the way Chris died—with dignity, intention, focus and finale! Chris's mother in bereavement reflected, "What a party we had on his last day! That visit was so special that I don't have words to express Chris's joy or my gratitude. The band allowed us to use their songs at Chris's memorial service. I know it wasn't written for Chris, but in my heart it is his song. I listen to it often and remember Chris's last day with love and gratitude." Chris's mother recounted:

> "A few months before Chris died, I was feeling very sad about the coming loss and began to cry. Chris asked me why I was crying. I told him that I was sad because he was leaving. He said, "You always knew it was going to happen." I said, "Yes, but it still hurts." He responded, "I'm not going anywhere any time soon." Later he rolled into to kitchen and said to me, "I know this is going to be hard on you, Mom, but you'll be okay. I also have his voice on CD and precious video of his last day on this planet to transport me back to my time with him."

Finale

To paraphrase fellow music therapist, Jane Edwards in a conversation we had in Ireland: I believe the first song on earth by humans is the one sung from a mother to their infant. To complete this circle and cycle of life by bring this chapter home, in finale, I would like to present two lullabies sung and recorded by a dying patient who had two small children. Mindy was a twenty-seven-year-old with metastatic desmoplastic round cell tumor, diagnosed in February of 2007. She died on January 3rd, 2009. She had two children at home, one three years of age and one eighteen months. The legacy themed intervention was to create lullabies for both children to create a consistent nightly ritual for coping and comfort.

With Mindy's country musical preferences in mind we were able to choose one song for each child. Mindy was from the south and had such a wonderful accent, perfect and sweet for lullabies. The three-year-old was a girl and Mindy chose "Baby Mine" from Dumbo sung by Allison Krauss. The eighteen-month-old was a boy and I presented the song "Godspeed" by the Dixie Chicks that Mindy exclaimed after hearing it for the first time, "This is perfect." Mindy was an artist and in between recording these songs she drew pictures to go along with them. Mindy recorded this introduction: For her daughter:

> *"Mommy knows how much you enjoy your little lullabies every night that you ask me to sing to you, so I thought that this one here was a beautiful lullaby and I thought it suited you perfectly and I thought this way if Mommy's not there you can have it with you always and you can listen to it how ever many times you want to baby to go to bed at night.*

And I hope you like it and hope you enjoy it cause' I love singing it for you, and I love you so very much!"

For her son:

"Mommy heard this song and the first thing I thought of was you...and I thought no matter where I'm at, no matter what you're doing, you can always have this with you to listen to and to hear at night and Mommy enjoyed so much making it so much baby, and I hope that you love it and hope you get to listen to it as much as often as you want to you. And I love you! Thank you babies!"

Using GarageBand, the original song was used to structure her vocals. Mindy was in so much physical pain due to her end-stage cancer and so much emotional pain from being away from her children that knowing that she was actively creating something that was going to alleviate some of this pain.

Both songs were edited using the same program. The original pre-recordings were cut and pasted throughout the final version to add strength and tiny finales at the end of the recordings. Mindy was very involved in this editing. The CD's were not burnt until they were "perfect." Many copies were made in hard cases to ensure that they would have extra copies if something would happen to the fragile discs. Recording this experience with Mindy was very important as a music therapist.

Music therapists have many roles: Composer, conductor, producer, performer, arranger, accompanist, artist, humorist, philanthropist, facilitator, supporter, educator, counselor, and documenter. These roles enable us to harvest our patient's emotions and find their voice and their home. Once this is accessed, we can create legacy through honoring their pain, their lives and their love—this is a symphony of life.

"Love is a very carefully cultivated or nurtured or protected approach to life. And love is also more like a rapturous adventure! But it's a strong regard for human life! I think as you get older, and you've had a lot of companions in your life who have died—they are very much still around and their love is around, and you're constantly nourished by their love. You're kind of imbibing it, taking it in. It's around you. It's influencing you."[14]

References

1. Dorak, MT. http://dorakmt.tripod.com/music/symphony.html, December 5, 2005.
2. Weidner, N. Personal Interview. Cincinnati, OH: Cincinnati Chidren's Hosptal Medical Center; 2008.
3. Mirriam-Webster on-line dictionary. 2006. http://www.m-w.com/dictionary/synergism. Accessed April 15, 2006.
4. Dileo C, Loewy JV, eds. Music Therapy at the End of Life. Cherry Hill, NJ: Jeffrey Books; 2005.
5. Rinpoche S. The Tibetan Book of Living and Dying. New York, NY: Harper-Collins Publishers; 1994.
6. Charpie M. A Magical Play of Love: Music Therapy as a Bridge between mother and baby in the neonatal intensive care unit.: Music Therapy Department, New York, University; 2002.
7. Keyes A. If I Ain't Got You. The Diary of Alicia Keys. New York, NY: J. Records; 2004.
8. Eminem. Beautiful. Eminem DP, trans. Relapse. 54 Sound, Effigy Studios; Ferndale, MI2009.
9. Laura Moncur's Motivational Quotes. Retrieved April 27th, 2006. http://www.quotations.com. Accessed April 27, 2006.
10. Cincinnati Children's Hospital. "Tell Me A Story". 2010 http://www.youtube.com/watch?v=JEXxVG550bs .
11. Pear Jam. "Release". Ten. Seattle, WA: London Bridge Studios; 1991.
12. Hughes J. Ferris Bueller's Day Off. 1986.
13. Stocco D. Music from a Tree. 2009. Accessed at http://www.youtube.com/watch?v=fY.
14. Robbins C. Personal Interview. Nordoff-Robbins Insitute, New York, NY2005.

CHAPTER 15

Audio-Communication: An Integrative Approach to Pain Treatment with Music Therapy

Iris Valentin BM

*"For those who do not love, disperses the music all hatred.
The restless are given peace, and those who weep are consoled.
Those who still do not know, find new ways
and those who reject everything win security and hope."*
Pablo Casals

Introduction

Music therapy in connection with pain treatment is usually understood as a nonverbal form of therapy, which enhances relaxation and regulates the imbalance of the parasympathetic and sympathetic nervous systems. The concept that I have developed, "Audio-Communication" is an empirically developed multi-modal therapy in which receptive-regulative music therapy is the main catalyst for an integrative approach to alleviating disturbing symptoms, does not only affect the stress-related symptoms but also focuses on the deeper psycho-social triggers which enhance pain. The most important aspect of this approach is the focus on a holistic perspective to pain. It is especially necessary to respect the interaction of all human levels that contribute to pain perception-the physical, mental and emotional state of the patient-in order to stabilize the health of the patient and give him the chance to deal with his pain so that he may himself influence his quality of life. This concept is based on the neuro-physiological model adapted to tinnitus therapy by Pawel Jastreboff[1] and the psychoneuroimmunology model of Ader and Cohen.[2]

When I started my work as a music therapist in an inpatient rehabilitation clinic in Germany, the majority of patients suffered from tinnitus. The word "tinnitus" derives from the Latin *tinnire,* meaning 'to ring,' and in English is defined as 'a ringing in the ears.' "Tinnitus is the conscious expression of a sound that originates in an involuntary manner in the head of its owner, or may appear to him to do so."[3]

I was asked to develop a form of therapy that would complement the existing program of sports therapy and counseling. Since "hearing" was the main topic, I built in different methods by which the patients not only considered their prime disturbance, but widened their perspectives to include the bio-psycho-social aspects of the situation. I learned that the tinnitus patient focuses on and may even obsess about tinnitus to the end of attributing his disorders solely to it. The ability to *listen* is disturbed. In this work it was important to redefine the act of hearing versus listening. Hearing is receiving information acoustically but listening is the awareness of what happens to one through what one hears. What better medium to activate self-awareness than music!

The concept needed a name: "Audio-Communication" was born. *Audio* focused on the hearing-listening aspect and *Communication* on the interaction between the group members. The latter additionally included focusing on the personal or internal dialogue between the different levels of perception: body language, emotional reaction and mental reaction.

As a whole then, this meant integrating group dynamics and sensitizing emotional awareness in a multi-faceted approach. Body awareness, relaxation strategies, elements of psychodrama and social therapy, and of course, music therapy all contributed to a concept that was developed to meet the needs of these individuals.

Stemming from this initial work with tinnitus patients, I became aware of common denominators in my work with oncology patients, namely, discomfort, distress and pain, and so I expanded the model to include this medical field. In the course of my clinical work the similarities of the disturbances that enhance pain became apparent. As a model underpinning the work with oncology patients, I implemented the theory of psychoneuroimmunology, which made the interaction between mind, emotions and body transparent. According to Ader and Cohen from the University of Rochester, "psychoneuroimmunology is the study of the interactions between psychological factors, the central nervous system, and immune function as modulated by the neuroendocrine system."[4] The psychoneuroimmunology model perceives the human being as a bio-psycho-social being and examines the 'network human being' at the molecular level.[5] David Spiegel from Stanford University goes a step further and defines illness as a communication disturbance between biological, psychological and social processes.[6]

So originating as a multi-modal group therapy, the framework based upon music receptive/regulative and active music therapy, lent well to the needs of both patients living with tinnitus and those with an oncology diagnosis. Patients acquiring an understanding as to the genesis of their pain experience can increase their ability to influence their perception of it, and immanently cope with their specific symptom-related, performance-inhibiting pain. The development and employment of new health-promoting and stabilizing strategies as occurs as a result of the counseling, self-experience and process of self-reflection inherent to Audio-Communication.

My development of Audio-Communication occurred as a response to human need, and so in presenting my work here, I hope to offer it as an effective method of pain treatment in both individual and group work. To better understand the impetus for the development of this approach, let us look at the specific relationship between pain and music.

Perspectives on Pain

The extension of Audio-Communication to a broader field of disorders brought up the point of defining pain, which is most often understood solely as a physically unpleasant sensation. According to the Merriam-Webster Dictionary, pain is defined as follows:

> a state of physical, emotional, or mental lack of well-being or physical, emotional, or mental uneasiness that ranges from mild discomfort or dull distress to acute often unbearable agony, may be generalized or localized, and is the consequence of being injured or hurt physically or mentally or of some derangement of or lack of equilibrium in the physical or mental functions (as through disease), and that usually produces a reaction of wanting to avoid, escape, or destroy the causative factor and its effects.[7]

Pain is the result of a biological reaction stimulated by an unpleasant experience, which in turn activates the autonomic nervous system, responsible for the life-saving stress reaction. It is important to understand that our stress reaction has two qualities: eustress and distress - and, accordingly, different hormone releases. Eustress releases the pain soothing endorphin and distress releases the pain increasing adrenaline. This reaction is autonomic and leads to the perception of pain, which is a result of neurological processing. Pain is not only an unpleasant sensory experience but also an emotional experience. Furthermore, pain is an important diagnostic feature and protects the body and spirit from further damage. Pain is not the enemy: The inability to alleviate and to counteract the distress reaction is the deficiency.

These facts open the door to possibilities of working with pain and activating compensatory processes, which are in our biological foundation, namely our so-called reptilian brain. If we are aware of the aspects that enhance pain perception, then it is possible to activate the counterpart in order to enable the pain victim to regulate his pain level. Further explanation of the concept helps to clarify what we are treating when working with pain.

Distress-Promoting Components:
Anxiety
Over- ambitiousness
Repressed grief
Dissatisfaction
Weakened self-image and self-esteem
Conflict avoidance strategies

Pain-Reducing Components:
Joy
Relaxation
Peace of mind
Understanding
Compassion

Another very important aspect in pain perception is the so-called "pain memory," which is the starting point for chronic pain. There was a time when people were told "be brave" or to "bite your teeth together" when painful situations arose. Today we know how dangerous these messages were: The brain does not forget. This memory is easily triggered by similar situations and can intensify the pain perception even when the pain stimulus is weak. The biological and emotional compensation for this is the plasticity of the brain as defined by Joseph LeDoux.[8] The brain compensates for damage by reorganizing and forming new connections between intact neurons. In order to reconnect, the neurons need to be stimulated through activity. We are capable of having new, pain-relieving experiences which lead to a reorganization of the brain.

The better we understand the source of pain and how many levels contribute to our perception of it, the better we can specifically employ music therapy to alleviate pain perception. Although the trigger for pain might be a physical stimulus, the subjective aspects that enhance the unpleasant perception are apparent and constitute the groundwork for the music therapeutic treatment.

To exemplify and specify the disturbances, described by Ader and Cohen, and Spiegel above, I constructed the iceberg model to illustrate the pain experience in both diagnoses. Both models can be seen in the Appendix at the end of the chapter. The table on the following page delineates the characteristics that are unique to both diagnoses.

TABLE 1

Disorders	Tinnitus	Oncology
Specific	acoustical deficiencies noise sensitivity balance disturbances	Side effects of: Surgery chemotherapy radiation
Physical	body tension restlessness nervousness	pain body tension nervousness
Emotional	sleeping disorders concentration problems anxiety depression	sleeping disorders grief anxiety depression
Social	Over-ambitiousness (burn-out) Weak self-protection skills (delimitation deficiencies) heteronomy conflict avoidance	Over-ambitiousness (burn-out) Weak self-protection skills (delimitation deficiencies) heteronomy conflict avoidance

Music and Medicine: Integrative Models in the Treatment of Pain

The Role of Music in the Treatment of Pain

Music has always been a medium with which mankind has enriched his life and subsequently influenced his well-being. Enjoying music is life-style, using music as a tool to specifically influence human processes is a benefit of music therapy. The greatest asset of music as a therapeutic intermediate is the holistic effectiveness. This is the bridge to the implementation of music in pain treatment.

    Fundamental to this idea is the use of specific components in pain-focused interventions. Rhythm and tempo have a direct influence on the physiological parameters such as the level of stress hormones, muscle tenseness, heart beat frequency/blood pressure, respiratory frequency and consumption of oxygen as well as metabolism. Harmonics and dynamics activate and enhance emotional vitality and trigger affects.[9] Mental-cognitive activity is aroused in the form of thoughts, memories and fantasies and confirm the congruency between Audio-Communication and the scientific underpinning of the Neuro Physiological Model and Psycho Neuro-Immunology. These aspects are integrated in the following music therapy graphic:

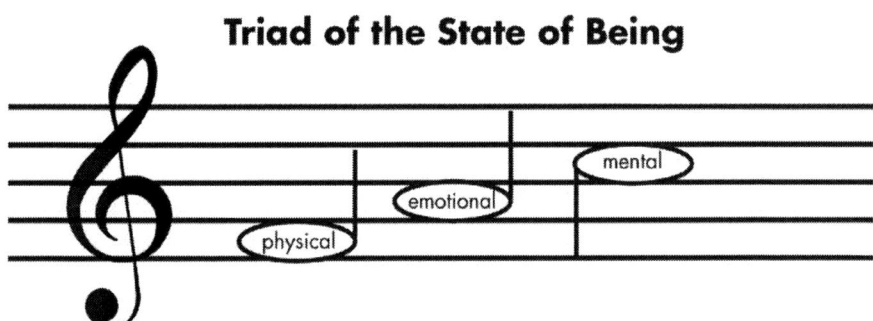

Audio-Communication: An Integrative Approach to Pain Treatment

Music as a Holistic Experience

Music has bio-physical and psychosocio-cultural components. Music is not a panacea, but a medium of communication and exchange. Music can appeal to the feelings of each person individually and cannot be generalized. The freedom of experience contributes to the special fascination of music.

An example of this understanding is reflected in the selection of the music pieces that are utilized in my sessions. I have been playing ' Morgenstimmung', from Edvard Grieg over a period of 12 years in many groups and am continuously amazed about the variety of experiences and reactions. Fantasy is triggered, creativity is activated. The ability to visualize is nurtured. Patients with minimal access to classical music and art, discover new talents in themselves which enhance life quality.

The individual feels emotionally understood and addressed to and is thus more willing and able to let his innermost feelings arise. Music can be regarded as a universal language; it has a catalyzing effect with respect to the coordination, integration and harmonization of the body -mind-emotion 'triad of perception.' Music is mainly perceived through the acoustical organ (the ear), whose physiological characteristic is constant reception, and whose function we cannot stifle or close at will either fully or partially, such as the eyes. Hearing fulfills the role of an "alarm bell" that can alert to imminent danger even during sleep.

The autonomic nervous system seems to be particularly receptive to musical and acoustical stimuli. Of all the human senses, hearing is most sensitive. The German language has an idiom which expresses the complexity of hearing: "ich fühle mich angesprochen " translated: "I *feel* spoken to." It is one of the first fully developed senses, functioning in the 18 week old fetus and the last sense to cease by death.[10] It is closely connected with our emotions, supported by the limbic system, responsible for emotional evaluation.

The Role of Classical Music

Many musical artists and scientists have detected an evident scientific basis for the holistic effect of music. Tonality is the organization of all tones and harmonies in a piece of music. European tonality is based upon the relationship of tones and harmonies to a tonic and has a particularly emotional element defined by the fact that all sounds are vibrations within a relationship. This is mirrored in particular in the fundament of the classical harmonic structures: the cadenza.

Music and Medicine: Integrative Models in the Treatment of Pain

Leonard Bernstein[11] claims that the 'dominant' interval is the key to the entire tonal system. It is dominant - "determining" - in relation to the prime. Above all, the dominant is the key to the resolution of the tension in the music: It comes from the prime and leads back to the prime! In the perception of overtones, the ear is very sensitive in the differentiation between harmonic and disharmonic sounds. The ear is a precise measuring instrument of integer, harmonic, vibration relations in contrast to complicated, disharmonic intervals.

What also makes the European tonality strong in the competition between different musical cultures is its simplicity, which is mirrored in the pragmatic symmetric scheme of the structure of simple beats and rhythm. Fundamental congruency between physical and physiological conditions promotes reception and effectiveness. The best example is the effectiveness of music as a sensual stimulation in the treatment of comatose patients.

Music therapy and Music Medicine are understood as adjunctive methods, which complement and support conventional medical treatment. Music may be used to divert attention away from pain by stimulating acoustical and tactile perception. Patients are given the opportunity to come in contact with their healthy resources, to win control over the state of being and thus re-evaluate their self-image. This in turn breaks the vicious circle of pain and diminishes fear and helplessness.

I also work on a palliative unit where pain is a main theme. With the integrated methods of Audio-Communication, the patient first learns to become aware of himself that is, of his breathing, his muscle tension and his fears. Through body-relaxing exercises such as Progressive Muscle Relaxation, developed from Edmund Jacobsen[12] and breathing awareness, he gains a feeling for himself outside of his pain perception. With many patients, I have experienced that the following insight led to stabilization, strengthened self-confidence and subdued pain perception:

> *I am winning a new perspective to myself and see myself as a person who is not defined through illness. I also possess health-promoting resources which enable me to cope with the situation and the pain which accompanies the illness.*

Acute pain is a time-limited perception of unpleasant sensations and deems as warning signal for disturbances. Music therapy supports the medical alleviation by activating the parasympathetic system, which induces pain-relieving reactions and enhances relaxation.

Audio-Communication: An Integrative Approach to Pain Treatment

In an outpatient oncology clinic, I treated patients during the chemotherapy sessions. By redirecting their awareness away from the unpleasant side effects of the treatment, to music and to group interaction, they experienced their ability to influence their state of being

Chronic pain is the result of prolonged pain perception in a stress-enhanced state. This leads to hypervigilance, an excessive alertness that is caused by a consistently heightened adrenaline level. This in turn enhances pain memory, which as stated before, can be counteracted through relaxation. Receptive music therapy and redirecting awareness to the inner state of being leads to relaxation and minimizes tension and anxiety. With active music therapy, repressed feelings can surface and find an outlet through nonverbal expression. This facilitates verbalization of these emotions, which often occurs, as the result of the group-dynamic process. Body movement to music is an important release for many patients: feeling the music, the flow and the pleasant interaction between themselves and the music contributes to reconciliation with their inner self and promotes self-esteem.

Finally, employing Audio-Communication as a long-term method encourages the re-conditioning of health-promoting strategies.
After the six-month program, one group wished to meet every three months. This led to a reinforcement of learned skills while promoting reflection competencies and the realization of transference dangers. Through regulative music therapy and employing more complex music pieces from the late romantic era, e.g. Brahms, Dvorak, the participants intensified their emotional vitality and gained control over affects that had induced repressive behavior in the past.

Audio-Communication in Clinical Practice

Group Work

As stated earlier, music therapy, being central to Audio-Communication, employs interventions across several domains to ameliorate the state of fixation on pain perception that often occurs. This hypervigilance is released through the experience of being able to perceive and feel music, which marks the starting point for the marginalization of pain perception. Through verbal reflection and exchange of experience, communication skills and conflict resolution strategies are developed and practiced. This form of therapy supports bio-psycho-social stabilization by increasing the awareness in health-retardant settings and promotes the cognizance of autonomous reactions.[13] As receptive, regulative and active music therapy approaches are most significant in Audio-Communication, they will be elucidated here for the reader:

Receptive Music Therapy is applied to enhance body awareness and to strengthen stress-reducing strategies. In order to influence body functions and to enhance relaxation, music pieces with stable rhythmic structures and balanced dynamics were played.

Regulative Music Therapy (C. Schwabe)[14] utilizes music as a catalyst for internal processes. This method includes psychotherapeutic components such as transference, countertransference and psychodynamics. It also focuses on the self-awareness of the group participants. The spectrum of music pieces is much wider and also includes works from the later classical/romantic era. This leads to an enhancement of emotional sensitivity and identification so that the patient experiences inner processes in a nonverbal form, and with the support of the group dynamic aspect, learns to verbalize his feelings and reactions. This is an important step in the detection and relief of pain augmenting factors. The music is chosen in relation to the current dynamic process of the group and acts as a nonverbal mirror for underlying conflicts such as exaggerated self-domination, heteronomy and repressed emotions.

Active Music Therapy is also integrated as a form of nonverbal communication as well as dance or movement therapy exercises by which underlying conflicts can emerge and be consciously approached. With an array of instruments such as the xylophone, drums, gongs, etc., the musical communication mirrors the quality of interaction between the group members and is very often a reflection of present conflict themes, such as repression of frustrations. Through reflection, new solving strategies can evolve. In the tinnitus field, active music therapy offers the possibility to reproduce the individual tinnitus sound with use of instruments such as bells, drums or other percussion instruments and leads to a confrontation and the chance of finding ways of reducing the disturbance level.

Structure of Audio-Communication Therapy

Introduction Phase
A brief welcome is followed by a short warm-up phase in which the patients share their current condition, if they wish. This often creates a relaxed atmosphere while activating spontaneity.

Redirection of Awareness Exercise
Through this exercise, our perception, or so to say antennas to the environment, are redirected from outer to inner awareness. This work unfolds in the following three sequential steps:

Audio-Communication: An Integrative Approach to Pain Treatment

1. Redirecting tactile perception through body awareness,
2. Redirecting optical perception through activating visualization,
3. Redirecting acoustical perception through breath flowing awareness.

Thus, the patient learns holistic self-perception and gains understanding for the complex processing of perception per say.

Music Phase
A piece of music from the classical / romantic era of about 5 to 10-minute duration is presented with a CD player.

Discussion Phase
The participants have the opportunity to share their quality of self-experience with the group and the therapist. This is initiated by the question, "*How* do you feel physically?" whereby the participant's awareness of his subjective perception is encouraged. The bodily sensations serve as a bridge to mood and emotional feelings as well as to thoughts and fantasies, so that the patient wins an integrative approach to his condition.

Listening Training
This is followed by a "*What* do I hear" perceptual phase in which the specific information *(e.g.*, volume, melody, rhythm, instrumentation, *etc*.) that was received is discussed by the participants. This specific form of hearing enhances the ability to objectify the acoustical experience. This is an important aspect in the tinnitus treatment, and deems as a fundamental step to neutralization of the disturbing tinnitus perception. The "*how* do I feel*",* becomes associated with the *"what* do I hear "perceptions. This leads to a *relationship* between listener and music piece. The participant wins awareness for the subjective-emotional as well as for the objective-informative messages. In this way the participants gain access to the "complexity of acoustical perception," (a prerequisite to understanding the neuro-physiological model) and also win a comprehensive insight to the complexity of perception per se.
    All the above can lead to an active group dynamic process. Emerging differences in perception and confounding factors become the groundwork for applying the learned relaxation techniques and for developing new conflict resolving strategies and communication skills.

Music and Medicine: Integrative Models in the Treatment of Pain

Second Listening Phase
The same music piece is heard again, thereby promoting integration of the experiences described above.

Goals
- to sensitize awareness of oneself through experiencing the stress-reducing effect of music in collaboration with relaxation and visualization methods.
- to strengthen both the internal resources and, in the long term, the immune system (dismantling of stress hormones) in context to **Psycho-**(emotions, affects)-**Neuro-Immunology** (bodily functions)
- to make the interaction between mental, emotional and physical state transparent
- to regulate physiological parameters (respiratory frequency, heartbeat *etc.*) through corresponding relaxation practices in order to counteract pain
- to enable access to emotional processes *(e.g.,* anxiety, sorrow, frustration, loss)
- to promote group dynamic processes in order to develop social and communicative competencies (*e.g.,* conflict-resolving strategies)

Tinnitus and Pain Treatment

The tinnitus patient defines his ailment as "pain." His suffering is expressed in his dwindling capacity to lead a normal life. In extreme cases, it can lead to suicidal tendencies.

Since my clinical work and up to the present, no concrete cause for the emergence of the tinnitus perception has been discovered. Since tinnitus is conscious information that is neurologically impressed in the memory, it has parallels to chronic pain. Tinnitus was the research topic of Pavel Jastreboff and Jonathan Hazell, and they developed the "Tinnitus Retraining Therapy",[15] which was based on well-established neurophysiological and psychological principles:

1. The main point of this tinnitus theory is the postulate that non-auditory systems, particularly the limbic system (involved in emotion), and the autonomic nervous system, which controls all body functions and triggers the "flight or fight" reaction, play an essential role in the subjective evaluation of tinnitus. The auditory pathways play a secondary role. According to this model, the *annoyance* of tinnitus is determined exclusively by the limbic and autonomic nervous systems.

2. The brain demonstrates high levels of plasticity and is capable of adapting to any neutral signal, once negative associations with the signal e.g. tinnitus, are neutralized.

In music I had the tool with which I could help the patient experience and understand how his sense of hearing functions and how he could learn to manage his perceptions and reactions.

As long as the patient defines his affliction as an acoustical phenomenon, he is doomed to suffer. As soon as he experiences the interaction between tinnitus and his symptoms, which are very often stress induced, he develops the ability to alleviate these symptoms with stress reduction and conflict management strategies. Subsequently, he wins self-regulation, more awareness and self-esteem.

Audio-Communication and Tinnitus

The initial clinical form of Audio-Communication was conceived as a three-week treatment program, consisting of two sessions per week. The quality control proved that this concept could only act as an impulse for further actions and not considered as a completed therapeutic process. The short time interval of three weeks did not allow for an integrative learning process. My decision to open an outpatient office was initiated through this shortcoming and the concept was extended to a six-month program with two phases. The intensive phase ran eight weeks with one session per week and the follow-up phase of four months in which monthly sessions were held to support the rehabilitation process. The advantage of this concept was confirmed in form of an evaluation project sponsored by the regional health insurance organization (BEK) and the German Tinnitus self-help organization 'Deutsche Tinnitus Liga.'[16]

Audio-Communication and Oncology

After opening my out-patient office I developed a wide spectrum of treatment concepts deriving from my clinical experience. I was subsequently contacted by an oncology team, and we began a co-operative group in their oncology outpatient office. It was conceived as a psycho-oncological complementary treatment to stabilize the condition of the patients and to alleviate some of the unpleasant side effects of chemotherapeutic treatment such as anxiety, nausea pain and fatigue. To illustrate the process that leads to pain alleviation I will present an evaluation of Audio-Communication in a psycho-oncology group process and a case study of a patient with a multi-morbidity diagnosis.

Music and Medicine: Integrative Models in the Treatment of Pain

Clinical Work

Group Work: Audio Communication and Psycho-Oncology

The initial group met in weekly sessions in the above-mentioned Oncology outpatient office, during which Audio-Communication was offered in different variations, relative to the music-therapeutic method that was deemed appropriate.

The group was constituted heterogeneously and all forms of cancer were represented. Additionally caregivers were invited to attend. Over a period of 2 years, several pharmaceutical companies were willing to promote this project through financial support. In the beginning the sessions were held in the treatment room, initiated as a compensation for the negative chemotherapeutic experiences. Although at first strange and unusual, the experience allowed patients to acquire the ability to redirect their attention and to neutralize certain aversions to things such as unpleasant odors and medical implements. The presence of the doctors (in the background) contributed to the promotion of a positive physician-patient relationship.

Audio-Communication as described above, was then implemented and in the phase in which the participants shared their perceptions and experiences, the question "How did you experience the music?" functioned as a bridge to self-reflection about the bodily- and sense perceptions, fantasies and memories. This initiated a group dynamic process of exchange and reflection out of which "key issues" surfaced, for example:

Dealing with Obvious Changes (e.g. hair loss, mastectomy scars) and with loss of responsibility.

Self-Image Verification: Identity re-evaluation

Self-Determination vs. Heteronomy: The majority of participants recognize their own demands on themselves and their striving for recognition as an attitude that often led to fatigue. The enhancement of self-esteem and acceptance of the illness strengthened the ability to redirect their focus to self-responsibility and enabled the development of a self-protecting attitude.

Dealing with Family and Social Environment: The frustration over the lack of understanding is a primary theme of the conversations. Through dialogues and the experience of solidarity, new strategies could be developed to withstand the incomprehensible attitudes of family member as well as the social environment.

Power Control: Re-evaluation of personal attitudes; for example, helplessness and dependency, and to enhance the perspective of self-control by activating health promoting competences such as relaxation and breathing techniques and health stimulating attitudes and visions (visualization á Simonton.[17])

Self-Protection Deficiencies: By means of the group dynamics and the constant "mirroring", the patients experience their ability to say "no" to the expectations of their environment.

Alleviation of Chemotherapy Side Effects: The correlation between listening to music and pleasant bodily response was made transparent and perceived as bringing relief from pain. Understanding the effectiveness and necessity of the chemotherapeutic action increased the acceptance. Accordingly, fears and inner resistances could be put into perspective.

Parting from Participants who Died (Death Anxiety): This aspect remains difficult, but experience shows that the process of consciously taking leave and dealing with private fears of death had a liberating effect. Rituals aided the process of "letting go." Being able to express their thoughts and fears concerning their own mortality encouraged many participants to consciously enhance their current quality of life.

Specific Role of Music
As described above, mainly three musical elements: pitch, rhythm and tempo regulated the physiological parameters. Melodic and dynamic elements triggered emotional awareness. This in turn activated mental energy in the form of memories, fantasies and thoughts.

Relaxation skills were conveyed and improved well-being through physical relaxation as a release of muscular tension. Emotional release was experienced as the discharge of unpleasant feelings, such as frustration, fear and sadness. Mental peace of mind was strived for by dealing with certain decompensating cognitive attitudes such as nurturing negative thoughts or brooding, thereby utilizing the group dynamic aspect in order to reevaluate their thoughts and premonitions and to develop new perspectives.

Encouraging and strengthening self-awareness was promoted through the targeted use of music in conjunction with daydreaming. Guided imagery was employed as preparation for visualization exercises.

By careful selection of the music pieces, subtle inner conflicts were addressed; e.g. dramatic and dynamic musical developments acted as a reflection of their own emotional reactions. Emotional verbalization was possible and led to a constructive debate as a counter-weight to repression.

Thus some participants gained the courage to confront and discharge underlying aggressive behavior.

An evaluation of the group process over a period of 3 months was performed by Marc Brueggermann,[18] a music therapy student from the University of Siegen in Germany. Brueggermann applied a specified Audio-Communication questionnaire as well as the standardized SPG (Skalen zur psychischen Gesundheit – A. Tönnies) questionnaire, a standardized psychological assessment tool for one's emotional and psychological well-being. The evaluation confirming the effectiveness of music therapy in the form of Audio-Communication in psycho-oncology, is expressed in the following excerpts:

> The analysis showed that significant gaps in the self-perception could be compensated. This factor is important. The oncology patient is often an outward-oriented individual who underestimates his own needs and limitations and thus adheres to the demands of others. The experience and realization of one's own well-being, both physical and emotional, is a prerequisite for dealing adequately with one's own needs and limitations.
>
> Through the group-dynamic process, the participants learn to recognize and express their needs for social exchange and understanding. Through the joint dealing with daily conflicts, they develop social skills; e.g. their ability to "give and take" empathy and advice. The experience of the liberating effect of verbalization of inner conflicts enhances their self-esteem.

The analysis from Brüggermann concludes that:

1. Oncology patients recognize music therapy in the form of Audio-Communication, as a measure with which they can influence and improve their quality of life significantly.

2. Oncology patients confirm that after participating in Audio-Communication, they have mastered pain-relieving strategies, developed greater self-determination, willpower and affirmation of life and thus have more competence to deal constructively with their situation. One aim of this method is to assist the patient in accepting his situation as it is rather than resigning and thus enhancing his suffering. The capability to identify and overcome heteronomy and to win self-esteem, through conflicts, if neces-

sary, is the prerequisite. This attitude can motivate the patients to set new goals in life which in turn enhance life quality and thereby stimulate recovery processes. Through Audio Communication patients learn that they can influence their own physical, emotional and mental well-being. They can build hope and confidence to live meaningfully, despite the disease.

Individual Work: Ms. R.

Set-up
Mrs. R. was recommended to me by her ENT doctor for music-social therapeutic treatment. In the first interview, she complained of intensely perceived tinnitus and dizziness. We agreed on a treatment plan over a period of 2 months.

The medical history revealed a congenital profound hearing loss in both ears. Meanwhile, the left ear is deaf and a severe hearing impairment of 90 dB HL exists in the right ear. In addition, Mrs. R. suffered from chronic tinnitus as a "head noise," which she described as painful, along with an increasingly high-frequency hyperacusis and vertigo. Hearing aids on both sides ensure the perception of noise for spatial orientation.

The Social-Biographical History
Ms. R. is a 56-year-old single woman, whose current social context consists only of the care of her bed-ridden mother and occasional visits to relatives. The hearing impairment was not recognized in childhood: As the second oldest daughter of seven children, her handicap was labeled a "conduct disorder." She learned to compensate the deficiencies by accepting responsibility within the family. She avoided talking and first started verbalizing when she went to school. Extremely difficult family circumstances (*e.g.* her father's alcoholism) resulted in reclusive behavior patterns. There were no psychological or medical therapeutic measures taken. Ms. R. excelled in sports and gained the qualifications to become a physical fitness teacher. During this time she worked closely with a speech therapist to develop her language skills and to learn lip reading. She practiced her profession in a special school until, at age 48; she retired due to her progressive hearing loss.

At the beginning of the therapy, Ms. R receded into her inner world, which was most profoundly reflected in her avoidance of eye contact with others. It was her trust in the ENT doctor, whom she had known over many years that empowered her to participate in the music-/social therapy service, called Audio-Communication.

Music and Medicine: Integrative Models in the Treatment of Pain

In Session

The first meetings were used to develop a therapeutic relationship. In view of her high level of distrust and anxiety behavior, this endeavor turned out to be a difficult task. First, relaxation techniques such as progressive muscle relaxation and breathing exercises were taught to solve the tense posture, which was a result of long-term fear.

With the support of headphones, that had been bought during a therapeutic "excursion into reality" with me, Mrs. R. could experience the physical effects of music through vibrations. According to the music (such as Boccherini – light Mozart divertimenti), she relaxed and experienced the emotional impact of music and learned to enjoy her well-being, which confirmed that she could deflect her tinnitus perception as well as the vertigo.

In conversations about everyday situations, Ms. R's behavioral overreactions surfaced, and they were brought in connection with her unprocessed anxiety. Traumatic childhood memories that were based on her upbringing, coupled with communication and socialization deficiencies, appeared sporadically. Ms. R. was increasingly overwhelmed by these memories due to the emotional revitalization. With the support of active music therapy, such as improvisations on the piano, she was able to express her frustration and anger. Subsequently, a reassuring piece from Bach, was played for her on the piano, and by feeling the vibrations of the piano, the soothing music helped her to regain inner peace and stability. This particular "Minuet in G major" was her "anchor piece," which carried her back to herself again and again. Ms. R. began to "think aloud" and to review her thoughts and their relationship to reality. Her self-image could be revised in accordance with the newly won insights. This led to an enhanced self-understanding and appeased her deep-seated self-reproaches, which resulted from negative biographical influences.

Notably, her intense facial expressions and body language were at times congruent with certain musical elements. Dynamic changes that affected respiratory rate and body tension, or lyrical passages that led to relaxation of facial and body muscle spasms, were at work within the music. Through these occurrences, non-verbal contact was established and the basis for a therapeutic relationship was laid.

Self-acceptance and self-esteem emerged due to her growing communication skills. Her initial tendency to run away, either by withdrawing or physically escaping incomprehensible situations, was counteracted through verbalization and insight. These behavioral changes strengthened her self-confidence and reflected a growing emotional stability.

Ms. R began to transfer her musical experiences to the interpersonal relationship with the therapist. She expanded her social activities through visits to concerts with relatives. Subsequently, painting with music (Pachelbel: Canon) was offered, in which an abstract colorful picture was produced. This opened the door to integrate older pictures that were drawn during the period of life in which Ms. R predominantly used reclusion as a protection strategy.

Two pictures illustrated her reclusion: the "Eskimo child" and "The Clown." These figures served as triggers for role-playing and integration. New musical experiences, won through improvisation and regulative music therapy sessions, enhanced the process. The important role of music is even more surprising, since an objective acoustic processing of sound waves is minimal. The effectiveness is due through the support of headphones and a strong emotional sensitivity and powerful imagination. She expanded the process by writing stories about these figures.

The fourth movement from the Brahms Symphony No. 1 activated the "Clown story." Many of her fears were expressed in the story, for example, that she would never speak again, as an expression of her fear of not being understood:. "I feel my grief - I've cried spontaneously a lot this week - I am the 'clown.'". The growing ability to express her frustrations, fears and grief liberated Ms. R. and a feeling of self-assuredness emerged. She expressed this very eloquently with the self-affirmation "I am I" The socialization process improved and Ms. R widened her social network to include distant relative and former colleagues. Her subjective pain perception diminished and she developed skills to alleviate the tinnitus perception and vertigo.

Shortly before the therapy was to be concluded, breast cancer was diagnosed. At that time I was on vacation. Upon my return, Ms. R. wished to continue the therapy. I was quite surprised how she had dealt with this new health crisis. Her ability to deal with the acute situation was a confirmation of her growing inner stability.

We extended the therapy and included specific psycho-oncological aspects. Ms. R. was capable of dealing with difficult situations that arose and the certitude that she had the possibility to reflect and to express her inner conflicts in the therapeutic setting, led to a strengthening of her self-confidence. Very often people with a hearing disability are marginalized and feel ignored. They experience a feeling of exclusion and are not capable of exerting themselves. This was not the case with Ms. R. She claimed respect and made demands in appropriate situations.

> *As Ms. R. looked at her appointment schedule for the radiation treatment, she realized that she would have to get up at 6 o´clock am and that would mean a 2 hour bus trip to the clinic. She explained this to the secretary and insisted on a*

change of appointments. She admitted to me that she would never have done that before.

These strategies supported the pain alleviation during the radiation phase. Through her relaxation strategies she could influence the grade of pain. Through free dancing, Ms. R. extended the benefits of therapy and experienced relief on a new level.

This case illustrates the holistic effect of music therapy and emphasizes its creative power. Music often activates impulses and affects that demonstrate what healing energy in the individual is and waiting to be integrated in the medical process. The inner acceptance and compliancy are basic attitudes that support and enhance the medical necessary treatment.

Conclusion

By describing my work and its underpinnings, I strive to demonstrate the congruency between music therapy and pain treatment. Through the holistic reflection, the term 'MusicMedicine' becomes transparent. The objective of medical treatment is the restoration of health. Interestingly, the definition of health given by the World Health Organization (WHO) is holistic: "Health is a state of complete physical, mental, and social well-being and not merely the absence of disease or infirmity."[19]

My experience verifies the pain relieving and health enhancing potential of music and the necessity to integrate it in our medical system. I emphasize the broader definition of pain and hope to support the insight that pain is a subjective, personal experience that cannot always be measured, but must always be taken seriously. How we treat it is the challenge.

The potential for music therapists in the field of pain treatment is immense and secures our position in the future expansion of medical treatment. We have the commitment to document our work in a way that the scientific aspects are transparent. Only then can we expect respect and acceptance from the established medical cultures. I am convinced that by sharing our experiences and underlining them with scientific methods, we can contribute to the validation of music therapy and promote the acknowledgment of the term MusicMedicine.

References

1. Jastreboff, P.; Hazell, J. A neurophysiological approach to tinnitus: clinical implications *British Journal of Audiology 1993, pp.73-94.*
2. Robert Ader, David L. Felten, Nicholas Cohen, *Psychoneuroimmunology, 4th edition,* Academic Press, 2006.

3. McFadden, D. *Tinnitus, Facts, Theories and Treatments.* Fischer Verlag, 1996 pp.34-42.
4. Ader,R.Cohen,N.*Behaviorally conditioned immunosuppression Psychosomatic Medicine,* Vol 37, Issue 4 333-340.1975
5. Miketta,G.*Netzwerk Mensch,*Trias Verlag,1996.
6. Spiegel,D. *Psychosocial Intervention in Cancer.* Jnl. of the National Cancer Institute,1993.
7. Merriam-Webster Dictionary, Merriamcompany,1977,p.824.
8. LeDoux, Joseph E. *The emotional Brain,*Touchstone, 1996.
9. Spintge,R.*The Functional and Therapeutic Effects of Music from a Medical and Neurophysiological Standpoint – Music as a Therapeutic Drug,*Villa Musica.1991 pp. 13-22.
10. Beherendt,J. *The world is sound.*
11. Bernstein,L.*The joy of music*Amadeus Press 2004.
12. Jacobson,E.. *Progressive Relaxation.* Chicago: University of Chicago Press,1938.
13. Valentin.I.*Audio-Kommunikation, eine multi-modale musiktherapie in der stationären Tinnitus Therapie,* Musik-therapeutische Umschau,Vonderhoeck &Ruprecht, 1001, Bd. 22.p.362.
14. Schwabe, C.Rohrborn,H.*Regualtive Musiktherapie* Fischer Verlag 1996 p.36-42.
15. See footnote 1
16. Willwoll, *Evaluation* von *Audio-Kommunikation-.Diplome thesis,* 2005.
17. Simonton,C. *Getting well again,* Tarcher, 1978.
18. Brüggermann,M. *Die Rolle der Musiktherapie in der onkologische Betreuung.*.Siegen, 2005.
19. World Health Organization, *Website.*

Music and Medicine: Integrative Models in the Treatment of Pain

APPENDIX

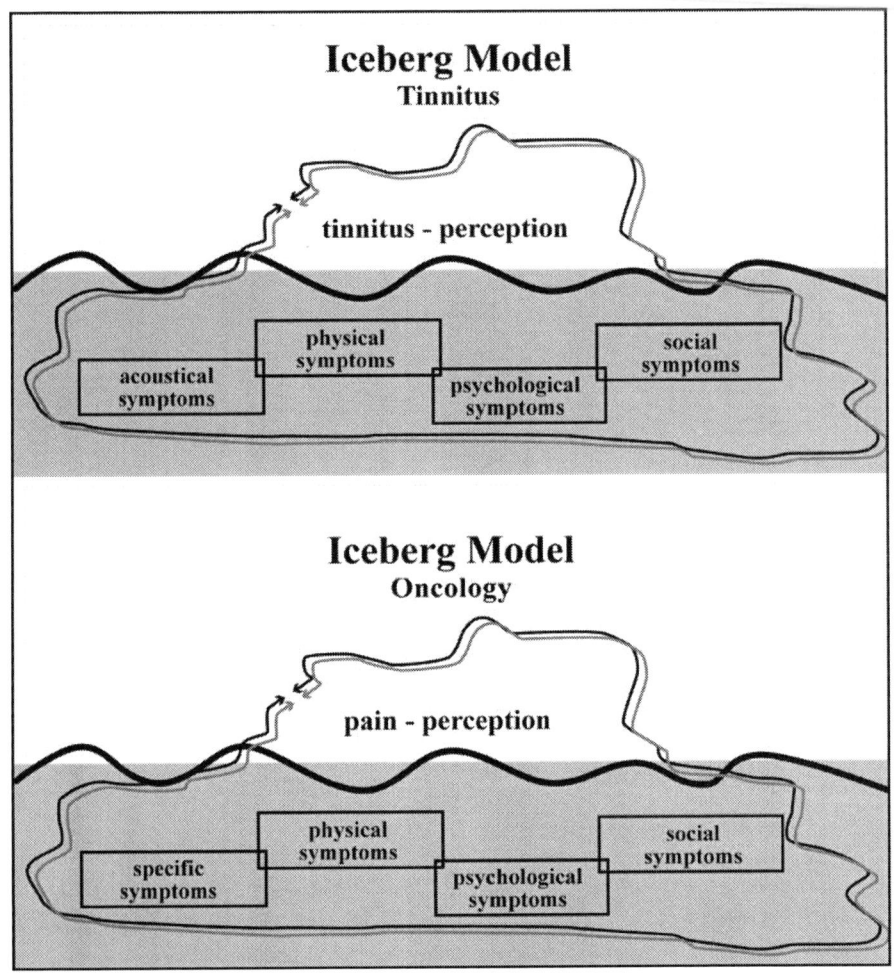

CHAPTER 16

Environmental Music Therapy: Rationale for 'Multi-Individual' Music Psychotherapy in Modulation of the Pain Experience

Andrew Rossetti MMT, MT-BC
Bernardo Canga MMT

"*Pain is as diverse as man. One suffers as one can.*"
Victor Hugo

Introduction

Pain is a complex multi-dimensional somatic experience.[1] It includes emotional and state elements as well as purely nociceptive or neuropathic features.[2] Though considerable controversy still exists as to how emotion may be defined, it is generally accepted that emotions have physiological as well as psychological aspects and that we experience emotion as a bodily awareness and judge the events that provoke emotions accordingly. Similarly, 'state' refers to one's subjective evaluation in the moment of one's entire being – mind and body. Focus on the complex psychological processes that regulate perception in such a subjective experience has led to novel approaches in pain management, and the subsequent research of their efficacy. One such approach is the use of music therapy as a form of psychotherapy in clinical practice with individuals, groups, caregivers, and the sound environment. This chapter offers several postulates that may provide a rationale and means for exploring the role and interaction of emotion and anxiety in the perception of pain, and will offer a foundation for Environmental Music Therapy (EMT) interventions that may influence and modulate the pain experience.

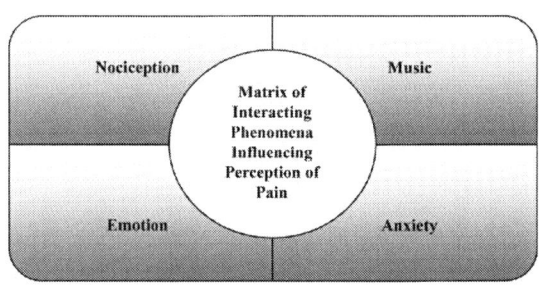

The postulates, which form our working hypothesis and rationale, provide the necessity for a working model of EMT. They are drawn from a number of cutting edge theories validated by research, clinical experience and our expertise in working within a 'multi-individual' group context. In this 'multi-individual' setting, the individuals are not necessarily collaborating with one another on common goals as in a group or even meant to be aware of one another. They are however co-habiting and sharing a space inclusive of personnel, circumstances, and - significant to the model- an audio environment that is meant to be safe and healing. This context has been shown to indeed have an apparent effect on the pain perception of patients as well an effect on affect states of caregivers and staff.

POSTULATES
1. Emotion is an integral part of the pain process
2. Anxiety is an exacerbating factor in the pain experience
3. Music can generate/modulate emotion responses
4. Music can modulate state anxiety
5. Noise is a noxious stimulus and potential stressor that can exacerbate state anxiety
6. The hospital can frequently be perceived as a hostile environment
7. Music can modulate perception of an environment
8. Prolonged time in waiting rooms where one might see or interact with other patients whose illness might be more acute or advanced, promotes anxiety and negative affective states

For several years we have been motivated in our clinical work with severely compromised patients in fragile environments to focus on the aforementioned postulates and have developed a working hypothesis for best practice interventions in delivering EMT to palliate pain. Our approach is to approach pain from a psychological standpoint rather than from a strictly physiological one. Pain treatment involves a perceptual process with respective associated awareness, selective abstraction, ascribed meaning, appraisal, and learning,[3] and specifically a condition in which emotional and motivational states are central to understanding its nature.[4]

The framework for the underlining emotional processes involved in pain perception has been identified by Price, where he found that the perception of pain is determined and expressed by a network of brain structures (anterior cingulate cortex, hypothalamus, insular cortex) and pathways (spinohypothalamic pathway, cortico-limbic somatosensory pathway).[5] In addition to relying on first hand observation and participation with years of patient referrals and treatments, we have gathered compelling theoretical perspectives on the likely interactions and co-relations of pain perception, emotion and affective states, and music. Examination of Melzack et al's Gate Control Theory and Neuromatrix Theory, Porges' Polyvagal Theory with music as vagal stimulation, Demasio's perspectives on emotion, and Hadjistavropoulos & Craig editors' Psychological Perspectives on Pain, along with many recent studies on music's effects on pain (which will be discussed below in this paper) have provided insight on its' complex mechanisms and theoretical ground upon which to build.

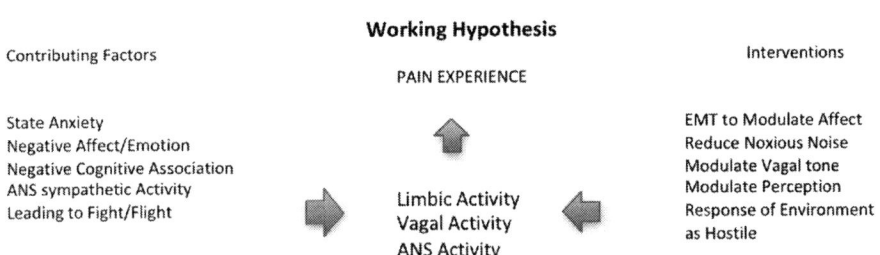

Personal Hermeneutic
As the researcher/clinician perspective of this topic involves highly focused attentiveness and observation, it may be useful to begin with a personal stance-of-the writer perspective. The clinician's personal history, belief and perspective about pain are undeniable touchstones that influence treatment throughout the entire trajectory of a hospital visit-from admission to discharge. This may be particularly true for a patient stay in an intensive care unit (ICU). It is also not far from a professional caregiver's experience where from the moment we evaluate and make an assessment to our final summary, we are using our evaluative expertise blended with our intuitive processes as 'therapists' to make clinical inferences. Our in-the-moment gut response and our subsequent professional adjustment provide a unique way of responding to the patient's experience. What is the essence of clinical music therapy practice in fragile environments such as hospital oncology settings and intensive care units? These environments are true petri dishes for various states of anxiety and emotional distress. As participants who have observed and provided numerous music therapy pain management interventions with fragile populations, specifically on Oncology environments both in-patient and in radiation and chemo therapy and within ICUs from the Neonatal Intensive Care Unit (NICU), Surgical Intensive Care Unit (SICU), Pediatric Intensive Care Unit (PICU), Medical Intensive Care Unit,

(MICU), and Cardiac Surgical Intensive Care Unit (CSICU), we have become acutely aware of the non-reported, but distinctly apparent yet subtle need within these environments. Patients' perception in general, and specifically changes in affect, emotion, and anxiety may color perception of the environment in and of itself, which is inclusive of the intrapersonal perceptions of patients, and interpersonal perceptions of patients, caregivers and staff. With regards to the concept of the apparent oxymoron 'multi-individual', personal experience in seeking to address individual needs of individual patients grouped together in a radiation therapy, chemotherapy waiting room, or within an ICU has lead to questions and the formulation of an approach that forgoes group therapy concepts and dynamics, but nevertheless does address the apparent needs within this distinct treatment area.

As Joanne Loewy commented; "Many people think music therapy in pain management is limited to individual work... but how does one work with a lone tree when confronted with an entire forest of ailing trees?" (personal communication, July 2012).

At Beth Israel Medical Center in 1998, a recognizable need in the hospital environment emerged when the struggle to treat an individual within a noisy ICU environment presented itself over and over again. There was an obvious difficulty in treating individuals with an aesthetically pleasing experience amidst a chaotic group environment. EMT as a concept and music psychotherapy intervention, was pioneered as a discipline. It has since continued to develop and its implementation is being researched in several hospital areas at Beth Israel as a provision for 'multi-individuals' who are being treated within this context.[6,7]

Clinical intuition can be seen as the motor that powers clinical improvisation in all aspects of music-based treatment, both musical and extra-musical. Intuition itself can be seen as that which is observed, but has not been processed into the cognitive mind. Psychologist, S.L.Hathaway provides the following discussion: clinical intuition denotes the process in which inferences have their source in cues or cognitive processes one is able to specify...or when the integrative powers of the percipient seem to exceed ordinary rational analysis.[8] Still, intuition is formulated on one's observations, and as such it colors decision-making and action on many forums and from distinct patient and caregiver perspectives both personally and professionally.

Theoretical Background

Music Psychotherapy
Music psychotherapy may be seen as a process in which change, a goal of all therapeutic interventions, happens within the relationship between patient

and therapist. Music serves to create a safe platform or context where painful feelings, perhaps too difficult to express in words, may be expressed in and through music. The process itself can be viewed as a patient's acceptance of the 'therapist as liaison'. Liaison to the inner workings of self, as well as to illness and treatment itself, and/or a liaison to the clinical team and treatment needs identified by the team. Music psychotherapy is provided within a continuum whereby the music therapist does not give answers or advice, but seeks to contextualize and provide avenues for the patient to gain perspective – literally 'seeing from two different points of view to gain depth of perception' – as the primary step in 'seeing' where change may occur, and moving towards it.

Music psychotherapy incorporates principals of psychotherapy and employs music and its elements as an integral part of the dynamic relationship. Thus music can be an agent of change as well as providing a context or 'space' for that change to occur. Transference and countertransference are manifested and worked through using improvisation, songs, and imagery in music. While many models of music psychotherapy are employed in practice, the model that serves as our basis is eclectic and draws principally from the philosophies of Ana Freud, Jean Piaget, Perls' Gestalt theory, as well as those of Maslow and Yalom.[9] Within the model, elements of psychodynamics as well as humanistic philosophy are incorporated and employed to seek and provide the patient with perspective on their unique patterns of relating to the world developed by each of us. Loewy states that music psychotherapy is exploratory in nature, and functions through assessment and processing of awareness of self, other and of the moment; thematic expression: listening, performing; collaboration; therapeutic relationship; concentration, range of affect; investment/motivation; use of structure; integration; self-esteem; risk-taking and independence.[9] Each of these concepts is active in the process of the music therapist attending to the sound environment, which will be expounded upon in the next section.

Environmental Music Therapy
The concept of EMT was originally conceived as a music therapy technique for addressing and modulating external ambient stressors in those hospital units where a state of "near medical emergency" is constant such as ICUs and Infusion Suites, where it has been observed as being particularly effective.[6,7,10] EMT seeks to modulate an environment perceived as being hostile, and convert it into a holding and soothing space. EMT is an interactive and dynamic therapeutic process in which the music is played in such a way as to create a "soundtrack" for the room that influences emotion and association in much the same way as the soundtrack of a motion picture does.

Music and Medicine: Integrative Models in the Treatment of Pain

Through the intentional use of music and sound to modulate the soundscape of a given area or room, a noxious sound environment is converted into one more conducive to healing and wellbeing by means of the interactive process between the person actively providing EMT and those actively receiving it. Through improvised and discerningly played pre-composed music, a soundtrack is constructed in such a way as to incorporate ambient noise as well as visual and aural clues from those present in a music experience. The experience may reduce stress responses and is conducive to more positive mood states. Musical motifs as well as pre-composed music that may reflect ethnicity, culturality, age group, and mood states of the staff and patients as well as visitors are used in the live music intervention. Recognition and changes, however slight, in mood states and affect are brought into play in the improvised soundscape. EMT may foster changes in the physical, psychological, social, and cognitive domains of the persons experiencing it by establishing a dynamic musical medium, which can address and modulate distress, anxiety, trauma, fear, isolation, and pain. It can also serve to ameliorate difficulties in communicating emotion through the therapeutic use of vocal and instrumental sounds that "convey a functional and metaphorical 'voice'" and "express emotional narrative".[11]

Our work is further being shaped by four (Institutional Review Board) IRB approved studies undertaken by the Louis Armstrong Department of Music Therapy research team. Two look specifically at EMT's effects on fragile hospital environments: The Effect of EMT on Anxiety Levels and Perception of Waiting Time in the Radiation Oncology Waiting Room and Environmental Music Therapy (EMT): A Pilot Study on the Effects of Music Therapy in a Chemotherapy Infusion Suite. The latter study has revealed positive effects on staff stress level and reduced the perception of noise in patients and caregivers waiting for chemotherapy treatment.[12] A third study, Effects of an Integrative Music Therapy Program on the Perception of Noise in the SICU: A Patient, Caregiver, and Physician/Nurse Environmental Study explores the effect of environmental music therapy on noise and the perception of patients as well as personal and professional caregivers. Few would argue that in fragile environments, noise may be thought of as a potent stimulus that fosters negative mood states. A forth study focuses on a protocolized live music psychotherapy intervention for state anxiety: The Impact of Music Therapy on Anxiety in Patients Newly Diagnosed With Cancer & Undergoing Simulation for Radiation Therapy. Parallel to measuring state anxiety pre and post intervention, pain is also measured on a Visual Analysis Scale (VAS) as well as on a Color Analysis Scale (CAS). These scales facilitate the gathering of descriptive data on each participant's pain experience, and can be found in Appendix A.

Physically Perceived Pain

Further exploration of the context in which the theory of EMT is being forged is served by additional elucidation of the phenomenon of pain itself as it occurs across various domains of the human experience.

Physically Perceived Pain

Gate Control and Neuromatrix Theories
It may be useful to think of pain as a percept, a pre-processed kind of music that only "becomes" distinguished as music in the brain when it is psychologically processed, and exists only as transmitted vibrations until it is processed on a cognitive level when we can make sense of it. In keeping with the Gate Control and Neuromatrix Theories of Melzack et al, indeed, transmitted messages that are not experienced as pain until cognitively processed, evaluated and "made sense of" perhaps do not exist or even denied from our feeling sense. Gate Control theory accommodates psychological perspectives to explain phenomena ignored by earlier sensory specific models of pain.[1] It identifies specialized systems in the cerebrum involved with distinct dimensions of pain – sensory discriminative, motivational/affective, cognitive/evaluative – and in doing so opens the gates on exploration on how these dimensions may be activated to modulate the pain response itself.

Melzack and Katz state that, regarding pain perception, the brain is a dynamic system filtering, selecting, and modulating input. This mechanism acts upon pain's psychological components, that is to say, attention, past experience, anxiety, affect, and the meaning of the situation.[3] This opens a pathway to the concept of modulation of pain itself through reduction of anxiety and modifying affect, which brings to mind a fascinating albeit simple and informal experiment I had become aware of and had undertaken numerous times with various groups of students.

The experiment consists of having a person place her or his hand in a bucket of ice water while listening to a recording of loud and unpleasant industrial sounds, and timing how long she or he could keep the hand submerged until the pain became too uncomfortable to bare. The unpleasant sound served to negatively modulate the subject's affective state while also producing a certain amount of anxiety. During the second part of the experiment, the subject was given time to dry the hand and allow it to return to its original temperature. He or she has been asked to identify a favorite piece of "relaxing" music. This recorded music was played while the other hand is submerged in the frigid water, and the response is also timed. While this is far from being a formalized research study, and the query was subject to a number of confounds, the majority of subjects were able to keep their hand submerged almost twice as long with "relaxing" music playing.

Music and Medicine: Integrative Models in the Treatment of Pain

The discovery that the dorsal horn is where 'central summation' of pain perception occurs, and is the 'critical determinant of pain' acting as a gating mechanism is of great interest to those using music as anesthesia. Descending inhibition results from gating.[3] This process further defines pain perception as a subjective multi-dimensional experience. Furthermore, endorphins contribute to descending inhibition of pain messages,[13] and tend to be activated by intense inputs[3] such as, perhaps, an interactive music experience.

The following is a hypothetical offering of the gate control theory mechanism as we understand it:

A patient, we shall call Zena is experiencing acute pain as a result of receiving radiation therapy. Nociception occurs in the area where tissue has been damaged. This initiates transmission of information along ascending neural fibers through an "open gate" to the dorsal horn which "relays" this information on to Zena's cerebrum. At the same time, Zena's cerebrum sends information about her emotional state (afraid or anxious, hyper-activated and vigilant, angry...) along descending neural fibers back through the gate. The combination of ascending nociception and descending emotional and cognitive information keeps the gate open and pain is continued to be perceived. If another stimulus is introduced, such as music, thus modulating her emotional state, the transmission of information about Zena's original unpleasant emotional state will be interrupted and exchanged for other "more pleasant" information, thus "closing the gate".

The Neuromatrix Theory may be seen as a continuation of the Gate Control theory. Again, the focus is on subjectivity. It differs from classical theory in which the qualities of experience are presumed to be inherent in peripheral nerve fibers and differentiates "pain" from "injury".[3] Subjectively, one is aware of the quality of pain experiences. This must not be confused with the physical event itself that leads to nociception. The qualities of experience are generated by structures in the brain. No external equivalents to the qualities we attach to the feeling of pain: throbbing, burning, stinging exist. Thus, once again, pain "becomes" pain in the brain, and its perception is dependent upon psychological mechanisms.

Psychology, Pain, and Emotion

Pain has long been of interest to the psychiatric community as evidenced by the Psychogenic Biomedical psychodynamic models of Freud (1895) Ellman, Savage, Wittkower, & Rodger, (1942); Scott, (1948) Pilowsky and Spence (1975), and Pilowsky, (1986).[14] However, in recent years psychotherapeutic approaches in palliating pain appear to have gained ground in clinical application. In following these approaches, pain may be defined as a complex, somatic experience with cognitive and emotional as well as sensory features.[15]

Pain models have moved away from the biomedical model, which is a uni-dimensional conceptualization, toward multidimensional conceptualizations that recognize the complex interplay between the physiological, psychological and sociocultural mechanisms that form the pain experience. While there are numerous systems of psychology- based thought on what pain is and how it can be palliated, many coincide in isolating two factors as especially significant: cognition and emotion. Cognition may be viewed as the interaction of attention, appraisal and attribution, and is linked to emotion in the pain process. "Persons in pain become emotional, not because reactions occur when the sensory message reaches the somatosensory cortex, but because nociception triggers multiple limbic processes in parallel with central sensory processes."[15]

It is worth noting that there are numerous discussions and dissent on what emotions are, and furthermore on how to differentiate between emotion, affect, and mood, and whether they are states or processes. It is not our goal or within the scope of our competency to 're-invent the wheel' of what constitutes emotion. We revert to a well used colloquial expression that is employed to categorize an observable event, infamously used by Supreme Court Justice Potter Stewart, in Jacobellis v. Ohio "I shall not today attempt further to define what I understand to be embraced within that description, and perhaps I could never succeed in intelligibly doing so. But I know it when I see it."

Anxiety's Role in Pain Perception

Anxiety is felt. It is the somatization of a diffuse unpleasant vague sense of apprehension or painful or apprehensive uneasiness of mind over an impending or anticipated ill.[16] It can be characterized by feelings of dread, trouble concentrating, feeling tense or jumpy, irritability, restlessness, hypervigilant watching and waiting for signs and occurrences of danger, an awareness of impending threat, and the sensation of your mind having gone blank.[17]

As Schmidt stated simply "anxiety exacerbates pain"(B.L.Smith, DDS, MD, PhD, Grand Rounds Beth Israel Medical Center, March 2012). A plausible line of thought is that the hypervigilence that accompanies anxiety may increase susceptibility to appraise nociception as being more acute pain than would be identified in low anxiety states. We have observed that time spent waiting for treatment is a strong contributor to anxiety in hospital patients. In a recently completed study, the emotional impact of waiting was measured through a 15-item questionnaire identifying moods and fears of 355 patients with cancer in an outpatient oncology clinic. It was suggested that the waiting room experience was distress-inducing and that the presence of aesthetic experiences during the waiting period contributed to a very different experience.[18] One such experience – Environmental Music Therapy – seeks to improve the psychological impact of waiting periods in threatening situations identified by patients-such as surgery, medical procedures and oncology treatments.

Of notable importance in the ongoing dialogue about the effects of music on state anxiety is the work of psychologist Stephen W. Porges, which will be discussed in the next section.

The Polyvagal Theory

Porges' Polyvagal theory provides phylogenetic and neuro-anatomic guidelines and a justification for the use of music therapy interventions to lower anxiety. In it he focuses on the vagus, the 10th cranial nerve, and how its myelinated section regulates sympathetic and parasympathetic activity of the autonomic nervous system.[19]

The myelinated branches of the vagus form a complex neural bi-directional pathway linking the brainstem to many organs. Of particular interest is that vocal intonation is mediated by vagal connections to the larynx. The orbicularis oculi, which is a muscle in the face that closes the eyelids and contributes to our forming a so-called "Duchenne" or authentic smile, and the stapedius muscle in the middle ear are also mediated by vagal connection. These areas are all involved in emotion and communication. The stapedius muscle along with the tympanic membrane can be activated by music. Thus, music can be employed as an effective tool for influencing vagal tone, and in doing so, influencing sympathetic and parasympathetic activity as well as emotion. This can lead to enhanced social engagement, which, as Porges explains, due to our phylogenetic make-up, is key to homeostasis.[19]

Furthermore, Porges also states "music may be used to calm, enable feelings of safety, and reduce the social distance between people….intertwined with emotion, affect regulation, interpersonal social behavior, and other psychological processes related to personal responses to environmental, interpersonal, and intrapersonal challenges. " Also, music "can elicit a variety of emotional experiences that are paralleled by adaptive psychological states" and "trigger the client's neuroception of safety."[19]

"Moreover, the neural regulation of the autonomic nervous system (ANS) is linked to the neural regulation of the muscles of the face and head, which signal our emotional state. These muscles of the face and head are involved both in actively listening to (i.e. the modulation of our middle ear muscles) and in producing of music whether by singing (i.e., the modulation of the laryngeal and pharyngeal muscles)."[19]

Music can be a precursor to social engagement by directly influencing vagal regulation - via stimulation of the tympanic membrane and the ossea - of the autonomic nervous system leading away from 'fright – flight – fight' responses toward homeostatic states.[11] Few would argue with the statement that feelings of safety are paramount to effective therapy. In accordance with the Poly Vagal Theory, music in and of itself, is a medium for fomenting feelings of safety.

Music and Emotion

The emotional experiences that music offers may well be one of the primary reasons for listening to music in the first place. Music is capable of communicating basic emotions universally across different cultures,[20-22] and provides for a sense of 'shared intentionality'.[23] Such shared intentionality in music may be seen as a basis for establishing trust and confidence – the foundation for the therapeutic relationship that must necessarily exist for the music psychotherapy process to thrive.

The communication of emotions by music has been a topic receiving a great deal of attention for quite some time, and empirical studies have described the role of individual features (tempo, mode, articulation, timbre) in predicting the emotions suggested or invoked by the music. Emotion is perhaps communicated through music by its metaphoric content – both literal (such as a low register melody in 2/4 time consisting of the tonic and a perfect fourth below in alternating quarter notes to conjure up the image of a huge lumbering animal) and figurative (such as Beethoven's Pastoral, which while it cannot be said that its sounds mimic anything in particular, still evoke a bucolic countryside). Musical elements of themselves play a strong part in the cues music gives us relative to 'what' we should feel. Harmonic tension is felt as tension. I imagine that our response to the climactic scenes of Hitchcock's "Psycho" would be quite different without the high-pitched minor seconds played on violin to warn us of impending horror.

Eerola states that emotions play a central role in human intelligence, and that it is clear that music is a system that can induce powerful emotions. Expectation in musical qualities provides a powerful mechanism for eliciting musical emotions that can perhaps contrast and nullify negative expectation such as that which precedes a medical procedure.[24] Music seemingly affects emotions in an immediate context, having the unique property to create and generate emotional experiences where they did not exist previously.[25] Emotional responses to music appear to be associative as well with the power to evoke images and metaphorical ideation.[26] It can be said that we think in words and images. Thus, music's ability to 'place' images in our minds represents a vastly powerful means of modifying mood, and directing affect, and has the capacity to express the deepest aspects of cognition and emotion.[27]

Researchers Coutinho and Cangelosi have developed novel models of the relationship between music perception and its emotional appraisal, that is to say the continuous emotional appraisal of music pieces (e.g., arousal and valence ratings). Specific psychoacoustic variables (e.g., tempo, mean pitch and loudness) play a key role in this process. In studies they have conducted psycho-physiological measurements (e.g., heart rate, skin conductance) are measured to view correlation with music-induced emotions. Such studies support the "emotivist" views on musical emotions, illustrating that music can directly elicit affective responses in the listener.[28,29]

Emotion's Role in Pain Perception / Studies on Music & Pain

Various studies have provided evidence of the effectiveness of music therapeutic methods in the treatment of distinct types of pain.[30-34] It may be more important to point out that while current music-based intervention studies provide evidence of feasibility and efficacy, their findings are far from homogenous. Meta-analyses suggest that the influence of music on pain relief, anxiety, and mood is highly variable, and found inconsistent effects that were partially explained by intervention type and practitioner methodology (e.g., health care personnel versus board-certified music therapists).[30,35,36]

The existing theoretical basis for the effects of music therapy interventions on pain perception we have chosen for our presenting model of EMT centers on change occurring in the music psychotherapeutic process, and its effectiveness is increasingly being under stood in terms of its connections to neurophysiological change.

The Nuts and Bolts of Environmental Music Therapy: Treatment Procedures

While this will not be an exhaustive "how –to" manual on how EMT is constructed and delivered, never-the-less, the following is a broad brush rendering of some of its more practice related concerns.

The EMT interventions we have provided for patients at Beth Israel Medical Center, in practice, have fallen into two broad categories: Those carried out on units, or in environments where ambient noise is a noxious contributing stressor, and those in environments (such as the majority of waiting areas) where the ambient noise level is low enough to be barely perceivable.

EMT is viewed as a multi-individual process in that those receiving it do not necessarily perceive themselves as forming part of a group and therefore are not interacting as such. Also the ongoing real time assessment and integration in the music of non-musical cues (speech, body language, gait cadences, facial expressions, observable muscle tension, ethnicity, assessed socioeconomic standing), observed mood states, and energy is carried out, in essence, on an individual level though they may be combined in the music as themes that encompass the whole of the unit or space.

These observed elements, both on a conscious level and as part of the clinical intuitive process combined in improvised (or in some cases pre-composed) music to create a holding space, which may facilitate interaction between patient and therapist and modulate mood state. A shift in the aesthetics of the space may occur, which may contribute to general relaxation, and brightening of affect. Gradual downward shifts in tempo from the base line calculated from observance of gait speed and general movement pattern frequency to which the Music Therapist entrains may contribute to like shifts in heart rate or respiratory rate and promote relaxation.

Musical metaphors produced in the music during Environmental Music Therapy may be employed to mirror and modulate the emotion the therapist perceives that those present are experiencing. These may be seen as agents for shared expression of those emotions and as a form of release that may contribute to lowering stress and promoting relaxation. Instrumental sounds " convey a functional and metaphorical 'voice'" ...and " express emotional narrative".[11] The information gleaned from observing the behavior and states of patients, professional caregivers, and personal caregivers as well as the "energy of the room" are used to determine the choice of music, and more importantly how this music should be played. A soundtrack is created in this process with the purpose of first "meeting" those present "where they are" and subsequently directing them through the metaphors present in music so as to meet the specific therapeutic goals set for that group.

Clinical Accounts

Journal Entry
The following is a journal entry account of a music therapist process recording of one particular EMT session carried out on a chemotherapy infusion suite at Beth Israel Medical Center:

"The music for the EMT interventions was selected based on the dynamics of the physical space, the level of noise in the room, and sporadic listener musical requests. The music was employed intentionally to match and reflect the environment in the moment, and was tailored to meet the needs and preferences of the patients, caregivers and medical staff as identified through the weekly surveys. Background noises, such as beeping monitors, pump sounds and talking, were addressed through the melding of tones and timbres in an otherwise often acoustically taxing environment. Violin, keyboard, guitar, and comfort sounds (Remo ocean drum) were utilized within a wide range of genres, including but not limited to classical, new age, R&B, gospel, reggae, world music and folk music. The intervention began with an improvisation utilizing a slow tempo, which served to explore simple movements of melodies that incorporated the sounds of the environment (in the natural surrounding of sounds, e.g. pump alarms, prosody of voices). These sounds were utilized as the basis for melodic and harmonic structure.

The opening improvisation provided a natural harmonic structure-base, which created opportunity for clinical improvisation. This became a basis for our ability to modify the tempo and other dynamics to effectively meld with the listeners' awareness. When we sensed tension through observation of listeners' facial expression and body gesture, we adapted our music in the moment to address it. Repetitive melodic patterns permit a high grade of anticipatory feeling and may communicate a sense of diminishing unpredictability that impairs the patients' quality of life. Additionally, through harmonic progressions and consistent rhythmic aspects of familiar tunes, the therapists provided the listeners with opportunities for tension release and a venue for a healing environment through auditory consonance. As staff members' listening became consistent, there was a trend towards their gradual familiarity with the music and therapists. As such, their participation in the sessions increased to the point where they were requesting songs that held personal significance, and there were moments of clear engagement in the music, actively and passively."[12]

Milieu Vignette: Radiation Oncology
This session takes place in the waiting area of the radiation oncology unit in one of the hospital's comprehensive cancer care centers. There is a mix of patients waiting to receive radiation therapy and their personal caregivers who have accompanied them, perhaps twenty-four in total. The people present range in age from their late forties to mid eighties. The majority of them are women. About three-quarters of them are Caucasian with the others being evenly distributed between African Americans, and Hispanics. No Asians are present during this session. Most of the patients present on this particular day, at this particular hour, have head and neck cancer, and as they become symptomatic from treatment, they will become susceptible to

experiencing considerable discomfort and pain (often acute) in the area being exposed to external beam radiation. A number of them are already receiving pain medication, and are carefully monitored and evaluated on the evolution of their pain experience. Some of these patients receive individual music psychotherapy sessions for pain management, and all of them received a protocolized music psychotherapy session targeting state anxiety prior to the simulation; a first step and planning session in external beam radiation therapy involving a CT Scan and fitting of the positioning device (a special mask molded on their face) that will be used during radiation therapy itself.

For this session I have chosen to use an extended range classical guitar that has four extra bass strings, and to use voice as well. I pick a spot, sitting down in the waiting area itself, and nodding in greeting to those people who make eye contact with me, I quietly tune the guitar. I scan the room on a conscious level taking in as much information as I can observe about the people there. I am also open to any intuitive 'feelings' I experience. Having 'read' the body language, facial expression, tension and 'energy' in the room, I create a clearing in my mind and allow outside energy and impressions to enter. As I recognize a thought and image of a holding space, a place where comforting may take place, I begin improvising. The music is lower medium tempo, with middle levels of intensity, contour, and harmonic complexity. Fragments of different melodies, and styles emerge.

During this process, I continue to observe and look for changes, cues and clues as to if and how the music is affecting people. My attention is drawn to one woman, mid-50's, Caucasian, jeans and a t-shirt, dressed in clothes that looked young for her seeming age. Her hair was long and untied and she was fidgeting in her chair with brow furrowed and arms crossed over her chest. She was un-comfortable looking and was visibly tapping her foot quickly, out of sync with the pulse of the music. I try entraining to the pulse she is beating with her foot, using it as a subdivision of pulse of what I am playing to no avail. As my rhythm starts to synchronize with hers, she changes it. It becomes evident that perhaps on an un-conscious level she avoiding this contact. She also does not make eye contact with me or say anything. A thought emerges, the rippling of an idea, a song….I fade out the music I am playing, and pause for a moment focusing on the movements of her foot (which she has not stopped tapping even though the 'music stimulus' has stopped). Changing intensity and volume I begin to play the intro to "Sweet Home Alabama" and come in singing on the first verse "big wheel keep on turning, carry me home to see my kin". The woman turns in her seat towards me with a look of astonishment on her face, begins tapping out the backbeat with her foot, and gradually, smiling, starts to sing along softly with me.

When the song ends, I walk over and introduce myself. In the exchange that ensued, she offered that, at first, she "wasn't aware of the music" because she was experiencing considerable discomfort, a "burning, sharp pain" in her throat. Coincidently, she explained that she was originally from the south, and had moved to New Jersey as a child, and "loved" southern rock bands like Lynard Skynard, the authors of the song we had just sung together. As we continued, she spoke about her difficulties with treatment, which I normalized and contextualized. Eventually, I asked her to rate the pain she was experiencing right at that moment. With a surprised look on her face, looking straight at me she replied, "well, close to none. I didn't even realize…"

Intuitively- I certainly had no idea that that particular song would be significant to her – a process unfolded, a person's affect changed as she became integrated in a music experience that began with my music instinct. With that change in affect, apparently, a change also occurred in the level of pain she had been experiencing.

Case Quotes-Patient and Staff Chemotherapy Infusion
Environmental Music therapy in the chemo infusion suite and waiting area involved an artistic medium utilized purposefully for interpersonal and emotional aesthetic expression while providing opportunity for discovery, experience, and transformation, particularly with aspects of the self in relation to the self, and within the environment, which is inclusive of others. The listeners can be transformed through musical experience. Music can increase the awareness of beauty and emphasize the creation of space for positive things, as reflected in the following comments made by patients:

> "It affected me greatly, before I was even aware of its effects- Good medicine."

> "I enjoyed my appointment more than ever. I'm really impatient and the music calmed me down."

> "Very unusual, I did not expect it. Relaxing. Takes your mind away from your thinking, if only for a while."

> "It was beautiful. Music is soothing and helpful when you are nervous about your treatment."[12]

Through continued observation and anecdotal commentary we found as well that the emotional burden on oncology care workers can be considerable. Oncology care can be very rewarding, but also can be stressful, as health care workers support patients and families through arduous treatments, unpredictable courses of illness, and sometimes death. Demanding schedules, lack of emotional support, and uncertainty of roles can make staff susceptible to dissatisfaction with their work and professional burnout.

Regarding this same study, staff reported the personally helpful effect of witnessing and momentarily engaging in the EMT sessions. Surveys indicated that music therapy helped staff improve their ability to care for patients through the skilled use of music and its impact on mood, feeling states, and degree of self-awareness.

Conclusion

This chapter has provided a rationale for the use of Environmental Music Therapy to palliate pain, which in turn may serve as a basis for a model of music therapy in fragile environments. The postulates formulated at the beginning of the chapter are based on clinical experience and treatment interventions. These were further synthesized through a blending of literature that was inclusive of varying perspectives of pain theories, including but not limited to gate control theory, neuromatrix theory, polyvagal theory as well as various psychology perspectives.

It is our hope that music therapists will begin to implement Environmental Music Therapy in an inclusive yet informed way. The clinical examples provided in this chapter are meant to explain the difficulties of this most challenging diverse population of patients. Caution should be exercised. While Environmental Music Therapy has the potential to bring harmony, it is equally at risk to create chaos. Future development and further research is needed to address the impact of improvisatorial live music that can foster a healing environment for patients, caregivers and staff. Since noise is an inevitable element of a working medical environment, music therapists must work intuitively yet systematically to integrate music in a way that fosters sensitivity, and aesthetic awareness. It is hoped that this chapter serves as a starting point for such development and query, as there is a dearth of writing and research on this important topic.

References

1. Hadjistavropoulos T, Craig KD. An introduction to pain. In: Hadjistavropoulos T, Craig KD, eds. *Pain: Psychological Perspectives*. Oxford, UK: Taylor & Francis; 2003.

2. Turk D, Melzack R. *Handbook of Pain Assessment.* Second ed. New York: Guildford; 2001.
3. Melzack R, Katz J. The Gate Control Theory: Research for the Brain. In: Hadjistavropoulos T, ed. *Pain: Psychological Perspectives.* Oxford, UK: Taylor and Francis; 2003.
4. Damasio A. *Emotion and reasons in the human brain.* New York: Grosset/Putnam; 1994.
5. Price DD. Psychological and neural mechanism of the affective dimension. *Science.* 2000;288:17769-11772.
6. Stewart K, Schneider S. The Effects of Music Therapy on the Sound Environment in the NICU: A Pilot Study. In: Loewy J, ed. *Music Therapy in the Neonatal Intensive Care Unit.* New York, NY: Satchnote Press; 2007:85-100.
7. Schneider S. Environment Music Therapy, Life, Death and the ICU. In: Dileo C, Loewy JV, eds. *Music Therapy at the End of Life.* Cherry Hill, NJ: Jeffrey Books; 2005:219-228.
8. Hathaway SR. Clinical intuition and inferential accuracy. *Journal of personality.* 1956;24(3):223-250.
9. Loewy JV. The use of music psychotherapy in the treatment of pediatric pain. In: Dileo C, ed. *Music Therapy in Medicine: Theoretical and Clinical Applications.* Silver Spring, MD: AMTA; 1999:185-206.
10. Mazer SE. Music, Noise, and the Environment of Care. *Music and Medicine.* July 1, 2010 2010;2(3):182-191.
11. Porges SW. The polyvagal perspective. *Biological psychology.* 2007;74(2):116-143.
12. Canga B, Hahm CL, Lucido D, Grossbard ML, Loewy JV. Environmental Music Therapy: A Pilot Study on the Effects of Music Therapy in a Chemotherapy Infusion Suite. *Music and Medicine.* October 1, 2012 2012;4(4):221-230.
13. Liebeskind JC, Paul LA. Psychological and physiological mechanisms of pain. *Annual review of psychology.* 1977;28:41-60.
14. Asmundson GJG, Wright KD. Biopychosocial approaches to pain. In: Hadlistavropoulos T, Craig KD, eds. *Pain: Psychological Perspectives*2003.
15. Chapman CR. Pain, perception, affective mechanisms, and concious experience. In: Hadlistavropoulos T, Craig KD, eds. *Pain: Psychological perspectives*2003.
16. Sadock BJ, Sadock VA. Anxiety Disorders. In: Sadock BJ, ed. *Kaplan and Sadock's Synopsis of Psychiatry: Behavioral Sciences/Clinical Psychiatry.* 10th ed. Philadelphia, PA: Lippincott Williams & Wilkins; 2007:579-583.

17. Anxiety attacks and disorders: guide to the signs, symptoms and treatment options. 2008. http://www.helpguide.org/mental/anxiety_types_symptoms_treatment.htm. Accessed March 3, 2009.
18. Catania C, De Pas T, Minchella I, et al. "Waiting and the waiting room: how do you experience them?" emotional implications and suggestions from patients with cancer. *Journal of cancer education : the official journal of the American Association for Cancer Education.* Jun 2011;26(2):388-394.
19. Porges SW. *The Polyvagal Theory: Neurophysiological Foundations of Emotions, Attachment, Communication, and Self-Regulation.* New York: Norton; 2011.
20. Peretz I. Towards a neurobiology of musical emotions. In: Juslin PN, Soloboda JA, eds. *Handbook of Music and Emotion: Theory, research, Applications.* New York, NY; 2010:99-126.
21. Bigand E, Vieillard S, Madurell F, Marozeau J, Dacquet A. Multidimensional Scaling of Emotional Responses to Music: The Effect of Musical Expertise and of the Duration of the Excerpts. *Cognition and Emotion.* 2005;19(8):1113-1139.
22. Peretz I, Gagnon L, Bouchard B. Music and emotion: perceptual determinants, immediacy and isolation after brain damage. *Cognition* 1998;68:111-141.
23. Cross I. Musicality and the human capacity for culture. *Musicae Scientiae.* 2008:147-169.
24. Eerola T. Modeling Listeners' Emotional Response to Music. *Topics in cognitive science.* Mar 2 2012.
25. Perlovsky L. Musical emotions, cognitive science, and art of music. *Physics of Life Reviews.* 2010;7(1):49-54.
26. Konecni VJ. The aesthetic trinity: Awe, being moved, thrills. *Bull Psychol Arts.* 2005;5:27-44.
27. Perlovsky L. Musical emotions: functions, origins, evolution. *Phys Life Rev.* Mar 2010;7(1):2-27.
28. Coutinho E, Cangelosi A. Emotion and Embodiment in Cognitive Agents: from Instincts to Music. In: Hexmoor H, Thompsom C, eds. *Proceedings of the 2007 International Conference on Integration of Knowledge Intensive Multi-Agent Systems (KIMAS'07)* Waltham, MA: IEEE Press; 2007:133-138.
29. Coutinho E, Cangelosi A. The use of spatio-temporal connectionist models in psychological studies of musical emotions. *Music Perception.* 2009;27:1-15.

30. Cepeda MS, Carr DB, Lau J, Alvarez H. Music for pain relief. *Cochrane database of systematic reviews (Online).* 2006(2):CD004843.
31. Schwoebel J, Coslett HB, Bradt J, Friedman R, Dileo C. Pain and the body schema: effects of pain severity on mental representations of movement. *Neurology.* Sep 10 2002;59(5):775-777.
32. Silvestrini N, Piguet V, Cedraschi C, Zentner M. Music and Auditory Distraction Reduce Pain: Emotional or Attentional Effects? *Music and Medicine.* 2011;3:264-270.
33. Voss JA, Good M, Yates B, Baun MM, Thompson A, Hertzog M. Sedative music reduces anxiety and pain during chair rest after open-heart surgery. *Pain.* Nov 2004;112(1-2):197-203.
34. McCaffrey R, Freeman E. Effect of music on chronic osteoarthritis pain in older people. *Journal of advanced nursing.* Dec 2003;44(5):517-524.
35. Bradt J, Dileo C, Grocke D, Magill L. Music interventions for improving psychological and physical outcomes in cancer patients. *Cochrane database of systematic reviews (Online).* 2011(8):CD006911.
36. Pelletier CL. The effect of music on decreasing arousal due to stress: a meta-analysis. *Journal of music therapy.* Fall 2004;41(3):192-214.

SECTION III

SPECIFIC POPULATIONS

Music and Medicine: Integrative Models in the Treatment of Pain

CHAPTER 17

Pathophysiology of Pain and Stress: Music Therapy Implications for Perinatal, Perioperative, and Chronic Pain Patients

Fred J. Schwartz MD

"Music training is a more potent instrument than any other, because rhythm and harmony find their way into the inward places of the soul."
Plato, The Republic

Introduction

The emotional and physiologic consequences of pain and stress are intricately related. Stress and pain become modulators for the extent of physiologic pathology. Part of this derangement is mediated through the autonomic nervous system. The two components of the autonomic nervous system, the sympathetic nervous system (SNS) and parasympathetic nervous systems (PNS), become out of balance. In most physiologic derangements, the sympathetic side is over stimulated in relation to the parasympathetic side, although the sympathetic system is necessary for an appropriate balance in the maintenance of body function, including blood pressure and flow, and cognitive function. Activation of the sympathetic side is a protective response to support blood pressure during hemorrhage during surgery. A sympathetic response increases performance during athletic competition as well as for the presenter in front of a group. The Chinese ancient medical paradigm views disease as an imbalance of Yin and Yang (sympathetic versus parasympathetic) and many of their treatments are geared to promote a more harmonious relationship between Yin and Yang.

Moment to moment changes in our stress levels are reflected by immediate changes in blood pressure, heart, and respiratory rates. While a therapeutic intention may bring about changes here, a stronger and more meaningful therapeutic music intervention will hopefully cause a decrease in the more enduring basal stress level. Heart variability (HRV) is a much more meaningful measurement of this basal stress level than the more transient patterns of blood pressure and heart rate changes. Variation of the time between heartbeats and other physiologic rhythms is a normal phenomenon. This variability is in general a sign of health and balance. HRV is computed by comparing the different heart beat intervals and analyzing their distribution.[1] The most meaningful information in HRV is contained in the high frequency component (HF), which reflects the relative balance between the PNS and SNS. When the benefits of an increased HRV are referred to, the author is usually talking about the HF component. A decrease in HRV corresponds with an increased risk of hypertension, cardiac disease, diabetic complications, and the overall mortality rate in the general population.[2]

Patients presenting for surgery are often treated with beta blocker drugs to inhibit the sympathetic component that contributes to hypertension and cardiac disease. If the sympathetic nervous system is allowed to be hyperactive during the perioperative period, morbidity and mortality are increased for as long as a year after surgery. It has been shown that in patients taking beta blockers, if this drug is not continued during and after surgery, there can be a prolonged effect on outcome.[2a] In the context of the compensatory stimulation of the SNS, the use of beta blockers during rapid hemorrhage can lead to a worse outcome.[3] In this situation the maintenance of blood pressure takes priority over the long terms effects of stress.

The goals of music therapy for perinatal, perioperative, and chronic pain states are to decrease stress, anxiety, pain, and inflammation, and bring a better balance between the SNS and PNS. The vagus nerve relays parasympathetic activity to and from the heart, lungs, and abdominal organs. Breathing and vocalizing are both ways to access the vagus nerve. This leads to opportunities to therapeutically access this with music and music therapy.

Perinatal Stress Reduction

An exaggerated stress response is often involved in pathophysiology during pregnancy and childbirth (see below). One of the goals of music and music therapy is to decrease this exaggerated SNS stress response.

Negative effects of Stress during Pregnancy
Miscarriage
PIH Pregnancy induced hypertension
IUGR Itrauterine growth retardation
Premature birth, low birth weight
Ineffective contractions during childbirth
Fetal distress
Increased incidence of cesarean section

Communication using music before and after childbirth strengthens the dialog between mother and the fetus and newborn. High risk pregnant women who are at bed rest for possible preterm delivery can achieve reduction in anxiety using music.[4] The use of music therapy during childbirth decreases the perceived length of labor, as well as decreasing pain and anxiety.[5] Music therapy improves postpartum depression and anxiety.[6a]

A recent Cochrane analysis concluded that "music can reduce pain intensity levels and opioid requirements during labor, but the magnitude of these results are small, and music should not be considered a first line treatment for pain relief." Music is frequently used during cesarean section under regional anesthesia. A Cochrane analysis concluded, that "music during planned caesarean section under regional anesthesia may improve pulse rate and birth satisfaction score. However, the magnitude of these benefits is small. More research is needed."[6]

Despite the lack of strong evidence in the literature, it is the author's experience that music can have a significant affect in improving the birth experience both during normal vaginal delivery and cesarean section.

Altered Fetal Brain Development

Fetal hearing begins at about 20 weeks gestation and the fetus senses the maternal heart beat rhythm via auditory and probably also through electromagnetic pathways. During pregnancy there is a dynamic communication between mother and fetus and besides neurohormonal mechanisms, this is likely conveyed by the fetus sensing heart rate variability from the maternal heartbeat as well as respiratory rhythms.[7,8] Over the last half of pregnancy there is entrainment of the variability of the maternal and fetal heart rhythms. Maternal fetal synchrony or coupling is an entrainment process that occurs between the maternal and fetal cardiac rhythms.[9,9a] This epoch synchronization is demonstrated by comparing segments of the HRV between the maternal and fetal heart rhythms and measuring the degree of similarity or synchrony. The emotional content within the maternal heart rate variability is sensed by the fetus. After birth the newborn can recognize emotional content contained in their own mother's heart rhythm, but not from other mothers.[10] It is intuitive that increased maternal stress would affect the maternal-fetal dialog. Chronic stress during pregnancy is associated with impaired long-term cognitive and emotional development in the newborn.[11] For the premature baby the early loss of this connection can affect the nurturing process.[12]

Music and music therapy can be used during pregnancy to enhance the maternal-fetal connection. Involving the mother in singing and talking to her unborn child increases the nurturing nature of this bond. Music has beneficial results decreasing the stress response for both mother and fetus.

Along with the early loss of mother's voice and heart rhythm, the preterm infant in the Neonatal Intensive Care Unit (NICU) is exposed to elevated light and sound levels. These altered sensory experiences in the NICU can cause stress in the premature baby. The consequences can be negative outcomes.

Negative Effects of Stress in the NICU
Increased oxygen and calorie consumption
Increased heart and respiratory rates
Sensitivity to pain
Impaired self regulation
Decreased weight gain
Miscarriage

Multiple studies have shown that the use of music and music therapy in the NICU has many potential benefits Among these are improved formula intake,[13] increased weight gain and earlier discharge from the NICU.[8,13-16] Less frequent episodes of oxygen desaturation and stress behaviors have been seen[13] as well as higher oxygen saturations and more time in the sleep state.[13,17] Music can decrease the stress response to heel sticks as evidenced by decreased heart rate and pain behavior.[18]

Perioperative Stress Reduction

The emotional aspects of the preoperative experience can negatively affect the patient experience. The preoperative use of music can decrease depression and sadness. Anxiety decreases and there is less preoccupation with pain and physical suffering. Feelings of withdrawal and defensiveness shift to warmth and depth in relating to others, and patients become more approachable to necessary procedures.

Perioperative music also can be helpful with the stress effects on physiology.

Physiologic Consequences of Perioperative Stress
Hypertension
Tachycardia
Peripheral vasoconstriction/low blood flow
Inflammatory response
Decreased immune function
Increased metabolism and oxygen consumption
Delayed healing
Increased anesthesia drug doses

The perioperative experience is associated with elevated levels of stress hormones. This is true under either general or regional anesthesia. Music can decrease this stress response when applied before, during, and after surgery.[19] When used during surgery under spinal or epidural anesthesia during music has been shown to blunt the intraoperative rise in cortisol levels.[16,19,20] The intraoperative use of music in sedated patients decreases sedative and analgesic requirements during surgery.[19] This effect continues after surgery. The exception is that during general anesthesia music doesn't blunt the intraoperative stress response and probably doesn't have any or much effect since general anesthesia blocks the central processing of auditory pathways.[21] This still leaves the pre and postoperative periods for the potential benefits of music in the patient undergoing general anesthesia. The use of preoperative music has been shown to decrease postoperative narcotic requirements when patients control their own intravenous dosage, as well as convey marked emotional benefits.[22] Preoperative music has been shown to lower anxiety measured by visual analog scale, as well as to increase heart rate variability.[23,24]

Stefan Koelsch and colleagues recently studied effects of music on propofol consumption and cortisol levels during spinal anesthesia at the University of Leipzig Clinic.[25] They compared preselected instrumental music compared with a control group exposed to soothing breaking sea waves. The music was started preoperatively and continued through the entire anesthetic. As shown in previous studies, cortisol levels in the music group did not rise as much as the control group throughout the surgery. During the surgery the patients were sedated with a controlled propofol infusion to a moderate level of sedation as measured by a BIS monitor (bispectral index). The BIS number is derived from brain waves and as BIS numbers decrease this reflects the continuum of increasing levels of sedation and general anesthesia.

The music group consumed significantly less propofol during surgery than the control group, and reached a deeper level of sedation with less propofol than the control group. The BIS number was compared to the level of sedation of both patient groups in order to derive a sedation ratio, and the music group had a large increased propofol effect, that is, the same amount of propofol caused more sedation in the music group (Figure 1).

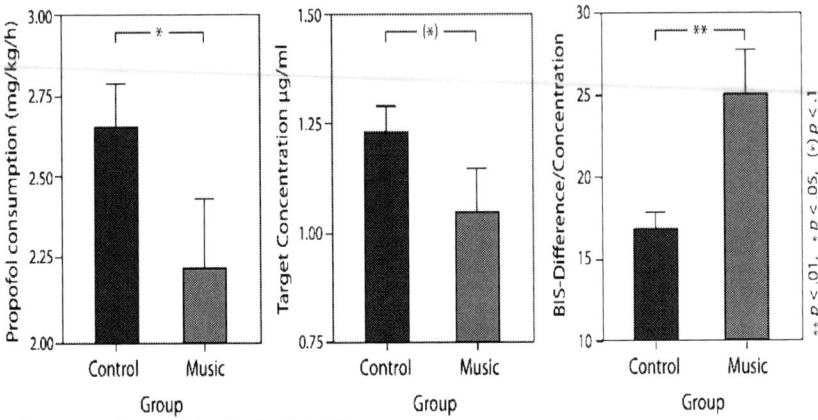

Figure 1 (from Koelsch, 2011)

Average propofol consumption (left panel), target propofol concentration (middle panel), and propofol concentration relative to the BIS-value (100–BIS-value/concentration, right panel), separately for the two groups (control group, music group). Particularly in relation to the BIS-values, propofol requirement was significantly lower in the music compared to the control group. Error bars indicate SEM.

Stress and Chronic Pain

Acute pain is often associated with a hyperactive sympathetic nervous system. With repeated episodes of pain, catecholamine levels are often increased even when there is no painful stimulus. This leads to hyperalgesia in that the threshold is lowered for inducing pain. The pain can become centralized, and pathways in the brain are activated and pain sensed even when there is no pain stimulus. Depression is often associated with chronic pain. It has been shown that the emotional component in chronic pain is a major factor in outcome.

Various Mechanisms by which Music Decreases Pain
Distraction
Stimulation of the dopaminergic system
Modulation of beta-endorphin levels
Increased oxytocin production
Increased growth hormone
Better autonomic nervous system balance

The number of well done controlled studies on music and pain are few. A Cochrane metanalysis concluded, that "listening to music reduces pain intensity levels and opioid requirements, but the magnitude of these benefits is small and therefore its clinical importance unclear."[26] Although there have been a paucity of well controlled studies on music and pain relief, some of the documented benefits have been decreased pain and anxiety, improvement in depressive symptoms, better quality of sleep, and less consumption of medications. A number of studies have shown non-significant reductions in blood pressure, heart rate, and respiratory rate. Despite the lack of strong evidence, it is the author's opinion that it is possible to achieve strong clinical benefits with the use of music. Inherent in this effect is the interaction of the healer and the patient, and how the music is used with the patient.

A recent study RCT showed marked benefits using music to treat chronic pain.[27] Dr. Stéphane Guétin, et.al. at Montpellier Regional University Hospital Centre in Paris, France, administered a customized instrumental music program from Music Care (http://www.music-care.com) through earphones, while the patients were wearing an eye mask, two times each day. This therapy was continued for 10 days in the hospital, and when the patients went home they were given access to the same music and the therapy was continued for another 50 days. Indices of pain, anxiety, depression, anxiolytic and antidepressant use were measured for a total of 90 days in order to see if there was a music effect after the 30 days of the music regimen. Both sedative and narcotic consumption decreased in a group of hospital inpatients, along with decreased indices of pain, anxiety, and depression compared to a control group. This effect was still present 30 days after the music intervention.

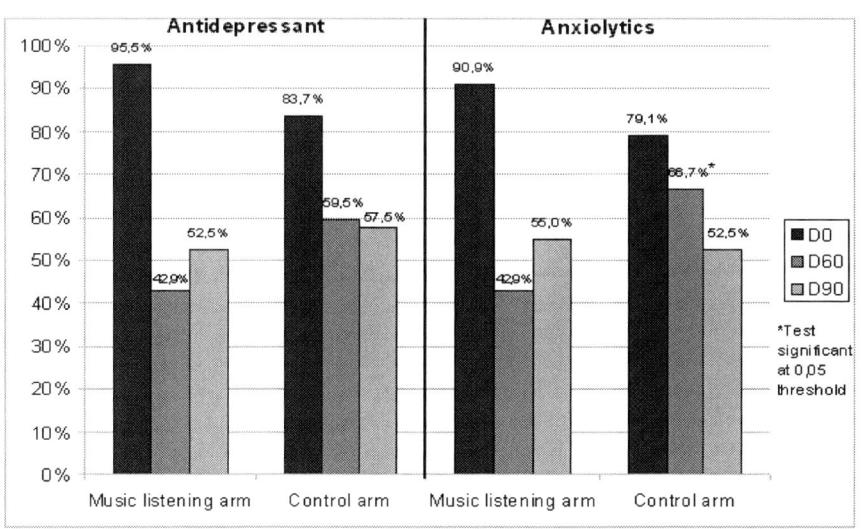

Figure 2 (from Guétin)

Music and Medicine: Integrative Models in the Treatment of Pain

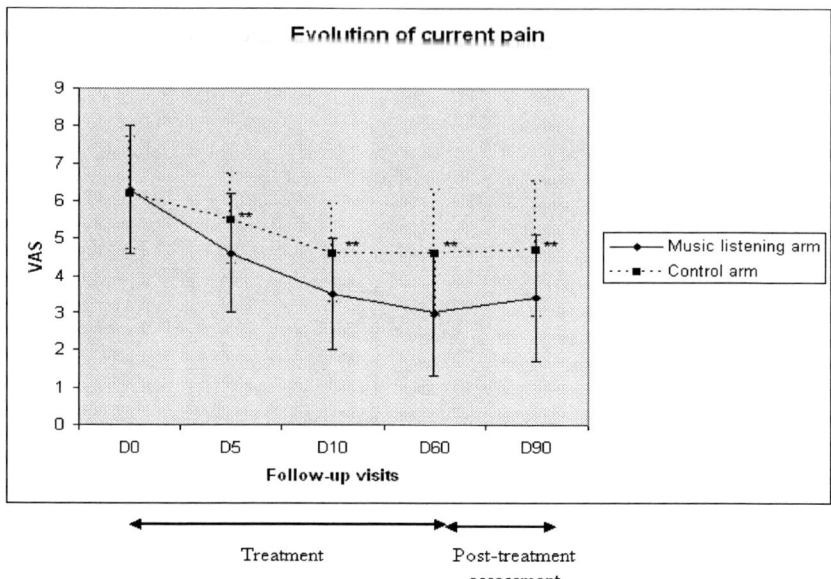

Figure 3 (from Guétin)

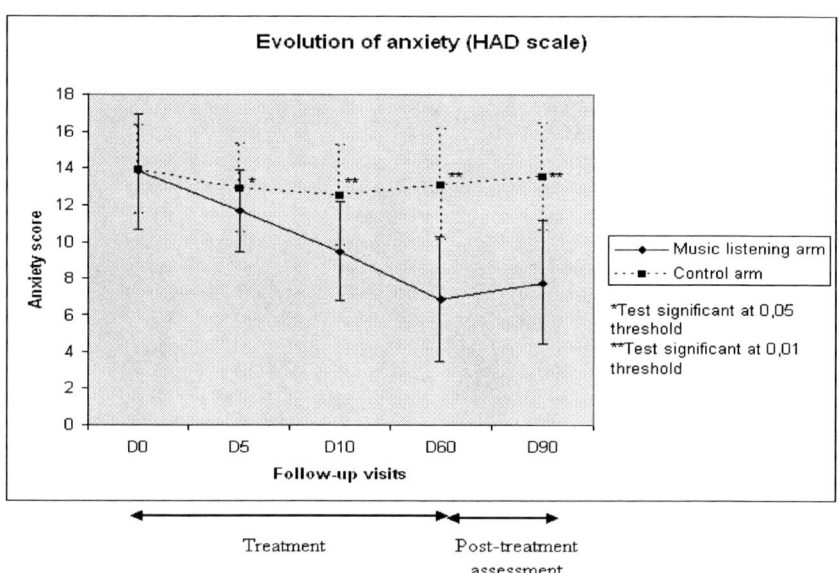

Figure 4 (from Guétin)

Conclusion

In summary, the stress response and autonomic balance are intimately associated with pathologic conditions in the parturient, premature newborn, surgical patient, and patients with chronic pain. The use of music is a modality that has the potential power to reverse some of this imbalance and promote healing.

References

1. Billman, G.E. "Heart rate variability - a historical perspective." *Frontiers in Physiology.* November 29, 2011. www.frontiersin.org (accessed April 6, 2011).
2. Thayer, J.F., Yamamoto, S.S., Brosschot, J.F. "The relationship of autonomic imbalance, heart rate variability and cardiovascular disease risk factors." *Int J Cardiol* 141, no. 2 (May 2010): 122-131.
2a. Mangano, D.T., Layug, E.L., Tateo, W.A. "Effect of atenolol on mortality and cardiovascular morbidity after noncardiac surgery. Multicenter study of perioperative ischemia research group." *n Engl J Med* 335, no. 23 (Dec 1996): 1713-1720.
3. Wallace, A.W., Au, S., Cason, B.A. "Association of the pattern of use of perioperative B-blockade and postoperative mortality." *Anesthesiology* 113, no. (Oct.2010): 794-805.
4. Yang, M.Y., Lingjiang. L., Zhu, H., Alexander, I.M., Liu, S., Zhou, W., Ren, X. "Music therapy to relieve anxiety in pregnant women on bedrest: a randomized, controlled trial." *MCN* 34, no. 5 (Sept/Oct 2009): 316-323.
5. Ranying, Z. "Effect of music therapy on the labor, anxiety and depression of primiparas." *Medical Journal of Chinese People's Health* 19, no. 9 (2007): 731.
6a. Xu, P., Hai, Y., Zhang, L. "The effect of music therapy on postpartum depression among 144 patients." *World Health Digest (Chinese)* 4, no. 5 (2007): 210-211.
6. Laopaiboon, M., Lumbiganon, P., Martis, R., Vatanasapt, P., Somjaivong, B. "Music during caesarean section under regional anaesthesia for improving maternal and infant outcomes." *Cochrane Database Syst Rev*, April 15, 2009: CD006914.
7. Schwartz, F.J. "Music and sound effect on perinatal brain development and the premature baby." In *Music Therapy in the Neonatal Intensive Care Unit*, by J.V. Loewy, 9-19. NY: Satchnote, 2000.

8. Schwartz, F.J. "Perinatal stress reduction, music, and medicalcost savings." *Journal of Prenatal and Perinatal Psychology and Health* 12, no. 1 (1997): 19-29.
9. Ivanov, P.C., Ma, Q.Y.M., Bartsch, R.P. "Maternal-fetal heartbeat phase synchronization." *Proc Natl Acad Sci* 106, no. 33 (Aug 2009): 13641-13642.
9a. DiPietro, J. "Psychological and psychophysiological considerations regarding the maternal-fetal relationship." *Infant Child Dev* 19, no. 1 (2010): 27-38.
10. Righetti, P.L. "The emotional experience of the fetus: a preliminary report." *Journal of Prenatal and Perinatal Psychology and Health* 11, no. 1 (1996): 55-65.
11. Talge, N.M., Neal, C., Glover, V. "Antenatal maternal stress and long-term effects on child neurodevelopment; how and why?" *Jnl of Child Psychology and Psychiatry* 48, no. 3-4 (March/April 2007): 245-261.
12. Krueger, C. "Exposure to maternal voice in preterm infants: a review." *Ad Neonatal care* 10, no. 1 (Feb 2010): 13-20.
13. Cain, J. "The effects of music on the selected stress behaviors, weight and formula intake, and length of hospital stay of premature and low birth weight neonates in a newborn intensive care unit." *Journal of Music Therapy* 28 (1991): 180-192.
14. Cassidy, J.W., & Stanley, J.M. "The effect of music listening on physiological response of premature infants in the N ICU." *Journal of Music Therapy* 32 (1995): 208-227.
15. Standley, J.W. & Moore, R.S. "Therapeutic effects of music and mother's voice on premature infants." *Pediatric Nursing*, no. 21 (1995): 509-512.
16. Amon, S., Shapsa, A., Forman, L., Regev, R., Bauer, S., Litmanovitz, I., and Dolfin, T. "Live music is beneficial to preterm infants in the neonatal intensive care environment." *Birth* 33, no. 2 (2006): 131-136.
17. Collins, S.K. & Kuck, K. "Music therapy in the neonatal intensive care unit." *Neonatal Network* 9, no. 6 (1991): 23-26.
18. Bo, L.K, Callaghan, P. "Soothing pain-elicited distress in Chinese neonates." *Pediatrics* 105, no. 4 (April 2000): e49.
19. Spintge, R., Droh, R. "Effects of anxiolytic music on plasma levels of stress hormones in different medical specialties." In *The fourth international symposium on music: Rehabilitation and human well-being.*, by R. Pratt, 88-101. Lantham, MD: University Press of America, 1987.

20. Koch, M.E., Kain, Z.N., Ayoub, C., Rosenbaum, S.H. "The sedative and analgesic sparing effect of music." *Anesthesiology* 89, no. 2 (Aug 1998): 300-306.
21. Migneault, B., Girard, F., Couinard, P., Boudreault, D., Prevencher, D., Todorov, A., Ruel, M., Girard, D.C. "The effect of music on the neurohormonal stress response to surgery under general anesthesia." *Anesthesia Analgesia* 98, no. 2 (Feb 2004): 527-532.
22. Bernatzky, G., Presch, M., Anderson, M., Panksepp, J. "Emotional foundations of music as a non-pharmacological pain management tool in modern edicine." *Neuroscience and Biobehavioral Reviews* 35 (2011): 1989-1999.
23. Lee, K., Chao, Y., Yiin, J., Chiang, P., Chao, Y. "Effectivenes of different music-playing devices for reducing preoperative anxiety: A clinical control study." Int J Nurs Stud 48, no. 10 (Oct. 2011): 1180-7.
24. Lee, K., Chao, Y., Yiin, J.,Hsieh, H., Dai, W., Chao, Y. "Evidence that music listening reduces preoperative patients' anxiety." Biol Res Nurs 14, no. 78 (2012): 78-84.
25. Koelsch, S., Fuermetz, J., Sack, U., Bauer, K., Hohenadel, M., Wiegel, M., Kaisers, X., and Heinke, W. Effects of music listening on cortisol levels and propofol consumption during spinal anesthesia. April 5, 2011. www.frontiersin.org (accessed Nov 15, 2011).
26. Cepeda, M.S., Carr, d.B., Lau, J. Alvarez, H. "Music for pain relief." Cochrane Database Syst Rev, April 19, 2006: CD004843
27. Guétin, S., Ginies, P., Siou, D.K., Picot, M., Pommie, C., Guldner, E., Gosp, A., Ostyn, K., Coudeyre, E., and Touchon, J. "The effects of music intervention in the management of chronic pain." Clinical Journal of Pain 00, no.00 (2011): 1-9.

Music and Medicine: Integrative Models in the Treatment of Pain

CHAPTER 18

Music Therapy for Pain and Stress in NICU Infants: A Developmental, Trauma-Informed and Family-Centered Approach

Angela Thompson MA, MT-BC

*On the night you were born,
the moon smiled with such wonder
that the stars peeked in to see you and the night wind whispered,
"Life will never be the same."*[*]
Nancy Tillman

Introduction

An infant is admitted to the Neonatal Intensive Care Unit (NICU), when they are born prematurely, or are born full term with medical complications including fever, physical abnormalities, low APGAR scores- which are indicative of a medical or genetic disorder, or abnormal vital signs. An infant who is classified as pre-term is less than thirty-six weeks gestation. Full term infants born with medical complications may be hospitalized for a short observation period and then released, unless there is a diagnosis of a medical condition or surgery is needed. Preterm infants may be hospitalized for several months depending upon their gestational age at birth, their diagnosis and their medical fragility.

Empathy is an important component of therapy. As a music therapist working with infants hospitalized in the NICU, I find myself trying to imagine what life is like for these infants; to come from a warm, safe regulated place out into a bright, loud unpredictable place, where pain and discomfort are a part of daily life. I think it must be like being in a warm,

---

[*] Tillman, *The night you were born*. NY,NY: Feiwel & Friends; 2005.

cozy bed on a cold winter's night, in a deep sleep. Suddenly, people come in, turn on the lights, remove your covers and begin moving and examining you, all the while your alarm clock is going off loudly. You feel cold and frightened, it's noisy, it's bright, and now someone is drawing blood and inserting an IV. This would be a difficult experience for a fully developed adult, but imagine being a small, premature infant who has yet to develop the capacity to regulate and recover from such an experience.

The NICU Environment

Infants hospitalized in the Neonatal Intensive Care Unit undergo pain and stress as a part of their daily lives. Whether infants are hospitalized for premature birth and its' subsequent complications, or for other medical reasons, necessary routine procedures can cause both pain and stress to an infant who has not yet had an opportunity to regulate to the outside world. The terms pain and stress will be used interchangeably throughout this chapter because for the dysmature infant, pain causes stress and stress causes pain in terms of physiologic parameters. Medical interventions stimulate a pain response and environmental stressors can further exacerbate that pain. For the preterm infant, non-painful stimuli such as noise, bright lights, and even touch or handling can be processed and perceived much in the same way that painful stimuli is processed and perceived.[1]

Although pre-term infant's systems are not fully developed, it should not be assumed their pain is less intense. Infants, both pre and full term, experience pain more intensely and have a prolonged reaction to pain as compared to adults. This is in part because the sensory nervous cells of an infant are more volatile and active than those of an adult, and therefore result in a more pronounced reflex when met with a pain stimulus.[1] The ability to modulate a pain response is not present in pre-term infants; as the nerves responsible for buffering pain have not yet been fully developed. As a result, pre-term infants suffer from a prolonged pain experience. Therefore, pre-term infants experience pain more intensely than adults, and with repeated exposure to painful experiences, the pain becomes more intensified.[2]

Routine procedures and medical interventions are necessary in the care and treatment of NICU infants however, the measures taken to ultimately improve and save an infant's life, can also cause tremendous pain, discomfort and stress. Infants in the NICU are subjected to multiple, and repeated painful procedures such as heel sticks, venipuncture, and endotracheal tube suctioning, as well as tube placements, tape removal, blood draws, IV and central line placement, and injections. Even routine exams such as eye exams, can cause an infant a tremendous amount of stress.

Naturally, frequency and type of procedure depends upon the infant's diagnosis and the medical interventions required to treat that diagnosis. All pre-term infants receive routine care, which even when non-invasive, can cause stress/pain depending upon weight and age. For young pre-term infants, whose skin is still developing; pain may result from simple forms of non-invasive care such as touching, examining and positioning.[3] Non-painful stimuli, such as lights and noise can be perceived as painful to the neonate because sensory input is not yet organized (into painful and non-painful) stimuli when it is transmitted along the spinal chord.[2]

Naturally, the youngest and smallest of infants are the most medically fragile and will therefore require more medial interventions than older preterm infants. Various research studies have been conducted to determine the average of painful procedures an infant receives during hospitalization. One study found that during NICU hospitalization, 10% of the youngest infants typically endured over 300 painful procedures.[4] Another study discovered that within the first two weeks of admission, infants in the NICU were exposed to an average of 14 painful procedures per day.[5] It was also observed that nearly 40 percent of the infants in the study did not receive any form of analgesia to cope with the procedures. Barker and Rutter conducted a study of fifty-four NICU infants and found that a total of 3,000 procedures were conducted, and nearly seventy five percent of the procedures were conducted on infants younger than 31 weeks gestation.[6] Grunau and colleagues,[7] conducted a study to determine the impact that painful procedures had on the stress levels of preterm infants. In the study, 136 infants between 23-32 weeks gestation were observed post heel stick and data was taken on the following: heart rate, behavioral pain reaction and state of illness. The study resulted in the conclusion that in preterm infants, recurrent exposure to pain resulted in the infants existing in a continuous state of stress.

Infants with untreated pain throughout their hospitalization have shown a propensity towards the following physiologic changes[3]: Hyperglycemia, increased protein catabolism, increased oxygen consumption, decreased gut motility, increased heart rate and blood pressure, decreased oxygen saturation, increased respiratory rates, changes in cerebral blood flow, and increase in secretion of adrenal stress hormones. When preterm infants undergo physiologic changes such as those mentioned above, precious calories, which could be used for growing and healing, are expended. In addition, secreting stress hormones as a result of untreated pain can cause infections, and poor healing.[7] These stressors therefore lead to a longer length of stay and increased medical complications. Untreated pain in neonates can also contribute to neonatal morbidity and mortality, particularly for the postoperative patient.[1,3] Current research is pointing to possible adverse outcomes later in life due to untreated pain such as: increased pain sensitivity and chronic pain conditions, anxiety disorders, hyperactivity/attention deficit disorder, impaired social skills, self-destructive behaviors and other neurodevelopmental, cognitive and behavioral disorders.[1,8-10]

It is imperative that pain is treated in NICU infants; those who experience untreated pain may require a longer length of stay in the hospital, as well as stunted development, both physical and psychosocial, and an impaired ability to self-regulate.[3] It is not the sensory experience of pain alone that attributes to stunted development and impairment of self-regulation; it is the hormonal stress response and experience of fear as well. Pain and stress provides unexpected stimuli and because the neonate's brain is not yet developed, it is forming under stressful conditions.[11] Neuroplasticity is the term defined by Puchalski and Hummel[11] to describe the ability of the normal brain of the neonate to undergo change based on exposure to unexpected stimuli. "The neonatal brain is in a period of rapid physical growth and development; the more premature the infant, the higher the risk that external stimuli can cause changes in that normal development including possible alterations to nervous system development."[11] Responding to an infant's pain, and providing comfort and stabilization during unexpected stimuli can ultimately "save the brain".

NICU Pain Assessment

Assessing pain and understanding how it is affecting an infant's development has become a vital part of NICU care, so much so that pain is now being referred to as the fifth vital sign.[12] In order to have a full, comprehensive assessment of a NICU infant, their level of pain/stress must be considered at all times, and requires formal assessment throughout the day.[12] Although measuring pain via a pain scale is an important aspect of understanding an infant's level of discomfort, true pain assessment must also take into account the full framework of the infant's diagnosis, needs, development and environment. The obvious difficulty when assessing pain in a nonverbal individual is the ability, as the assessor, to miss-interpret behavioral cues or signals. Pain in neonates and newborns is typically observed via behavioral signals such as the brow bulge, gaping mouth, and cry face.

There are significant differences between the way pre-term infants and term infants respond to pain. Full-term infants typically respond to pain with an increase in crying and body movements as well as an increase in blood pressure and tachycardia.[1,13] When pre-term infants experience pain they may become lethargic and unresponsive versus active. This response to pain is not due to the preterm infant's lack of feeling or experiencing pain but rather it's attributed to "a failure of the central nervous system to mount a response to pain."[1] It is as thought the pain is overwhelming the infants' systems. The consideration that infants (and possibly other non-verbal) patients may be experiencing pain without exhibiting clear signs caused the International Association for the Study of Pain to revise the standard definition of pain to reflect this consideration: "The inability to communicate in no way negates the possibility that an individual is experiencing pain, and is in need of appropriate pain-relieving treatment".[14]

As a music therapist working with infants hospitalized in the NICU, it is vital to be aware of the variability in pain responses. Pain scales are one aspect of assessing pain in NICU infants, and there are a variety of scales in existence. Typically, pain assessment tools are effective for a particular population, but are not comprehensive across all populations and situations. As previously mentioned, infants experience pain differently depending on gestational age, and many tools do not clearly distinguish pain behaviors from generalized stress behaviors. The majority of pain scales also lack the ability to distinguish acute and chronic pain. Being well versed in how to use each pain scale is ideal as is selecting a pain scale, which examines both behavioral responses and physiologic parameters.

The Attia Behavioral pain scale assesses the infant's behavioral response in relation to a pain stimulus. The quality of the infant's cry, facial expression, motor activity and tone, quality of suck, sleep, consolability, sociability and excitability are examined and rated on a scale of zero to two, with zero being the most severe reaction, or level of discomfort.[15] When using this scale it is important to note that the infant's gestational age is not taken into account, and therefore a differentiation of pain response between young pre-term infants and older pre-term infants is not made solely using the scale. The Premature Infant Pain Profile (PIPP) is specific to the preterm infant population and is used with infants aged twenty-eight weeks to thirty-six weeks gestation. "Taking gestational age into account, the PIPP accommodates the recognition that the youngest and smallest infants may not be able to mount or sustain a response to pain in the same fashion as an older infant. Therefore, these infants are given points toward their overall profile based on their gestational age."[3] The PIPP is comprehensive in that it examines both the infant's behavioral state, as well as their physiological parameters. The PIPP score is calculated by scoring each individual area on a scale of zero to three and then adding the total score so that a score of six or less is indicative of minimal to no pain, a score of seven to twelve indicates mild to moderate pain and a score of twelve or higher moderate to severe pain.[16]

The CRIES Neonatal Pain Scale, like the PIPP assesses both behavioral and physiological responses to pain. CRIES is an acronym which assesses the following vital signs and behaviors:
CryingRequiresO2 for Sat >95Increased vital signsExpressionSleeplessThe CRIES is specified to assess pain post-operatively in neonates and assists the medical team in determining when an infant should receive pharmacological intervention to aide in pain relief.[17]

In situations where the music therapist is without access to the physiological profiles of an infant, for instance, when an infant is briefly taken off the monitors, the NIPS- Neonatal Infant Pain Scale, is a useful tool. This particular tool examines behavioral signals but does not include psychological parameters. Behavioral cues such as movement of extremities, facial expression, state of arousal, breathing patterns, and quality of cry are assessed.[18]

The Échelle Douleur Inconfort Nouveau-Né, Neonatal Pain and Discomfort Scale (EDIN) assesses for signs of prolonged pain in neonates. Facial activity, body movements, quality of sleep, quality of contact with nurses and consolability are rated on a scale of zero to three and then a total score is calculated with higher numbers indicated higher levels of prolonged pain.[19]

Music Therapy for Pain

Music therapy for pain relief has been well documented in the literature[20-25] and research has indicated that music can counteract the negative physiologic effects that pain and stress may cause. The literature shows benefits of both live and recorded music however, the focus of this chapter is on live, interactive and in the moment music which can be entrained to the infant in order to achieve maximum potential for self-regulation. Studies across populations further demonstrate the effects music has on specific physiological parameters. Figure 1. below contrasts the physiologic responses pain has on neonates with what is shown in the literature to be the physiologic responses music therapy can incite across various populations:

PHYSIOLOGIC EFFECTS OF PAIN AND STRESS ON NEONATES:	PHYSIOLOGIC EFFECTS OF MUSIC:
Elevated Heart Rate[26,27]	Lowered Heart Rate[29-33]
Elevated Blood Pressure[11]	Lowered Blood Pressure[33,34]

Elevated respiratory rate[28]	Lowered respiratory rate[33]
Decreased OT Saturation[28]	Increased OT Saturation[33,35,36] Decrease in overall pain response[37,38]

Figure 1. (continued)

In addition to the physiologic effects music has on pain, music also has a known effect on affect and emotion. Music counter-stimulates the afferent fibers of spinal mechanisms involved in pain modulation. Music also stimulates endorphins, which may activate the endogenous system of pain modulation.

Research continues to emerge specific to music therapy, pain and the NICU population. In a study done in 2000, Butt and Kisilevsky[30] observed fourteen neonates receiving music therapy during heel stick procedures. Infants over thirty one weeks gestation were able to return to their baseline parameters in terms of behavioral state, heart rate and facial expressions. Infants in the study who were less than thirty-one weeks took longer to return to baseline post heel stick despite receiving music therapy. This result illustrates the difficulty younger; dysmature infant's systems have to regulating in general. In another study, infants who received music therapy in combination with non-nutritive sucking during heel stick procedures displayed increased oxygen saturation levels and a decrease in pain behaviors.[31]

Music therapy, in conjunction with EMLA (Eutectic Mixture of Lidocaine and Prilocaine) during circumcision was studied on a sample size of twenty-three neonates. The infants receiving this combination of treatments displayed signs of pain relief as opposed to the non- music therapy group.[32]

Music therapy can be used to address pain from a developmental, trauma-informed and family-centered approach. As previously mentioned, NICU infants are developing on a different trajectory than they would be if they were born full term. They are discovering the world through a very different environment when contrasted with the comforting buffer of the mother's womb. Full term infants hospitalized immediately following birth can also have compromised development as a result of separation from caregivers and being in a hospital versus a home environment. Developmental approaches to NICU care are becoming immensely popular, as trends in later-in-life diagnoses have emerged. The NICU infant often experiences delays in reaching developmental milestones post discharge, along with other physical and psychological complications.

Music and Medicine: Integrative Models in the Treatment of Pain

Stewart[39,40] has developed PATTERNS (Preventive Approach to Traumatic Experience by Resourcing the Nervous System), a trauma-centered approach to music therapy with NICU infants and their families. As a music therapist working in the NICU, it is important to realize that a pre-term birth, or medically complicated birth, and subsequent hospitalization, is traumatizing to the infant and their fragile systems both physically, and in many ways emotionally. Understanding how trauma, and particularly trauma which is rooted in painful experiences, affects these infants and their development will, inform the music therapy approach and subsequent interventions. Families of NICU infants often suffer trauma: their infant is medically fragile, they are separated from their infants, and the role they expected to have upon their infant's birth has shifted, they are now secondary caregivers. Families of NICU infants often feel helpless, and suffer feelings of loss, anxiety, depression and stress.

Understanding that pre-term infants in particular, regulate off of their caregivers, stabilizing the parents of these infants is an important music therapy treatment goal. Parents, who are physiologically and emotionally regulated, will thus be able to provide physiologic and emotional stability for an infant experiencing pain. This stability can promote regulation and reconstitution following painful procedures, as well as comfort and safety amidst chronic pain.[41]

Developmental Approach
When working with an infant in pain, I am always trying to envision how exposure to pain at such a young and fragile age might affect their development and how I can counteract the pain with music and contact. As important as the music is in music therapy, the contact and relationship are equally as important. Through the relationship, contact and the music, the therapist is able to support the infant(s) as they continue on towards healthy development.

"A developmentally supportive approach to caregiving is essential in the NICU and is an important adjunct to effective pain management".[1] Developmentally supportive care is focused on relational care and the way the infant is responding to non-invasive care such as touching and holding. The literature cites a variety of non-pharmacological treatments, which are developmentally supportive in nature for pain relief in the NICU infant. These include: music therapy, sucking,[42-44] holding and rocking.[1] Newcastle, states that integrating a developmentally supportive approach to caregiving "reduces noxious stimuli from the environment while promoting the infant's own coping abilities, thereby possibly reducing pain and stress."[1] Caregiving, which is developmentally focused, can also improve weight gain, decrease length of stay, and improve neurodevelopmental outcomes.[46]

The Newborn Individualized Developmental Care and Assessment Program (NIDCAP)[47] is a specific developmentally-focused program, which focuses on relationship-based caregiving. NIDCAP provides a model for the neurobehavioral development of the premature infant. A defining attribute of NIDCAP is the understanding that the infant is both the recipient of, and an active participant in caregiving.[46,47] In the framework of music therapy, this attribute provides the therapeutic rationale for basing music therapy interventions around an infant's vial signs.

This approach views the music of the infant as valuable, and heard by the music therapist. The music of the infant is entrained and mirrored within the music of the therapist. The music of the infant includes the rhythm both of the breath and heart rate, the infant's vocalizations and cries. The therapist's music is not only entrained to the infant's vitals, it is also in tune with the surrounding environment.

The other goals of NIDCAP include comprehensive consideration of each infant's comfort level as well as their capacity to cope with painful procedures, and a focus on enabling the infant's ability to self-regulate.[46] Assessing behavioral cues, and implementing individualized interventions, are key components of the NIDCAP program in order to reduce infant's stress behaviors and increase the ability to self-regulate. Facilitating these goals has resulted in improved medical and developmental outcomes for NICU infants.[47]

Deanna Hanson-Abromeit developed a model marrying the theories of NIDCAP with music therapy.[48] Hanson-Abromeit states that "The outcomes of NIDCAP studies have demonstrated very similar benefits as those identified in research regarding the therapeutic use of music for young infants." Because of this parallel, particularly with both NIDCAP and music therapy being relationally focused, the two models compliment one another therapeutically.[48]

Another area of overlap between the two is the family-centered aspect of care. One of the goals of NIDCAP is to support and nurture the parent's cherishing, of their infant and their confidence in caring for them and taking pride in supporting their infant's development. This treatment goal should also be present in music therapy as music can support bonding and loving interactions between infants and their parents.

Trauma-Informed Approach
Having a trauma-informed approach to NICU music therapy, involves understanding the infant from the perspective of being traumatized in a multi-layered way. There is traumatic birth (be it early or full term) where something has occurred which requires hospitalization and medical intervention. Then there is the emotional trauma of separation from the womb,

and the parents. There is the physiologic trauma of no longer having the regulatory systems of the mother with which to organize oneself, and instead developing in an unpredictable environment, which can be perceived as hostile and painful. In both NIDCAP and Stewart's[39,40] music therapy trauma model, the importance of timing, environmental adaptations and gradual initiative taking when working with NICU infants is emphasized. Particularly in moments of acute pain, it is important to understand that the infant's systems can be on overload and therefore, it is all the more important to layer interventions with time for observation (both of behavioral cues and the infant's vitals) in order to promote recovery and organization.[39,40] Music interventions which are slow, steady, simple and repetitive will offer the optimum potential for "taking in", particularly after a painful procedure.[39,40] Familiarity is also a key element of music which can provide comfort during stressful times. Ideally, if music therapy can be provided while mom and dad are present, they can take an active role in musically comforting their infant.

Often times parents are not permitted at the bedside during procedures, the music therapist has the unique role of being able to "be there" for the infant before, during and after painful procedures while offering stimuli that is comforting to counteract the painful stimuli.

Family-Centered Care
The NICU can be an intimidating place to families who are already feeling overwhelmed and traumatized. In order to help families feel empowered and supported, Meyer, et.al.[49] developed a program whereby individualized, family-based interventions were applied to families of NICU infants. Families were first surveyed via a variety of questionnaires, which assessed their foremost areas of need. Areas of need varied from understanding infants' medical status, to the effects of limited social support, and subsequent marital tension. Interventions were tailored to meet the various areas of need through education, counseling, and assisting families in the transition from hospital to home. The study found that family-based psychosocial interventions offered throughout the families' NICU experience positively influenced parental adaptation and early parent-infant connections.

COPE (Creating Opportunities for Parent Empowerment) is a NICU program focused on introducing and implementing behavioral and educational strategies designed to empower parents of NICU infants. COPE consists of four phases, which all revolve around providing parents with information. The information provided to parents focuses on recognizing and understanding the behavior of premature infants, and on providing means of participating in the care of their infant. Specific parenting activities are prescribed to enable parents to participate in their infants' care as well as to further infant development. The phases are timed to provide parents with education and instruction throughout the hospital stay, during the transition to home and then finally in the home one week after infant discharge.

Implementing programs such as COPE, enable the NICU to be a supportive, empowering place for parents as opposed to one that is frightening and unknown. Music therapy can also play a significant role in supporting and empowering parents of NICU infants. The music therapist can show parents how to assess cues, and responses to music. The music therapist can provide education to the families regarding music for transitional support and in particular pre and post painful procedures. In order to support and empower families, they should be involved in music therapy sessions whenever possible. This will also facilitate bonding and provide them with healing experiences. Music can provide a tangible way for parents to feel connected to their infant, while also providing them with a way to care for and interact with their infant.

Marrying the Principles of Trauma, Bonding and Family-Centered Care within NICU Music Therapy

As previously mentioned, music therapy can promote bonding in the NICU where it is disrupted due to physical separation itself as well as the ensuing stress, anxiety and fear experienced by the parents. Parental involvement in their infant's care is paramount to strengthen bonding and ultimately promote healing. Music therapy can assist in facilitating this bonding through a variety of interventions. Non-music therapy research has shown how physical interaction such as rocking, holding and kangaroo care (skin to skin contact) as well as breastfeeding before, during and after procedures can minimize the pain response of neonates.[51,52] Music therapy in conjunction with these effective parent interactions may further minimize pain responses as well as provide support, relaxation and an environment of care for parents during this time.

I often provide environmental music therapy for moms when they first begin breastfeeding. Breastfeeding with a pre-term infant can be a slow and sometimes frustrating experience for mommies, as the infants have not yet developed the strength and coordination necessary to do so. For NICU moms, this can feel like an additional barrier to normalized parenting. They want so badly to participate in their infant's care, to nurture and nourish them with their milk. When providing environmental music therapy, I am attuned to the environment of the NICU and providing music that encompasses the mood and energy around me. Often times, parents will request songs and so I attempt to weave the families' preferred music into the music

I am providing. It is not uncommon for parents to become emotional during our sessions as well as during environmental music therapy.

Recently, a mom became quite emotional while I was providing environmental music. I made the clinical decision to end the music and offer her support as she sat at the bedside holding her infant. She apologized for crying but said, "I couldn't help it, the music is such a stark contrast to the hospital environment that it really touched and moved me". Sometimes simply providing respite for the parents from the pressures of breastfeeding or feeding, from hearing the alarms, from watching an infant leave and go home while theirs is still hospitalized, is a treatment goal in and of itself.

Another important goal for music therapy in the NICU is to assist the parents in becoming grounded, which can ultimately impact the infant's ability to self-regulate. Assessing the level of trauma in both parent and infant is imperative to the grounding process.[39,40] Parent-infant interactions, which are loving, grounded and stable, can prevent the infant from physiologically and neurologically developing under a constant state of trauma. Music therapy can foster this relationship thus lessening the impact of pain and stress on both baby and family. "The perception of safety is the turning point in the development of relationships for most mammals. The perception of safety determines whether the behavior will be developed as pro-social or defensive".[53] "Safety trumps fear"[53] therefore, providing an atmosphere of safety despite a painful procedure, via musical (and non-musical) relationship can provide corrective experiences and thus ultimately impact development. "The nature of the attachment relationship is as a buffer to stress."[46]

Infants are capable of perceiving energy from interactions with caregivers and then registering these interactions physiologically. This phenomenon has been illustrated in the well-baby literature. In one study in particular, mothers suffering from depression had infants who tended to be more irritable, less self-regulated and more withdrawn. The infants in the study exhibited these tendencies due to the their exposure to the mother's biochemical imbalance.[54,55]

Painful stimuli and an overwhelming environment may cause the NICU infant to neurologically wire defensively. Instead of wiring in such a way as to be able to regulate experience, they are in a frequent state of "fight, flight and freeze."[56] Porges developed a model of social engagement, which is derived from the Polyvagal Theory.[56] The Polyvagal Theory highlights the development of neural circuits, which are capable of supporting social engagement as well as fear responses such as fight/flight/freeze. Loving, grounded and developmentally supportive interactions can therefore cultivate the neural circuits, which support social engagement. Music therapy can support the infant's caregivers to interact from a place of engagement and developmentally supportive behavior rather than from a place of fear or anxiety. This in turn will positively impact the infant's ability to regulate more quickly from pain experiences and move towards a place of positive, healthy development.

Clinical Interventions and Casework

Jack
"Jack" was born at twenty-seven weeks gestation. He was his parents' first child and as a result of his pre-term birth his parents were naturally anxious. The NICU staff referred Jack's parents for music therapy shortly after his birth to support coping, promote bonding and decrease anxiety and stress. It became evident after an initial session with Jack's parents that in addition to anxiety, his mother Emily appeared to be additionally suffering symptoms of post-traumatic stress syndrome. At the bedside, I regularly bore witness to Emily's suffering. If an alarm went off, she would jump up, yell for a nurse, pace, leave the room, return, shout "is he ok, is he ok?!", begin crying and frantically tap on the isolette calling Jack's name. Despite the nurses' assurance that Jack was stable or that it was a monitor malfunction, Emily seemed unable to register such information. She would remain in a state of daze and disconnection. While speaking, Emily transitioned anxiously from topic to topic, and had difficulty focusing or answering questions. Jack's parents wanted to do everything "right", they asked countless questions about music and development and wanted to know what more they could do to help Jack. They expressed feelings of helplessness, loss of control, fear and stress. They also seemed locked into a cycle of repeatedly asking "why?" "Why had Jack been born so early?" "why wasn't mom able to carry him to full term?", and "why weren't they able to celebrate his birth like they had planned?".

My main goal with Jack's parents in music therapy sessions was to provide them with tools to feel grounded. The nurses caring for Jack began to express concern for Jack's well being when his mom was visiting. They reported that her anxiety was so palpable that whenever she interacted with him he began to exhibit stress behaviors, which were manifested physiologically. Jack would frequently have episodes of de-saturation and bradycardia when his mother was at the bedside. Acknowledging and processing the trauma the parents were going through was a key element in supporting their ability to become grounded and ultimately be there for Jack.

When Jack was receiving a painful routine procedure such as a blood draw, or IV line placement, the nurses felt it would be detrimental to Jack for his parents to be there as it would only cause all of them more stress and ultimately impact his ability to recover. I was routinely present at the bedside during such procedures, offering music therapy interventions focused primarily on toning and singing lullabies to comfort Jack and assist him in reconstitution. Jack's parents and I (as well as the rest of the NICU staff) had many discussions regarding self-care. We encouraged his parents to rest, to take time away from the bedside to eat and visit with friends and family who were there to support them. They began to understand that their well-being impacted Jack's well-being. Even in brief bedside sessions, we would focus on breathing and on the importance of feeling the ground under one's feet. Education regarding Jack's status, self-care, breathing, and articulating their feelings became the important tools Jack's parents needed to become grounded.

As Jack grew and became more medically stable, his parents began to feel more comfortable interacting with him. One of the most beautiful moments, which illustrated how "far" they had come, was when Jack was moved to the step-down unit. The step-down unit is for the infants "on their way out the door", as the staff likes to refer to it. The staff had begun discharge planning and Jack was to be going home in a matter of days. As I entered the unit, Emily was sitting in a rocking chair holding Jack who was sound asleep in her arms. The picture was one of harmony and contentment. I approached her to check-in and she reported Jack had had his eye exam earlier in the morning and was feeling "wiped out" as a result. She explained, with a smile on her face that the only thing he wanted to do was sleep in her arms for comfort.

With the support of friends and family, a caring NICU staff and music therapy, Emily had been able to process her journey, resolve the trauma she was experiencing and become the grounded presence Jack needed to facilitate his healing and recovery.

Music therapy Interventions for Pain in NICU Infants

When an infant is referred for music therapy for pain, whether chronic or acute, there are specific music therapy interventions that can address their needs. "Music therapy can provide an environment of safety during painful procedures".[41] Music therapy can also address the need of the infant prior to medical intervention, and post procedure. The principle of entrainment is vital to effective music therapy especially for those dis-regulated infants who are unable to reach a state of self-regulation post procedure. The music and the music therapist can provide a regulating presence. Ideally the parents of the infant are present and involved during the music therapy session, as the infant will derive optimal comfort and regulation from the parents and the music combined. Undoubtedly seeing their infant in pain, can create a stress response within most parents. In such scenarios, music can provide regulation and stability for both the parents and their baby.

Vocalizing, singing the infant's name and toning, when specifically matched to the pitch of the infant's cry, can afford the perception of the pain experience to be altered.[41] To further support pain relief and regulation, the music therapist should entrain to the meter of the infant's breath. Music therapy, and entrainment to the infant's vitals can distract the infant from attending to the painful stimuli.[41] Loewy states, "Music can assist the infant in reconstitution at post procedure time."[41] Reconstitution is a key factor to self-regulation, which is an important music therapy goal when working with pre-term infants.

Preterm infants have left the mother's womb prior to fully developing and must finish their development in the care of medical professionals while hospitalized, at times for months. The comforting and predictable sounds of the mother's heartbeat, the fluids heard in utero and the mother and father's voices are replaced with unpredictable and unfamiliar sounds and voices. Offering womb sounds during music therapy can re-create the calming, comforting, familiar and predictable environment of the womb when environmental factors and sensory stimulation, such as pain is unpredictable.

The predictable and stable qualities of music afford many benefits across populations. Interventions, such as entrained womb sounds (entrained to the infant's vitals) were researched in a multi-site study involving[11] Northeastern NICUs.[57] Infants had a positive physiological and behavioral response to womb sounds, specifically the Remo Ocean Disk which was used to simulate the fluids heard in the mother's womb[58] as well as the gato box, which was played to replicate the mother's heartbeat.[58] Re-creating the womb environment during a time of pain and distress can assist the infant in reaching a state of self-regulation as well as offer feelings of comfort and safety.

Not all infants emerge from a comforting and predictable womb environment. Some infants have been exposed to narcotics, alcohol and prescription drugs while in utero. Exposure to such substances can sometimes induce a painful period of withdrawal after delivery. For these infants, music's predictability can afford the possibility of achieving moments of self-regulation, and a decrease in pain. The therapeutic relationship that develops in music therapy can provide the infant with loving and caring interactions, and a corrective experience.

Music therapy has been proven effective to incite a sedation response prior to medical intervention and at times, in place of pharmacological intervention.[59] Music therapy for sedation can be offered pre medical intervention, or post intervention, to enable the infant to achieve a state of deep sleep in order to recover from the procedure. Sleep enables pre-term infants to conserve calories. This in turn promotes growing, healing and at times dis-charging faster from the hospital. Sleep also promotes uninterrupted neurologic development.

Song of Kin[60] and Lullaby

"The Song of Kin is a well-known tune from the patients tradition; from popular repertoire, or from their cultural/religious heritage. This song has special meaning for the patient. When a family member is unable to connect with the patient, the music can bridge the distance between them. The sound waves travel to a place where the words may not be permitted to reach.[60] For NICU infants and their families; the Song of Kin becomes an "orienting theme, which accompanies them through transformation."[60] By accompanying the family throughout their NICU journey, the Song of Kin essentially becomes a transitional object; "An inanimate object adopted and utilized by an individual to aid in maintaining a psychophysical balance under conditions of more or less strain."[61] The Song of Kin can be an existing song, which is adapted into a lullaby, or an original song written for the infant by the family with the support of the music therapist.

Transitional objects allow an individual to develop the ability to control inner states of tension. For NICU infants, the song of kin can function as this object by providing comfort, and lessening the impact of painful experiences. Psychoanalyst Donald Winnicott studied and developed the concept of the transitional object and its' role particularly in an infant or child's life as vital for fundamental development.[61] Winnicott describes the transitional object as a fantasy for the infant or child in that it represents the mother, her breast and thus comfort and security.[61]

McDonald,[62] expands the idea of musical idioms as transitional objects and specifically names lullabies as transitional tunes. McDonald cites Winnicott's acknowledgement of the auditory sense as a transitional object.[61] An infant often needs a song or tune to transition to sleep therefore, McDonald draws the conclusion that music is essentially functioning as a transitional object.[62] The song, word or tune, is functioning transitionally, and additionally acts as anxiety prevention for the infant or child.[62] Most often the song or tune takes on the principles of a lullaby as it acts to lull and comfort an infant to sleep ("bye") at a time of separation. "Because musical experiences frequently promote associations and imagery, music as a transitional object can support the integration of positive associations and imagery for controlling anxiety and discomfort."[63]

With regards to music therapy for infants in the NICU, the lullaby can act as a transitional object for the family. The family song or lullaby holds the fantasy of a normalized interaction between family and baby (home and healthy) and sustains the family as it transitions between two phases. Infants or children clinging to a transitional object are wavering between two phases: finding a balance between his/her own needs and accommodation to others. [61] This is not unlike NICU families vacillating between the dream of a healthy baby and typical transition home, to the adjustment of a hospital setting and the infant's fragility. The transitional experience, as described by Winnicott,[61] is the phase whereby the infant can develop his or her creative self while still feeling protected.

Michael
One infant I worked with for several months Michael was diagnosed with Zellweger syndrome at birth. The diagnosis was a shock to his parents, as Michael was their first baby and the pregnancy had been without complication. Complications from Michael's disorder caused him to need a tracheotomy as well as a gastrostomy during hospitalization. He was hospitalized for several months during which time he endured many procedures. His prognosis was a life expectancy of less than a year. His parents were lovingly devoted and at the bedside daily. They fully participated in his care and they used music therapy as a means for self-care as well as to enhance bonding and normalize their experience. Their song of kin was "Our House" by Crosby, Stills, Nash and Young. One day as I was processing the case in supervision, my supervisor pointed out the significance of their song of kin. The lyrics highlight aspects of "normal life", and for this family, life was anything but normal.

Their song of kin truly held the fantasy and dream of a normal family life. They used the music to process what had become their new definition of "normal" - being at the hospital daily, learning about the complex medical diagnosis of their son, bonding and looking forward to bringing him home while also consulting with hospice services. Above Michael's hospital bed, they placed a decorated sign that said his name, birth date, and how he loved music and loved music time with mommy and the music therapist. Music and music therapy became a way for the family to give Michael an identity other than that of his diagnosis.

Hallie
Hallie was born full-term with a diagnosis of Vein of Galen Malformation. Following heart surgery she continued to face a difficult recovery, sustaining a seizure, which caused a hemorrhage in her brain. As a result, her parents and the medical staff recognized that her responsiveness and social engagement seemed compromised. Hallie had to undergo a number of procedures while in the hospital, which included preforming frequent "taps"

to drain her head of the excess fluid, which had accumulated after the bleed. She also had to have a shunt implanted to relieve pressure.

One of the difficulties with assessing pain in infants, who have experienced brain injury, is that their response to pain may not be a typical one. Both the medical staff and Hallie's parents felt that she must be experiencing pain as a result of medical intervention in spite of it not being displayed in a typical fashion. Hallie rarely cried and her lack of response upset her parents. They knew she must be in pain, but weren't sure how to comfort her.

In spite of her increased complications, Hallie's parents were excited for her to have music therapy. They expressed a desire for her to have stimulation, which they hoped would aid her recovery to her "old self", pre-seizure. Music therapy sessions focused on being present for Hallie before, during and after procedures. Although her parents were anxious for Hallie to receive stimulation which they felt would best support development, the medical team felt that there was a delicate balance of over-stimulating an infant who was in pain but unable to show it. Because Hallie was full-term, her parents desired for her to have musical interactions such as playing and expressing through songs. Their hope was that this type of stimulation would restore some of the functioning that had been lost. In Hallie's case however, it was important for her parents to understand that the safest way to approach stimulation with Hallie was through simple and predictable means. This was due to the fact that there was an assumption of pain and a need for Hallie to heal from an ongoing regimen of medical procedures. Simple, predictable music such as toning, or singing the melody of the song of kin on "ah" can provide safe structure that can comfort and soothe infants experiencing pain. Such were the interventions that I regularly utilized when working with Hallie throughout her care.

Rhythmic Entrainment of Non-nutritive Suck

Non-nutritive suck is a widely used intervention for pain with NICU infants.[42,43,64] Providing a predictable rhythm on an instrument such as the gato box, as well as modeling a suck response, can support the infant in engaging in non-nutritive suck for pain relief. At a time when the infant may be feeling overwhelmed due to medical procedures, creating a rhythm into which they can lock and entrain can provide refocusing from other stimuli. Gently humming or singing the infant's name while providing a stable rhythm for sucking entrainment can further provide contact and comfort during a distressing time. This intervention is particularly helpful for infants who are unable to coordinate the suck response, sometimes due to gestational age, other times due to poor muscle tone as a result of a genetic disorder, or at times after a prolonged intubation.

Mohammed

Mohammed was born at just twenty-six weeks gestation. His family was from Pittsburgh but had been in New York on vacation, visiting friends when Mohammed's mother went into labor and spontaneously delivered. Mohammed was his parents' eighth child.

Once his mother had recovered, both parents returned to Pittsburgh to attend to un-wielding responsibilities. For Mohammed's father, this meant a demanding schedule as a medical student, and for his mother, the demands of seven other children. Pleased with the care Mohammed was receiving in New York, his parents opted not to have him transferred to a closer hospital. He was hospitalized for a total of 164 days and during that time they tried to visit as much as they could, typically about once a month.

Music therapy was referred when Mohammed reached thirty-two weeks gestational age to aid in self-regulation, support transitions as well as to comfort and soothe him. As Mohammed grew and developed treatment goals shifted and music therapy was used to enhance development as well as foster social engagement. Coordinating times of procedures with music therapy was important as Mohammed was learning to self-soothe and self-regulate without the presence of his parents. During routine blood draws and heel sticks, I would hold Mohammed, offer a pacifier and entrain a melody to his suck pattern. He developed a strong and coordinated suck as he matured and non-nutritive suck brought him much needed comfort. When paired with music therapy in the form of either singing or toning, Mohammed's pain response would be minimal. The nursing staff often remarked that the integration of music therapy during procedures was ideal and induced an almost sedative effect on him.

Conclusion

Music therapy for stress and pain in NICU infants involves assessing pain with a comprehensive understanding of development, level of trauma and impact of environment; in particular the impact separation from caregivers has on an infant physiologically. Music therapy prior to painful procedures can provide a sedation effect, as well as stabilization of physiologic parameters for faster reconstitution post procedurally. During painful procedures, and particularly when parents are unavailable, music therapy can offer safety and comfort whilst acknowledging and mirroring the infant within the music, either via vocalizing, toning or offering womb sounds for regulation.

Music and Medicine: Integrative Models in the Treatment of Pain

Music therapy can assist NICU families in feeling bonded to their infant by providing a forum in which support and empowerment can be provided.

Experiencing the powerful way that music and their own voices can affect the infant physiologically further empowers and connects the parents to their infant. As they witness their infants in pain, parents can foster a feeling of being grounded with the help of music therapy. Their use of the soothing qualities of music to reconcile their own feelings of helplessness and displacement can allow them to be fully present and physiologically organized for their infants.

References

1. Mountcastle K. An ounce of prevention: Decreasing painful interventions in the NICU. Neonatal Network. 2010; 29(6): 353-358.
2. Anand K J S, Arnada JV, Berde CB, Buckman S Capparelli E, Carlo W, et. al. Summary proceedings from the Neonatal Pain-Control Group. Pediatrics. 2006; 117: S9-S22.
3. Verklan MT & Walden M. Core Curriculum for Neonal Intensive Care Nursing: Fourth edition. St Louis, MO: 2010.
4. Stevens B, McGrath P, Gibbins S, Beyene J, Breau L, Camfield C, Finley A, Franck L, Howlett A, McKeever P O'Brien K, Ohlsson A & Yamada J. Procedural pain in newborns at risk for neurologic impairment. Pain. 2003; 105(1): 27-35.
5. Simons SHP, van Dijk M, Anand KJS, Roofthooft D, va Lingen RA & Tibboel D. Do we still hurt newborn babies? Archives of Pediatric andAdolescent Medicine. 2003;157: 1058-1064.
6. Barker DP, Rutter N. Exposure to invasive procedures ineonatal intensive care unit admissions. Archive of Dieases in Childhood: Fetal and Neonatal. 1995;72(1): F47- F48.
7. Grunau RE, Holsti L, Haley DW, Oberlander T, Weinberg J, olimano A, Witfield MF, Fitzgerald C & Wayne Y. Neonatal procedural pain exposure predicts lower cortisol and behavioral reactivity in preterm infants in the NICU.Pain. 2005; 113(3): 293-300.
8. McClain BC & Kain ZN. Procedural pain in neonates: The new millennium. Pediatrics. 2005; 115: 1073-1075.
9. Wolke D. Psychological development of prematurely born children. Archive of Diseases in Childhood: Fetal and Neonatal. 1998; 78: 567-570.
10. Anand KJS, Phil D, Hiey PR. Pain and its effects in the human neonate and fetus. The New England Journal of Medicine. 1987; 317: 121-1329.

11. Puchalski M, Humel P. The reality of neonatal pain. Advances in Neonatal Care. 2002; 2(5): 234-244.
12. Gallo AM. The fifth vital sign: Implementation of the Neonatal Infant Pain Scale. Journal of Obstetric Gynec ologic and Neonatal Nursing. 2003;32: 199-206.
13. Johnston C, Sevens B, Craig K & Grunau R. Developmental changes in pain expression in premature, full-term, two and four-month-old infants. Pain. 1993; 52: 201-208.
14. International Association for the Study of Pain (2011). IASP Taxonomy. International Association for the Study of Pain Newsletter. Retrieved March 2, 2012, from HYPERLINK "http://www.iasppain.org/AM/Template.cfm?Section=Pain_Definitions"
15. Attia J, Amiel-Tyon C, Mayer NN, Shnider SN & Barrier G. Measurement of postoperative pan and narcotic administration in infantsusing a new clinical scoring system. Anesthesiology. 1987; 67(3): A532.
16. Stevens B, Johnston C, Peryshen P & Taddio A. Premature Infant Pain Profile: Development and initial validation. 1996; 12(1): 13-22.
17. Krechel SW & Bildner J. CRIES: A new neonatal postoperative pain measurement score. Initial tesing of validity and reliability. Paediatric Anaesthesia. 1995; 5: 53-61.
18. Lawrence J, Alcock D, McGrath P, MacMurray SB & Dulberg C. The development of a tool to assess neonatal pain. Neonatal Network. 1993; 12(6): 59-66.
19. Debillon T, Zupan V, Ravault N, Magny JF & Dehan M. Development and initial validation of the EDIN scale, a new tool for assessing prolonged pain in preterm infants. Archive of Diseases in Childhood: Fetal and Neonatal. 2001; 85: F36-F41.
20. Lictenszteijn M. The clinical use of piano with patients suffering from breathing distress related to pain. In Azoulay R & Loewy JV, eds. Music, the Breath & Health: Advances in integrative music therapy. New York: Satchnote Press; 2009.
21. Loewy JV. Music psychotherapy assessment in pediatric pain. In Dileo C, ed. Applications of music in medicine vol. II: Theoretical and clinical perspectives. Silver Spring, MD; AMTA; 1999.
22. Tan X, Yowler CJ, Super DM & Fratianne RB. The efficacy of music therapy protocols for decreasing pain, anxiety, and muscle tension levels during burn dressing changes: A prospective randomized crossover trial. Journal of Burn Care Research. 2010; 31(4): 590-597.

23. Leari S, Pietroleti R, Angeloni G, Necozione S, Ranalletta G & Del Gusto B. Randomized clinical trial examining the effect of usic therapy in stress response to day surgery. British Journal of Surgery. 2007; 94(8): 94-947.
24. Walworth D, Rumana CS, Nguyen J & Jarred J. Effects of live music therapy sessions on quality of life indicators, medications administered and hospital length of stay for patients undergoing elective surgical procedures for the brain. Journal of Music Therapy. 2008; 45(3): 349-359.
25. Magill L & Berenson S. The conjoint use of music therapy and reflexology with hospitalized advanced stage cancer patients and their families. Palliative and Supportive Care. 2008; 6(3): 289-29.
26. Johnston CC & Strada ME. Acute pain response in infants: A multidimensional description. Pain. 1986; 24(3): 373-382.
27. Johnston CC & Stevens BJ. Experience in a Neonatal Intensive Care Unit affects pain response. Pediatrics. 1996; 98(5): 925-930.
28. Craig KD, Whitfield MF, Grunau RV, Linton J, Hadjistavropoulos HD. Pain in the preterm neonate: behavioral and physiological indices. Pain. 1993; 54(1): 111.
29. Tse MM, Chan MF & Benzie IF. The effect of music therapy on postoperative pain, heart rate, systolic blood pressure and analgesic use following nasal surgery. Journal of Pain and Palliative Care Pharmacotherapy. 2005; 19(3): 21-29.
30. Butt ML & Kisilvinsky BS. Music modulates behavior of premature infants following heel lance. Canadian Journal of Nursing Research. 2000; 31(4): 17-39.
31. Bo LK Callaghan P. Soothing pain-elicited distress in Chinese neonates. Pediatrics. 2000; 31(4): 17-39.
32. Joyce BA, Keck JF & Gerkensmeyer J. Evaluation of pain management and interventions for neonatal circumcision pain. Journal of Pediatric Health Care. 2001; 15(1): 53-61.
33. Arnon S, Shapsa A, Forman L, Regev R, Bauer S, Litmanovitz I & Dolfin T. Live music is beneficial to preterm infants in the neonatal intensive care unit environment. Birth. 2006; 33(2): 131-136.
34. Chafin S, Roy M, Gerin W & Christenfeld N. Music can facilitate blood pressure recovery from stress. British Journal of Health Psychology. 2004; 9: 393-403.
35. Kennon G. Analysis of music therapy research report. Kentucky Nurse. 2007: 55(3); 12.
36. Collins SK & Kuck K. Music therapy in the neonatal intensive care unit. Neonatal Network. 1991; 9(6): 23-26.

37. Sendelbach SE, Halm MA, Doran KA, Miller EH, Gaillard P. Effects of music therapy on physiological and psychological outcomes for patients undergoing cardiac surgery. Journal of Cardiovascular Nursing. 2006; 21(3): 194-200.
38. Stouffer JW, Shirk BJ & Polomano R. Practice guidelines for music interventions with hospitalized pediatric patients. Journal of Pediatric Nursing. 2007; 22(6): 448-456.
39. Stewart K. Patterns- A model for evaluating trauma in NICU music therapy: Part I- theory and design. Music and Medicine. 2009; (1): 29-40.
40. Stewart K. Patterns- A model for evaluating trauma in NICU music therapy: Part II- treatment parameters. Music and Medicine. 2009; 1(2): 123-128.
41. Loewy JV. A clinical model for music therapy in the NICU. In Nocker-Ribaupierre M, ed. Music therapy for pre and newborn infants. Gilsum, NH: Barcelona, 2004.
42. Shiao SY, Chang YJ, Lannon H & Yarandi H. Meta-analysis of the effects of nonnutritive sucking on heart rate and peripheral oxygenation: research from the past 30 years. Issues in Comprehensive Pediatric Nursing. 1997; 20(1): 11-24.
43. Blass EM & Watt LB. Suckling and sucrose-induced analgesia in human newborns. Pain. 1999; 83(3): 611-623.
44. Carbajal R, Chauvet X, Couderc S & Olivier-Martin M. Randomized trial of analgesic effects of sucrose, glucose and pacifiers in term neonates. British Medical Journal 1999; 319: 1393-1397.
45. Als H, Lawhon G, Duffy FH, McAnulty GB, Gibes-Grossman R, Blickman JG. Individualized developmental care for the very low birth weight infant: Medical and neurofunctional effects. Journal of the America Medical Association. 1994; 272: 853-858.
46. Als H. NIDCAP Program Guide: Changing the Future for Infants in Intensive Care, NIDCAP Federation International 2010 HYPERLINK "http://www.nidcap.org/file.aspx?fileid=pg"
47. Als H. A synactive model of neonatal behavioral organization: Framework for the assessment and support of the neurobehavioral development of the premature infant and his parents in the environment of the neonatal intensive care unit. In Sweeny JK, ed. The High-Risk Neonate: Developmental Therapy Perspectives. Physical and Occupational Therapy in Pediatrics. 1986; 6(3/4): 3-55.
48. Abromeit D H. The Newborn Individualized Developmental Care and Assessment Program (NIDCAP) as a model for clinical music therapy interventions with premature infants. Music Therapy Perspectives. 2003; 21: 60-68.

49. Meyer EC, Garcia CT, Lester BM, Boukydis CFZ, McDonough SM, & Oh W. Family-based intervention improves maternal psychological well-being and feeding interaction of preterm infants. Pediatrics. 1994; 93(2): 241-246.
50. Melnyk Mazurek B, Feinstein NF, Alpert-Gillis L, Fairbanks E, Crean HF, Sinkin RA, Stone PW, Small L & Gross S. Reducing premature infant's length of stay and improving parent's mental health outcomes with the creating opportunities for parent empowerment, (COPE) Neonatal intensive care unit program: A randomized, control trial. Pediatrics. 2008; 118(5); 1414-1427.
51. Gray L, Watt L & Blass EM. Skin-to-skin contact is analgesic in healthy newborns. Pediatrics. 2000; 105(1): e14.
52. Gray L, Miller LN, Phillip BL & Blass EM. Breastfeeding is analgesic in healthy newborns. Pediatrics. 2000; 109(4): 59-593.
53. Porges SW. Social engagement and attachment: A phylogenetic perspective. Roos of Mental Illness in Children, Annals of the New York Academy of Sciences. 2003; 1008: 31-47.
54. Cambel SB & Cohn JF. The timing and chronicity of Postpartum Depression: Implications for infant development. In Murray L, Cooper P, eds. Postpartum depression and child development. New York, New York: Guilford Press. 1997: 165-197.
55. Winberg J Mother and newborn baby: Mutual regulation of physiology and behavior- A selective review. Developmental Psychobiology. 2005; 47(3):217-229.
56. Porges SW. Asserting the role of biobehavioral sciences in translational research: the behavioral neurobiology revolution. Developmental Psychopathology. 2006; 18: 93-933.
57. Heather on Earth Multi-Site NICU music therapy study, in publication.
58. Decker-Voigt HH, Maetzel FK. Cardiovascular Complaints Music and Health.
59. Energon: The scientific-medical music program (book and CD's), 1997; PolyGram GmbH, Hamburg, Germany.
60. Loewy J, Hallan C, Friedman E & Martinez C. Sleep/sedation in children undergoing EEG: A comparison of Chloral Hydrate and Music Therapy. American Journal of Eletroneurodignostic Technology. 2006; 46(4): 343-355.
61. Loewy JV. Music therapy in the neonatal intensive care unit. New York, New York: Satchnote Press; 2000.
62. Winnicott DW. Transitional objects and transitional phenomena. International Journal of Psycho-Analysis. 1953; 48: 368-372.

63. McDonald M. Transitional tunes and musical development. In Feder S, Karmel RL Polock GH, eds., Psychoanalytic explorations in music, First Series. Madison, CT: International Universities Press, 1990. (Original work published 1970).
64. Nolan P. Music therapy improvisation techniques with bulimic patients. In Hornyak LM & Baker EK eds., Experiential therapies for eating disorders. New York, New York: Guilford Press 1989.
65. Liaw JJ, Yang L, Ti Y, Blackburn ST, Chang YC & Sun LW. Non-nutritve sucking relieves pain for preterm infants during heel stick procedures in Taiwan. Jnl of Clinical Nursing. 2010; 19(19-20): 2741-2751.

Music and Medicine: Integrative Models in the Treatment of Pain

CHAPTER 19

"Hear My Song":
Giving Voice to Adolescents with Sickle Cell Disease

Maya Charlton MA, MT-BC

Frustrated, in pain
My mind is going crazy
They don't know how to confiscate it
It just keeps going on and on and on
I'm falling in this hole that's made for me to feel defeated
I'm falling in this trap that keeps me suffocated
Please free my pain, I am breaking
Patient living with Sickle Cell

Introduction

The above words were written by a 16 year-old girl, admitted to Children's Hospital Oakland (CHO) for an acute sickle cell pain crisis. Her words echo those of many patients with Sickle Cell Disease (SCD) who live with chronic and acute pain and accompanying feelings of helplessness, powerlessness and defeat.

This chapter presents case examples to explore the clinical application of music therapy for adolescents with SCD. Music therapy offers an age appropriate and culturally sensitive approach to treating both the physiological and psychosocial aspects of SCD and in supporting resiliency, communication and advocacy.

Sickle Cell Disease

SCD is a genetic blood disorder that afflicts approximately 1 in every 500 individuals of African Ancestry in the United States.[1] The SCD gene causes an abnormality in the iron-rich protein hemoglobin that is responsible for carrying oxygen through the blood and giving blood its red color. The abnormal hemoglobin causes cells to become "sickle shaped" resulting in irregular blood flow.[2] The red blood cells can stick and block the flow of blood to the limbs and organs resulting in recurrent severe pain episodes, organ damage, and chronic anemia. Despite improvements in survival rates, life expectancy for those with sickle cell disease remains shorter than the general population and their quality of life is severely impaired by their illness.

Pain in Sickle Cell Disease
The hallmark feature of SCD is frequent, unpredictable and severe pain episodes, termed vaso-occlusive crises (VOC's). Pharmacological treatment of SCD VOC's typically includes non-steroidal anti-inflammatory drugs, opioids, and adjuvant medications.[3] Blood transfusions are needed sometimes in patients with chronic and severe pain.[4]

Sickle cell related pain typically increases in intensity and frequency in adolescence and adulthood.[5] Overall, patients show an inconsistent response to pharmacological interventions, particularly during adolescence, creating a challenge for both clinicians and caregivers. Because the majority of adolescents cope with pain at home or through visits to the emergency department, once a patient is hospitalized, he/she is usually in severe pain. For some teens these hospitalizations may be recurrent and prolonged, resulting in profound interruption in development. The additional impact by outside psychosocial factors is also of concern.

Patients with SCD frequently report feelings of inadequacy regarding their care, as well as feeling profoundly misunderstood by non-sufferers. Barriers to adequate pain management include the fact that most individuals with SCD in the United States are African American, and many are of lower socioeconomic status. When adolescents with SCD seek treatment for acute pain in an emergency department, there is great potential for racial stereotyping, mistrust, and uneasy physician-patient communication.[6] These factors may result in a negative pain management experience.

These factors along with related psychological and emotional stressors can complicate the progress and perception of physical pain. Thus the need for more targeted psychosocial interventions for this age group.[7] How adolescents approach pain management and experience the health care system may have a significant impact on how they transition into adulthood and the probability of medical compliance. Helping adolescents developing effective pain and stress management strategies is key to helping them manage the transition to adult services more effectively.[3]

Psychosocial Issues for Adolescents with SCD
Health related quality of life (HRQOL) outcomes in children and adolescents with SCD are poor[8] and teens are particularly at risk for significant psychosocial maladjustment. Studies show adolescents with SCD to be at risk for depression, anxiety, low self-esteem, social isolation, poor academic performance, behavioral issues, poor family relationships, and social and economic issues.[9]

Coping with SCD may impinge upon a teen's independence as they remain dependent on caregivers and medical personnel. Repeated or prolonged hospitalizations can also increase the risk of an individual missing the developmental tasks of adolescence. Compliance with medical regimen can be problematic due to the frequent and natural tendency during adolescence towards rebellion as a demonstration of independence. Additionally compounding the challenges in treating this age group is that teens are often aware of their prognosis and of its impact on their future.

It is of great significance that SCD is unique in that there are no similar chronic diseases that affect primarily those from an impoverished, minority background. Patients with SCD in the US report feeling "different" from their peers and face the stigma of a "black" disease. Health-related stigma can have detrimental effects on the lives of teens and their families. The credibility or trustworthiness of young African American patients with SCD is often questioned by health care providers who may label patients as malingerers, manipulators, or even drug seekers.[6] Notably for patients with challenging home situations there may also be secondary gains from hospitalization such as increased attention and support.

Psychosocial support for patients with SCD includes cognitive behavioral therapy, biofeedback, self-hypnosis, coping skills/self-regulation training, educational programs, support groups, and family counseling. However there has been a lack of targeted interventions specific to teens with SCD, as there are many challenges to working with this population. The most effective interventions are those that are culturally sensitive and family centered. Crucial as it may be, engaging African American adolescents and families in psychosocial interventions can be challenging. In developing culturally sensitive interventions, it is important to acknowledge the importance of the extended family in African American culture and to choose interventions, which empower the family to work together. Effective management of SCD related pain during adolescence may be contingent upon the success of this intervention. Studies point to significant family /caregiver stress and examine its impact on patient care and on family relationships.[10,11] While psychosocial support empowering both patients and their families is of great value, specific attention given to the unique needs of the adolescent is crucial. To this end, teen patients are enabled as active participants in their medical treatment to the greatest extent possible.

Ultimately psychosocial interventions need to support adolescents in developing coping skills and pain management tools that they can use independently. Supporting them in their own self-advocacy can contribute favorably to improving patient/provider communication, and supporting a patient's sense of identity and self esteem.

Music Therapy Interventions for Adolescents with SCD

At Children's Hospital Oakland (CHO), a specialized center in the treatment of sickle cell disease, music therapy referrals received for inpatient adolescents are most often targeted at pain management, or to address behavioral issues, non-compliance and/or support of coping skills. Patients may be seen for a single session or, over the course of multiple admissions. Sessions are patient directed and integrate cognitive behavioral techniques such as deep breathing, mindfulness and positive thinking, with a range of music therapy techniques including music assisted relaxation, clinical improvisation, therapeutic drumming, therapeutic voice work and songwriting.

Treatment Goals

- reduce pain and anxiety
- promote resiliency & coping strategies
- provide opportunities for control, decision making and independence
- provide outlets for emotional expression
- increase self esteem, positive body image and sense of identity
- facilitate family and peer relations/ socialization
- support family relationships
- empower patients with the skills to advocate for themselves
- offers positive coping tools

Music therapy holds great potential in offering a developmentally appropriate treatment modality that can be both patient and family centered as well as culturally sensitive. Especially suited for adolescents with SCD, music therapy can be effective in supporting patient empowerment, resiliency and advocacy. While engagement of adolescents in more traditional therapeutic models can be challenging, there is a large evidence base in the music therapy literature attesting to the effectiveness of music therapy interventions with this age group. Patient preferred music offers a gateway into the culture of our patients in general, but music as an expression of identity can be especially central to the lives of many teens.

The primary psychosocial goal is to encourage patients to take an active role in their care, to address emotional and social difficulties, and to give them tools to be used at home. Individuals with chronic pain often perceive their pain to be something unique to their case, and therefore feel increasingly isolated and powerless. Music therapy can empower patients and offer them a sense of control by promoting active engagement with the experience of pain. This work is effective in helping individuals attune to their pain and in developing mind-body awareness. Teens with SCD identify on many levels with their pain not only as defining who they are, but also in determining how others view them in terms of their disease.

The music therapy process is one of reaching out to patients, and meeting them where they are, with the intention of helping them to identify their own strengths and resiliency. Music therapy supports patients in gaining a sense of control and independence in addition to promoting self-expression in music and ultimately in their lives. Music making creates a positive sense of embodiment, wholeness, identity, strength, and resilience.

Additionally, music therapy sessions promote engagement, which can decrease a patient's sense of isolation by providing a space where he/she feels heard and witnessed throughout the process. It transcends barriers of communication, and helps facilitate self-advocacy by increasing a patient's sense of independence. Through the use of audio/video recording, and performance when appropriate, music therapy can provide opportunities for an individual diagnosed with SCD to be heard and viewed by the medical staff as more than just another patient. Such opportunities enhance the patient sense of control, and provide him/her the possibility to be heard, seen, and acknowledged by the staff.

Inclusion of family members in music therapy sessions such as family jam sessions, drum circles, group improvisation or collective songwriting can be important in supporting the present needs of the patient. Such music therapy sessions can also support family members in gaining a sense of empowerment through engagement. Provided with a forum in which they too can be heard, such intervention can positively impact relationships within the family unit. Inclusion can strengthen family communication, support healthy family resilience, support overburdened caregivers, and support the teens in navigating their shifting relationships and roles of autonomy and independence.

While engaging the family in the creative process can encourage new modes of communication and support, playfulness, confidence and advocacy can also be reignited. Music therapy in this capacity can additionally play an effective role in bridging the communication gap between patient and family, and between the family and healthcare professionals. As a father rapped, in the midst of a family music therapy session, "This is what we need, this is how we can get our stress out".

Music and Medicine: Integrative Models in the Treatment of Pain

Clinical Work

Y, 16 yrs
"I want all the doctors to hear my song so that they know what it's like to live with sickle cell disease."

Y met the music therapist for the first time when she came to join the weekly teen music therapy group. She was in acute pain and spent the group time curled up on the couch. With support from the music therapist she composed song lyrics about her pain and distress. (see lyrics at beginning of this chapter). Through her lyrics Y expressed openly her frustration with the medical team, the inadequacy of medication in treating her pain, and her perceptions of not being heard or understood by her doctors.

> *You don't know how it feels*
> *to be let down so many times*
> *You can't even bear a mile in my shoes for a while*
> *I'm falling in this hole that was made for me to feel defeated*
> *I'm falling in this trap that's kept me suffocated*
> *You can't even tell through the smile on my face*
> *that I'm dying inside*
> *Please help me, free my pain.*
> *I am breaking.*

The song clearly described her experience of feeling "broken", a similar theme for many people living with chronic pain. The lyrics additionally reflect the lack of having a cohesive sense of self or of wholeness. In addition she describes the sense of defeat, hopelessness and isolation and specifically of being let down and repeatedly misunderstood. The songwriting and recording process became a catalyst of transformation for Y. Through the process of writing and recording this song, from the initial sessions to the time of our final recording, I saw profound changes in Y's physical appearance. Her initial presentation of being curled up in inward fetal position because of the acute pain she was experiencing, shifted to being outwardly engaged, fully in her body and empowered.

While she sang about her pain and isolation, the act of songwriting transformed her experience of pain on multiple layers. Through the act of singing and rehearsing, Y found her voice, and reclaimed her identity. She freed her own pain, both physical and psychological, and regained a sense of control and hope. What began as a cry for help out of frustration and desperation became empowering and transformative. The song itself served as a testimony of her experience and a direct invitation for others to understand her pain.

The potential value of voice work with adolescents with SCD is enormous as the act of singing promotes deep breathing and muscle relaxation, while increased vocal strength and flexibility can lead to a greater sense of control and a stronger sense of identity. Vocal techniques have long been used for healing purposes in many cultures across the globe. I frequently incorporate vocal toning into my work with teens with SCD with the goal of reducing pain and supporting a patient's sense of embodiment. Vocal toning is described by Austin as "the conscious use of sustained vocal sounds for the purpose of restoring the body's balance. Sound vibrations free blocked energy and resonate with specific areas of the body to relieve emotional and physical stress and tension".[12]

The building of resilience and strengthening of coping skills can be accomplished through creative songwriting and recording. Through songwriting teens can share their own unique experience in their own voice. For a teenager, the value of recording and more so performing can be pivotal in strengthening a patient's coping skills and giving him a sense of achievement. Themes that have emerged in songwriting with adolescent sickle cell patients include control vs. powerlessness, independence vs. dependence, loneliness vs. support, hope vs. fear, and feeling "broken" vs. strength and resiliency. Issues of identity often emerge, focusing on the questions: "who am I and who will I be beyond my illness and my pain?"

Through recording a CD of this song Y created her own legacy at CHO where her song is a regular part of music therapy in services for resident doctors, facilitating awareness of and dialogue about the very real struggles of the patients they treat. In one such presentation a young doctor commented, "We often feel frustrated with these patients because we don't know how to treat their pain adequately and they are angry with us".

T, 17yrs
"The future is only what I can dream."
The psychosocial stressors faced by many SCD patients are complex and cannot be ignored in our work with this population. Given the urban nature of CHO, song lyrics written in music therapy sessions often reflect themes of social isolation, violence, poverty, struggle, lack of social support, and family conflict. It is a tragic reality that in Oakland the leading cause of death amongst teen male sickle cell patients is gun violence. This reality is reflected in the song lyrics of many of these patients.

I met T for a brief single session after referral for medical non-compliance and verbal and behavioral outbursts toward the staff. When I met with T, her mother was present at the bedside and appeared overwhelmed and frustrated by both her daughter's behavior and the impact of an extended hospitalization. Despite presenting as a tough, streetwise teen, T shared within moments of meeting me that she wrote poetry. It was during this initial session that she wrote a poem titled "Me":

> *So here's the thing*
> *I've been in the hospital for about 2 weeks*
> *But that's not stopping me from dreaming*
> *Last night I dreamt of a place where it's just me*
> *and nobody can cause me to shed tears...*
> *Life is like a fairy tale; is what you see real or is it a nightmare?*
> *When you wake up on a block*
> *where there's more police lights than street lights*
> *and you can't face the truth of another fallen soldier, RIP ____*
> *The future is only what I can dream*

From her words I gained valuable information, which was that alongside coping with SCD and frequent hospitalizations this young girl had lost many friends and relatives to gun violence. Not only did she live with the physical experience of pain and the reality of a life limiting medical condition, but she lived in a place where there were few prospects and where the threat to basic survival was felt on a daily basis.

Based on T's musical preference, I created a melodic/rhythmic hip hop style pattern on guitar. T read the poem aloud over this loop, and her mother provided back up vocals. From a family-centered perspective, T's mother's participation allowed her to connect with her daughter's most vulnerable sides, while providing a nurturing and supportive presence in the music. In many ways, her own needs as a mother were honored, held, and witnessed as she felt pride in her role in the final recording.

I also gained insight into T's resiliency and the important role that her creativity played in bringing it to fruition. I had only a single session with T but in this session her story had been heard. She left the hospital that week with a recording of her song in hand, and a positive memory of her experience in the hospital.

D, 14 yrs
"One minute I was in pain, next thing I had a song out of it."
D, 14yrs, was labeled as a "problem patient". D had been coming to CHO her whole life for treatment of SCD and had a complex psychosocial background. Some developmental and possible mental health issues impacted her ability to cope with hospitalization or to follow good self-care practice at home. Furthermore, she lacked an involved caregiver to help support her at home and through her hospitalizations. During hospitalizations, D presented with high anxiety, behavioral outbursts, and was fre-

quently non compliant. D was additionally seen as receiving secondary gains from hospitalization and showed negative attention seeking behavior.

Music therapy was consulted for support of coping skills and pain management. Her relationship with the music therapist became one of the significant factors in providing support of her coping skills during admissions. In music therapy sessions D participated in music-guided relaxation aimed at reducing pain and anxiety and in creative songwriting aimed at helping her develop coping skills. She was enthusiastic in engaging in music therapy sessions and jumped readily into creative songwriting through the use of "fill in the blank" songs. As an assessment tool, I used the "Hospital Blues" - a standard I,IV,V structure providing familiarity, repetition and containment. I learned of D's strengths and struggles regarding hospitalization, and was able to gain insight into her profound loneliness and sense of abandonment. As a result of her earlier life experiences, these feelings continued to negatively impact her current experiences of hospitalization.

MT: I got those blues, those hospital blues
D: Those lonely feeling hospital blues
MT: Well, the hardest thing about being here is...
D: Getting shots in the morning
MT: It makes me feel...
D: Feel so unwanted

Using the ocean drum, while I supported on the guitar, D used music and guided visualization to create and record a song about being by the ocean with her loved ones. Feeling the cool breeze of the wind in her hair, and the water on her skin was a powerful component of the visualization. Such imagery was directed at decreasing pain; for example the image of feeling "the breeze in my hair, and the cool cool water" was powerful for her during intense flare-ups, as it counteracted the burning sensation she experienced during acute pain flare-ups. Retrieval of such imagery helped support D in reducing her pain perception. By visualizing her (imagined) support of family and friends being with her at the ocean, D helped reduce her feelings of isolation. This was mirrored in her building a therapeutic rapport with the music therapist and finding new means of support through music itself. For a patient such as D, music can act as a support of ego strength. To this end, it was noted that D used her patient controlled analgesia (PCA) pump less often during and shortly after music therapy sessions, and generally reported a decrease in pain when engaged in music therapy.

Because D was so frequently hospitalized and there were many secondary gains of hospitalization for her, it was particularly important to have clear boundaries around frequency of sessions and regarding the use of our time together. Goals remained focused on helping her integrate positive coping skills that she could also use independently at home. D went on to compose and record many songs during our sessions. While the process was therapeutic in the moment, many of the songs also served as transitional objects that provided means of support between sessions and hospitalizations as well.

Conclusion

As the music therapy literature and research on addressing pain in an integrative manner expands, it is my expectation that the awareness of the social and cultural issues that arise for patients living with pain have to be incorporated in their management. Chronic illness and pain are inclusive elements of these issues, and sickle cell disease deserves greater and more specific attention. As a particularly vulnerable group, adolescents will benefit from the culturally sensitive and age appropriate interventions that music therapy can offer, giving them a voice and helping them shift from a sense of defeat and hopelessness to one of empowerment and resiliency.

References

1. National Heart L, & Blood Institute. 1996.
2. National Heart L, & Blood Institute. NHLBI;2010.
3. Benjamin LJ, Dampier CD, Jacox AK, et al. APS Guideline for the management of acute and chronic pain in sickle cell disease. Glenview, IL: APS; 1999.
4. Styles LA, Vichinsky E. Effects of a long-term transfusion regimen on sickle cell-related illnesses. Journal of Pediatrics. 1994;125:909-111.
5. Platt OS, Thorington BD, Brambilla DJ, et al. Pain in sickle cell didease: rates and risk factors New England Journal of Medicine. 1991;325:11-16.
6. Jenerette CM, Brewer C. Health related stigma in young adults with sickle cell disease. Journal of the National Medical Association. 2010;102(11 November):1050-1055.
7. Chen EC, Cole SW, Kato PM. A review of empirically supported psychosocial interventions for pain and adherence outcomes in sickle cell disease. Journal of pediatric psychology. 2004;29:197-209.
8. Palermo TM, Schwartz MT, Drotar D, McGowan K. Parental report of health related quality of life in children with sickle cell disease. Journal of Behavioral Medicine. 2002;25:269-283.
9. Edwards CL, Scales MT, Loughlin C, et al. A brief review of the pathophysiology, associated pain, and psychological issues in sickle

cell disease. International Journal of Behavioral Medicine, United States. 2005;12:171-179.

10. Palermo TM, Riley C, Mitchell B. Daily functioning and quality of life in children with sickle cell disease pain: Relationship with family and neighborhood socionomic distress. Journal of of Pain. 2008;9(9):833-840.

11. Mitchell MJ, Lemanek K, Palermo TM, Crosby LE, Nichols A, Powers SW. Parent perspectives on pain management, coping, and family functioning in pediatric sickle cell disease. Clinical pediatrics. 2007;46(4):311-319.

12. Austin D. The theory and practice of vocal psychotherapy: Songs of self. London: Jessica Kingsley Publishers; 2008.

Music and Medicine: Integrative Models in the Treatment of Pain

CHAPTER 20

GIM: Deprivation and its Contribution to Pain in Eating Disorders

Annie Heiderscheit PhD, MT-BC, LMFT

> "Music expresses that which cannot be said and on which it is impossible to be silent."
> Victor Hugo

Introduction

Every day in the United States we are inundated and surrounded with images and messages on focused beauty, fashion, thinness, body image, and losing weight. From magazines, commercials, billboards, and pop-up ads, we have become acculturated to this obsession with weight. It is not only present in the media, but in daily conversations. Go out to lunch or dinner and listen to the food-focused conversation. You may hear someone comment, "I can't eat that, it will be on my hips for a month" or "I love to eat fries, they are my guilty pleasure". We have labeled foods good or bad, healthy or unhealthy, rather than see all food as fuel for the body and utilizing a model of balance for living.

While research does not demonstrate a casual link between media and eating disorders, it does show that the body type portrayed in advertising as the ideal is possessed naturally by only 5% of American females.[1] Research also reports that 47% of girls in 5th-12th grade reported wanting to lose weight because of magazine pictures, while 69% reported that magazine pictures influence their idea of a perfect body shape.[1] The current literature indicates that 80% of American women are dissatisfied with their body and appearance,[2] and also suggests that over one-half of teenage girls and nearly one-third of teenage boys use unhealthy behaviors to control weight. These include skipping meals, fasting, smoking cigarettes, vomiting, and taking laxatives.[3] Struggles with body dissatisfaction serve as an opening to the development of eating disorder. Living each day feeling unhappy and displeased with one's own body is a painful and difficult experience. When this focus becomes so strong, changing the appearance of the body to align with these images seems like a reasonable solution to resolving these feelings. The journey into the world of life with an eating disorder begins an odyssey of treating the complexities of the psychological and physiological stresses, as well as the barriers to treatment a patient may encounter.

The fact that the eating disorder impacts the mind and the body necessitate an approach that encompasses simultaneous attention to both entities. The Bonny Method of Guided and Imagery and Music (BMGIM) is an approach that fosters the psychotherapeutic use of music and imagery to access and address issues underlying the eating disorder. The dynamic unfolding of images through the music is experienced not only in the mind but in the body as well. This allows integrative healing through mental, emotional, physical and spiritual aspects of the patient. This chapter will describe and illustrate the painful complexities of eating disorders and the use of the BMGIM to treat the psychological and physiological pain eating disorder patient's experience. These will include the struggles that lead the patient to develop an eating disorder, as well as, the difficulties the patient experiences as a result of it.

Eating Disorders Statistics

In the United States, as many as 10 million females and 1 million males are diagnosed with an eating disorder, including anorexia or bulimia. Additionally, approximately 25 million Americans are struggling with binge eating disorder.[4-8] A review of literature demonstrates a significant increase in the incidence of anorexia nervosa from 1935 to 1989 and from 1988 to 1993 the incidence of bulimia tripled.[8,9] While the majority of those diagnosed with eating disorders are girls and women, males are often less likely to be diagnosed early with an eating disorder. Physicians are often less likely to diagnose eating disorders in men and boys as it is often considered a female disorder.[7] Research regarding males hospitalized for eating disorder treatment reported feelings of shame for having a disorder that was stereotypically associated with being a female disorder.[7,8] Research reports that eating disorders have the highest mortality rate of any mental health disorder.[10] Recent research reports the following mortality rates for the various eating disorders: 4% for anorexia nervosa, 3.9% for bulimia nervosa, and 5.2% for eating disorder not otherwise specified.[11] Patient mortality as a result of eating disorders, is attributable to heart failure, organ failure, malnutrition or suicide. In many cases, the medical complications of a death are reported rather than the eating disorder, which ultimately compromises an individual's health.[12] These medical complications clearly identify the physiological distress that patients with eating disorders encounter as a result of the severity and prolonged course of the disorder.

GIM: Deprivation and its Contribution to Pain in Eating Disorders

Diagnostic Characteristics

This section will provide hallmark characteristics of each eating disorder diagnosis rather than complete diagnostic criteria. The full diagnostic criteria can be reviewed in the Diagnostic and Statistical Manual IV or in the upcoming DSM-5. Note that Binge Eating Disorder was included in the DSM-IV as a provisional diagnosis, but in the DSM-5 will be an official diagnosis.

Anorexia Nervosa (AN) is characterized by unwillingness to maintain a normal or healthy weight, pursuit of thinness and can result in emaciation from ongoing malnutrition. The extreme weight loss associated with anorexia is often achieved through dieting, restricting food and compulsive and excessive exercise, self-induced vomiting, or misusing/abusing laxatives, diuretics or enemas. A distorted body image, and intense fears surrounding weight gain foster these obsessive thoughts and compulsive behaviors. The significant weight loss associated with anorexia also leads to irregular or the absence of menstruation.[13]

Bulimia Nervosa (BN) is characterized by hallmark symptoms of bingeing and purging. This includes recurrent and often frequent episodes of eating large quantities of food, followed by a behavior that compensates for the binge, this may including purging, excessive use of laxatives or diuretics, fasting or engaging in excessive exercise. While individuals diagnosed with bulimia often fall within a normal weight range, they still encounter a fear of gaining weight and are dissatisfied with body image. The symptoms of bulimia are often in secret, as individuals feel shame and disgust about the purging behaviors.[13]

Eating Disorder Not Otherwise Specified (ED-NOS) is the diagnostic category for individuals who do not meet the criteria for anorexia nervosa or bulimia nervosa, but still have significant struggles with eating behaviors or patterns and body image. This can mean that an individual that demonstrates all of the symptoms of anorexia nervosa, but who still has a normal body mass index (BMI), normal weight range, and menstrual cycle would be diagnosed with ED-NOS. ED-NOS differs from BN in that frequency of binge and purge episodes does not meet the diagnostic criteria for BN.[13]

Binge Eating Disorder (BED) is characterized by cravings for that can occur any time of day or night. The binge behaviors are often carried out in secret, as patient's feel a great deal of shame about eating such large quantities of food. Bingeing eating behaviors are often rooted in feelings low self-esteem, poor body image, using of food to deal with stress, or connected to other distorted or dysfunctional thoughts. While binge eating is also characteristic of bulimia nervosa, purging or compensating for the binge does not occur with binge eating disorder. Therefore, individuals with BED are likely to be overweight or obese.[13]

While the diagnostic criteria differ for each disorder, there are common issues among them. Individuals living with an eating disorder struggle with their relationship with food and weight and utilize a set of symptoms and behaviors to deal with these struggles. Eating disorder symptoms can lead to a wide variety of physical and medical complications. It is important to remember that while eating disorders are considered a mental health diagnosis, there are serious medical complications that can arise as a result of symptom use. These two aspects of eating disorders can make them complex to treat. It is vital that the treatment approach address the psychological and physiological aspects of these disorders.

Psychological Distress
Distress is a response to a stressor or demand that is detrimental to an individual.[14,15] Psychological distress is the emotional discomfort experienced in response to the stressor or demand that can result harm to the individual. Researchers have described five characteristics that define psychological distress: one's perceived inability to cope effectively, change in emotional status or mood, expression or communication of the discomfort, and harm from the impact of stress on the system.[14,16] Research also suggests that individuals experiencing psychological distress also experience the following: pessimism toward their future, self-depreciation, isolation and social withdrawal.[17]

Patients diagnosed and living with eating disorders experience a variety of issues that cause psychological distress. Those diagnosed with eating disorders are often diagnosed with various comorbid mental health issues. Research demonstrates that well over half of women diagnosed with AN, BN, and BED are also diagnosed with an anxiety disorder.[18-20] Clinical studies also suggest high prevalence rates of depressive disorders, post-traumatic stress disorder, and substance use disorders for individuals with eating disorders.[18,20] Coping with multiple mental health diagnoses is a stressful and a distressing process for a patient.

Patients with eating disorders persistently struggle with body dissatisfaction, anxiety and discomfort regarding the level of closeness in relationships. This can result in increased depressive symptomology, a frequent need for approval, and difficulty forming and maintaining relationships.[21,22] These challenges persistent and intensify throughout the course of the disorder and often until patients reach recovery.

Research suggests that poor emotional processing, emotion dysregulation, and emotion avoidance further perpetuates and intensifies eating disorder symptomology.[23-26] These issues surrounding emotional processing and silencing one's emotions, also foster negative thoughts and maladaptive beliefs.[24] Therefore, in order to interrupt symptom use these underlying issues need to be addressed as a part of treatment.[23]

There are many barriers that eating disorder patients encounter with regards to treatment. Research indicates that only about 30% of individuals with AN receive mental health treatment while only 6% diagnosed with BN receive any mental health care.[20] Additionally there are limited treatment facilities that provide specialized eating disorder treatment, which can require patients to travel a great distance to receive the specialized care. Unfortunately, this leads to only about 45% of patient's diagnosed with an eating disorder receiving treatment that is specific to eating disorders, leaving the majority of patients to receive care that does not adequately meet their needs.[20]

There are several psychological struggles patient's encounter due to living with an eating disorder. The symptom use surrounding eating disorders is often conducted in secret due to shame, which can lead to withdrawing from relationships and fostering greater struggles in the family and various interpersonal relationships. Comorbid mental health diagnoses bring an additional challenge to managing not only the eating disorder, but all other stressors as well. Navigating these struggles is also complicated by the difficulties with emotional processing, emotion dysregulation, and avoidance. Lastly, the complications of obtaining specialized and sufficient treatment to effectively treat the eating disorder and comorbid diagnoses is often the largest obstacle to overcome. Each of these issues becomes a compounding factor to increasing the impact of psychological distress. While the psychological stressors are many, eating disorders also have physiological complications and issues associated with the disorder.

Physiological Distress
While there are a myriad of psychological stressors, patients with eating disorders also face physiological distress. There are many medical and physical complications that arise as a result of and in conjunction with the eating disorder. Frequent and chronic eating disorder symptom use negatively impact every system of the body. The longer an eating disorder persists, the greater the effect of physiological distress on the body as well.

Restricted nutritional intake and purging behaviors can cause renal and electrolyte imbalances and abnormalities, which can lead to cardiovascular issues as well as gastrointestinal complications.[27,28] Patients also encounter endocrine and metabolic abnormalities as a result of symptom use, which lead to problems in thyroid functioning. These issues can lead to increased cortisol (stress hormone) levels, interruption of the menstrual cycle, and loss of bone density.[28]

Decreased oral intake and malnutrition also impact the neurological system. Imaging studies illustrate loss of gray and white matter, leading to structural and functional complications in the brain.[29] These changes in the brain then manifest into impaired cognitive functioning.[28] As long as nutritional intake is restricted, cognitive functioning is compromised. When the body begins to receive the nutrition it needs to function optimally, functioning can begin to stabilize.

The immune and hematological systems are also impacted by the eating disorder. This can result in suppressed immune system response leaving the body susceptible to illness and infection.[27] There are a variety of dermatological issues that arise as a result of eating disorder symptom use: hair loss, brittle nails, dry skin, acrocyanosis (bluish coloring in the fingertips), hypercarotenemia (orange discoloration of the skin). Dental complications also occur as a result of ongoing purging behaviors. Over time enamel from the teeth is eroded and gums are irritated and this can lead to tooth loss.[28]

The medical complications associated with eating disorders are serious as they can be fatal.[30] Additionally, the physiological issues that arise as a result of the eating disorder are many and can lead to serious medical complications. While physiological distress associated with eating disorders manifest throughout the entire body, the myriad of psychological stressors need to be addressed to treat the complexities of the disorder. Effectively treating an eating disorder requires an approach that can attend to the needs of the mind and body, as the disorder compromises both aspects of the individual.

The physiological and medical complications reviewed in this section do not provide a comprehensive review, rather a brief introduction. This review provides a brief overview of the impact of the eating disorder on the body. For a more complete understanding of the medical and physiological complications associated with eating disorders, the reader is encouraged to consult an eating disorder sourcebook.

The Bonny Method of Guided Imagery and Music (BMGIM)

The Bonny Method of Guided Imagery and Music is the use of imagery evoked by a relaxed state and music, to foster self-understanding, insight, and personal growth[31]. It is a depth-oriented form of music psychotherapy, which encourages exploration for the purpose of developing and gaining a deeper self-awareness.[32,33] Bonny developed the method in the early 1970s, as a part of her work at the Maryland Psychiatric Research Center.[31] She found the music allowed patients to achieve a deep relaxed state, relinquish control, and fully enter into the therapeutic experience.[34]

GIM: Deprivation and its Contribution to Pain in Eating Disorders

While the BMGIM has been utilized in a variety of clinical settings, currently there is no published literature documenting its use in eating disorder treatment. Research surrounding the BMGIM has however been conducted addressing both psychological and physiological issues, including immune function, interpersonal problems, and ability to cope.[35] Patients with eating disorders struggle with similar physical and psychological issues, therefore it is reasonable to explore the use of the BMGIM in eating disorder treatment.[36]

The BMGIM in Eating Disorder Treatment

The author has implemented the BMGIM with patients diagnosed with various eating disorders in many different levels of treatment, including its use to address both psychological and physiological issues pertaining to the eating disorder. These include: explore interpersonal and intrapersonal relationships, perfectionism, fears, body dissatisfaction, discover and process latent or repressed emotions, feelings, uncover issues underlying eating disorder, address and face fears, reconnecting with one's own body, symptom use, and trauma.[37,38]

The remainder of the chapter will provide case illustrations utilizing the BMGIM with patients in eating disorder treatment. The cases will demonstrate how the BMGIM is implemented to address various psychological and physiological issues that patients encounter as a result of their eating disorder and through the course of treatment. Additionally, comments from patients regarding their experiences and images will also be included in these case illustrations.

The following case illustrations are from sessions the author conducted with eating disorder patients during the course of their treatment in various levels of care. The names of the patients and identifying details have been changed to protect their identity. The BMGIM was a part of their multi-disciplinary treatment.

It is important to note that various music therapy methods were utilized during their treatment and the BMGIM was introduced when it was evident that this method was warranted and the patient was amenable to this therapeutic approach.

Each case illustration will help demonstrate how the BMGIM was implemented to address various aspects associated with psychological and physiological distress. Excerpts from session transcripts show how these issues are represented and processed within the imagery. Each transcript illustration includes the BMGIM program that was utilized during the session from the Music for Imagination by Barcelona Publishers. In the illustrations each transcript will include the dialogue to occur in the session.

Music and Medicine: Integrative Models in the Treatment of Pain

This dialogue includes the questions I asked as the guide and the descriptions of the imagery and experiences of the patient. The questions asked are in parentheses and the responses of the patient are not.

Clinical Work

Case of Caitlin: Facing Perfectionism and Fear

Caitlin was a college sophomore at a prestigious university when she entered residential treatment for her eating disorder. She had struggled with anorexia nervosa since her junior year in high school and had consequently been followed in outpatient treatment during this time. Transitioning to college, her check-ins with her outpatient therapist occurred only during breaks. While she continued to use and struggle with symptoms through this transition, it was during her sophomore year that her symptom use intensified. Caitlin began to restrict her nutritional intake even more, as well as increase her level of exercise. Due to this increased symptom use, Caitlin lost a significant amount of weight and began to experience lightheadedness, had difficulty focusing on her schoolwork, and eventually was required by the university to leave campus and enter treatment.

Caitlin began taking dance lessons when she was 3 years old and continued throughout high school. She described herself as a perfectionist and she would practice for hours to perfect a routine. She discovered early on that doing well at a competition, earned her the much desired approval of her parents. This soon became her motivation; do well in everything in order to receive their approval. This began her journey into perfectionism. She began restricting in high school in order to be the perfect weight and have the perfect body for dance. In time she would begin to use symptoms as a way of punishing herself if she didn't do as well as she believed she should. If she didn't do something perfectly in her eyes, then she didn't deserve to eat.

As the pressures of college intensified, she found it more difficult to be perfect and deal with her feelings of disappointment. Her symptom use continued to serve as a means of punishing herself and as a way of numbing or turning off her feelings. If she was hungry and focused on restricting, then she could not feel her feelings of shame. She was stuck in a cycle of never feeling good enough, then not feeling deserving of food, and immanently not having the energy to complete her schoolwork. This vicious cycle resulted in a significant weight loss and the need for a more intense level of treatment. When Caitlin arrived in the residential treatment program she was aware of her perfectionistic tendencies, but she was not connected to her feelings or to her body. She was very much a thinker and in her head. If she were asked about her feelings she would think. If she were struggling with eating a meal, she would try to think of a solution. Ultimately, she was unable to identify her feelings. Her process in music therapy included utilizing other approaches as Caitlin needed to begin to process her experiences before she could identify and feeling her emotions. After she had been in treatment for about six weeks and had restored some weight, her ability to process information had also improved. Additionally, at this point I had also developed a rapport with her and could begin to explore the idea of deepening the therapeutic process. So after six sessions of processing Caitlin's life story through her song autobiography, I introduced the idea of the BMGIM.

Caitlin and I discussed what the process of the BMGIM entailed, how the music fostered the imagery and how the imagery was a projection of her inner experiences. I shared with her why this approach was recommended, as it would allow her to connect with her body, explore her feelings, and address her perfectionism. Caitlin felt it was important to address these issues and was interested in exploring this approach; she also expressed her apprehension about feeling her feelings. I gave her an information sheet about the approach as well as encouraged her to give it more thought and they would discuss it further the following week. When we met the next week, Caitlin shared that she wanted to begin some sessions utilizing the BMGIM. Again I described the process of the session and asked if Caitlin had any additional questions. Caitlin shared she felt ready to begin. Caitlin was invited to get comfortable in a recliner while I prepared the music. When she was comfortably situated, I began to guide her through a brief relaxation induction to help her focus during the experience. What follows below is the details and transcript from Caitlin's first BMGIM session.

Session #1
Induction: Deep breathing, with focusing image of a path
Program: Relationships

Chopin: (What do you notice?) No response from Caitlin. (What are you experiencing?) I don't know, nothing. (What are you aware of?) No response from Caitlin. (What are you feeling?) No. (Let yourself be with the music.) Music continues allowing image to develop. (What do you notice now?) Caitlin opens her eyes, sits up and begins to sob. She begins to say I don't know how to do this, I can't do this and continues to sob.

Postlude
I processed Caitlin's experience and her feelings around this session. Caitlin felt she had failed as she thought her image should have appeared sooner.

When it didn't appear right away, she began to feel she could not do this perfectly, which kept her stuck in her thoughts about not being good enough, not being able to do this. I reiterated that there is not just one way to image and that each of us images differently. Therefore, essentially there is no wrong answer. This concept did not seem possible to her. She just felt as if she'd failed. At the end of the session, I encouraged Caitlin to spend some time journaling about her experience and feelings and affirmed that we would meet again the following week.

During the interim, I had grown concerned that due to her perfectionism, Caitlin would be unwilling to continue with the imagery sessions. However, when she arrived she shared that she wanted to continue with the imagery sessions and was motivated to try again. This proved to be a turning point in Caitlin's therapeutic process. She had a tendency to avoid anything she did not feel she could do perfectly, but now she was willing to try to change this pattern. So, we discussed how to proceed for the second session. Caitlin shared her need to return to the image of the path, because she'd felt it was significant for her to explore. The second session began with the relaxation experience and a return to the image of the path. Below are excerpts from Caitlin's second session.

Session #2
Induction: Deep breathing, with focusing image of a path
Program: Pastorale
Debussy: (What is happening?) I am walking down the path. I don't know where I am going. I am looking for something. No one is with me. (How do you feel as you look?) I feel confident and strong. I can find what I am looking for even though I am alone. I see a fork in the road. One path is clear and the other path goes into the woods. I can barely see that path; it twists and turns in the trees. I am not sure which way to go. One path is straight and clear, it seems like the best way to go. I can see ahead on this path and it is a dead end. There is a brick wall at the end of the path. (A brick wall.) I want to look at it. I am walking down the path. The wall is too high. I can't go around it. I am looking for a way through it. This was the wrong way. (The wrong way.) The other path looks scary. I don't want to go down that path. I go down the clear path again. It's still a dead end. I can't go anywhere here. (Can you touch the wall?). Yes, it's a solid wall. The bricks are thick and rough. I can't get through it. I walk back to the fork in the road and then I walk back to the brick wall. Part of me wants to find a way through this brick wall. (How does that feel?) I feel a sense of hope and then frustration. (Frustration.) I walk back to the fork in the road. I walk back to the wall again. What else is there? (What else?) I keep looking back and forth to both paths. I realized I should try the other path, but it's scary. I

have to remember that this path is a dead end. (It's a dead end.) I am walking on the path in the woods, I keep walking through, but I can't tell where I am going. It must be the right way. I don't see anything yet. I am fighting my way through. (How do you feel?) Nervous, I don't know where I am going. I can see a little bit of sunlight coming through the trees at times. I am still determined to make it through. (Still determined.)

Liadov: I have reached the edge of the woods. I found my way out. (Found your way out.) There is a huge open field. I see the blue sky. I think about all the possibilities, it is so open and so free. (How do you feel?) I can breathe here. I can breathe the fresh air. This is what I was looking for. I am no longer stuck on that path. (No longer stuck.) I can look across the field and see the brick wall, that wasn't the way to go to get here. It wouldn't work. This path was harder, but it got me here. (It got you here.) I realize how happy I am here and I am glad I gave up on the other path. I could have been stuck a long time. It wasn't the right way to go. (How does it feel to be here?) I am happy, smiling, I am proud of myself for being brave enough to go through the woods. (Let yourself take in those feelings.)

Postlude

During this session the path that Caitlin wanted to be able to take was a dead end. She continued to try to make it work only to continue to get stuck there. When she became frustrated she was finally able to face her fear and go down the other path. Following the session, we processed her imagery experience. Caitlin recognized how the dead end path was representative of her eating disorder. While she continued to engage in using her eating disorder to cope day to day, it was actually keeping her stuck. She was able to acknowledge that facing her fear of the unknown allowed her to get to where she needed to go. She was able to take this message and lesson into her treatment and recovery process to help her face her fears. Caitlin continued with a series of BMGIM sessions in which she faced her fears, worked through feelings of sadness, anger, shame, and discovered her inner strength and empowerment as a result. Her ability to decrease her emotional distress, allowed Caitlin to no longer avoid her feelings, but instead experience and manage them.

Case of Kate: Symptoms and Underlying Emotions

Kate developed her eating disorder her junior year of high school when she began restricting her food intake and engaging in compulsive and excessive exercise. These symptoms persisted for about three years and then she began to purge as well. Over the years she was in various levels of treatment from inpatient to intensive outpatient, residential, and eventually outpatient. She has had multiple stays in various levels of care over the years. In addition to her eating disorder, Kate was also diagnosed with generalized anxiety disorder, major depressive disorder, borderline personality disorder, and post-traumatic stress disorder. It wasn't until her fourth experience with residential treatment that she began to address her feelings associated with her traumatic experiences. Once she began to deal with these multiple traumas, her symptoms stabilized and she could begin to manage in outpatient treatment.

At this point in her treatment, Kate was 25 years old and had been living with her eating disorder for nearly 8 years. Kate had become accustomed to managing her emotions with her symptoms. When her emotions became too intense, her practice was either to restrict or purge. Either symptom would numb her feelings and allow her to avoid dealing with them. In residential treatment, Kate had worked at developing her coping skills, so symptom use was not her way of managing her feelings. When she transitioned to outpatient treatment, she continued to process her traumatic experiences utilizing the BMGIM, a process she began in residential treatment. Kate was often unable to talk about the traumatic experiences in verbal therapy would only be able to write. The BMGIM to help her connect with her body, process through her traumas, and explore unexpressed feelings. While Kate was not able to process the trauma verbally, she was able to do so through the imagery. She soon discovered her ability to image, and subsequently achieved a sense of safety and comfort in the imagery process.

Kate was doing well in her outpatient treatment where she continued to process through her trauma. She had even returned to work, feeling as though life was normalizing. When a family health crisis emerged bringing a flood of emotions, these intense emotions were difficult for her to manage. She arrived for her session appearing extremely anxious and agitated. When I inquired about what she was feeling, she reported that she needed to throw up. I sat next to her and asked if she felt she could explore how she was feeling in her body. Kate thought she could. I encouraged her to get comfortable, like she had for many other BMGIM sessions. I guided her through a brief relaxation experience to help her calm and focus. The transcript below includes excerpts from the session that focused on exploring the symptom and the feelings connected to it.

GIM: Deprivation and its Contribution to Pain in Eating Disorders

Session #2
Induction: Deep breathing, Focus on the feeling in stomach
Program: Positive Affect

Elgar: (Let yourself connect with your stomach and how you are feeling there.) (Allow an image to come into your awareness that represents how you are feeling.) (What do you notice?) I see a thick, blue, tar like substance all throughout my stomach. It fills up most of my stomach. There are some small pockets of where the food is, but most of the area is filled with the blue thick tar. (What do you need?) I need to get the food out of there. I can't get the thick tar out of there, it is too thick. I have to get the food out. (Is there anything else you can do?) I don't know. I need to throw up. (Can you ask your stomach what it needs?) I don't know. (Try to ask it what it needs?) What do you need? There is no answer. (Can you ask again?) What do you need? It needs to release the blue thick tar. That thick tar is all the sadness and grief. When I express my feelings the tar dissipates. When I don't share or hold onto my feelings the tar builds up and then I need to release the tension by throwing up the food. (Can you give your stomach what it needs?) I need to release my sadness. Tears begin to roll down Kate's cheeks. She begins to sob. (Let yourself release the sadness.) Kate continues to sob. (What do you notice?) As I let myself feel the sadness, the thick tar begins to thin out. It becomes less sticky. I can begin to breathe easier. The thick tar is disappearing. (How does that feel?) I don't feel like I need to throw up anymore. (Let yourself breathe, just breathe.)

Postlude
Kate was able to be with the discomfort and feelings that were prompting her urges to engage in symptom use. In the imagery, she was able to experience and explore her discomfort and discover how to resolve it. She recognized that the thick, blue tar represented her unexpressed sadness and grief. The longer these feelings went unexpressed the thicker the tar would become.

Case of Ana: Processing Poly-Trauma

Ana first entered inpatient treatment her senior year in high school. She began restricting her food intake and compulsively exercising her junior year of high school, but by her senior year it had become so severe she was emaciated and medically unstable. Over the years she continued to struggle with anorexia nervosa spending time in and out of treatment. She continued to restrict, compulsively exercise and in time began to binge and purge as well. Throughout this time she was in various levels of treatment from inpatient, and outpatient, to residential.

In her late 20's Ana did achieve approximately about a two-year period when her symptoms subsided. During this time she married and had her son. Shortly after her son was born she began to struggle with symptoms again and subsequently entered residential treatment. Now 30, Ana felt defeated to be back to struggle with symptoms. At this point in her treatment she was diagnosed with anorexia nervosa, major depression, generalized anxiety disorder, post-traumatic stress disorder, obsessive-compulsive disorder, and borderline personality. Ana's trauma history included multiple traumatic events. She was raped the summer before college and just a few days before her wedding she'd had an abortion. Additionally, she felt that something had happened to her when she was a child. Suspecting sexual abuse, but having no conscious memories of such episodes. Ana felt conflicted about whether or not anything had actually happened at all.

Beginning our work together during this residential treatment episode she Ana was able to identify issues she had worked to address in previous treatment episodes. She also shared that she was continuing to notice feelings she did not want to feel and that her anxiety seemed to be higher, which increased her symptom use. When Ana came into residential treatment her weight was quite low and she needed to restore some weight for her cognitive processes to stabilize. When her thought processes were clearer, I began a series of BMGIM sessions to address the issues and feelings underlying her symptom use.

Through the series of BMGIM sessions, images, memories, and feelings related to Ana's various traumas surfaced. The excerpts from sessions below help to illustrate the images representing and relating to her traumatic experiences. She began to process her feelings as she uncovered memories and feelings from the various moments in her life. It is important to note that excerpts included in this case illustration do not include the intense or graphic images as I felt it would be inappropriate to include them.

Session #4
Induction: Holding something in your hands
Program: Nurturing

Britten: (What do you notice?) I am holding a doll. She is a rag doll. She is so tattered and worn. Her dress is torn and dirty. There is dirt on her face, legs, arms, and hands. Her hair is messy, tangled and snarled. (How do you feel as you see her?) I feel sad for her it looks like no one cares enough about her to take care of her. (No one cares about her.) I see my sister's doll sitting on her bed. Her doll is beautiful. She is clean, very neat and well taken care of. My rag doll used to look nicer; she didn't always look tattered and dirty. (How does it feel to hold her?) I feel sad for her, I want to wash away the dirt and make her clean again. (Want to make her clean again.)

Walton: (What do you notice now?) I see my sister. We are young. I miss her and my brother too. He took me away. He picked me. He said I was different, that I was better than my sister. He took me to the bathroom. I didn't want to go. (What do you see?) His face is not clear to me. His face is fuzzy and I can't see it clearly. He is holding my hand to tight. (How do you feel?) Afraid. (Do you feel it in your body?) It is hard to breathe; my throat and chest feel tight. Feel like I'm suffocating. (What do you need?) I want to put a big bubble around me so no one can touch me. I don't know how to heal these wounds. There are so many layers. I can't get all the dirt washed off.

Postlude
In the discussion following the imagery session, Ana shared she felt like the rag doll. She felt worn, tattered, and dirty. She recounted that throughout her childhood she had often felt different from her sister and brother and that she felt a need to protect them. She recognized she often felt these feelings growing up, and believed these feelings were a result of her doing something that was bad or wrong. She continued to feel unsure about whether something actually happened, or if these were memories or only childhood imagination. We discussed not needing to make a decision regarding these images, but to allow them to occur. I felt that without editing the process Ana would eventually discover her answer.

Session #6
Induction: Chair
Program: Relationships

Chopin: (What do you notice?) I am sitting in a chair and there is a dog in my lap. He is hurt and whimpering, his paw is hurt. There are people dancing in a ballroom. The dog is growling and wants to fiercely attack them. He doesn't trust them. It is all a façade. (How do you feel?) I feel mad, sad, angry, confused, disgusted, and worthless.

Rachmaninoff: (What is happening now?) I am on the leash and the dog is pulling me. No one understands that I was raped. Everything is forgotten because of my parent's drama. No one knows how to help me. No one wants to deal with it. (How do you feel?) I feel like I have to go where they want me to do, do what they want me to do. No one listens to what I need, so I have to go and do what they want me to do. It all just feels like a lie.

Postlude
Following this session, Ana was able to recall that shortly after she was raped, it was revealed her father had had an affair. Subsequently, he left her family and was unable to help her. She felt she needed to act as if she was fine in order to keep things calm. Ana shared that her parents never talked with her about the rape and that she did not receive therapy for this trauma. She developed the belief that she was supposed to live this façade and reported that she needed her eating disorders symptoms to push back the feelings of the rape. This resulted in her restricting even more and increasing her compulsive exercise. She shared that these symptoms helped to numb her feelings.

Session #10
Induction: Holding a box in your hands
Program: Emotional Expression I

Brahms: (What do you notice?) I am putting the box on a shelf in a dark room. This room is full of boxes. The boxes are stacked on top of one another and covered with dust. There are memories in them. (How does it feel to be there?) I feel sad and that this is my place to protect. There is a box sitting alone on a shelf. I grab that box and go sit in the corner. This box holds something very precious. (How do you feel as you hold it?) I feel a deep sadness. (Do you feel that in your body?). I feel it in my stomach. It is a dull ache, like a hurt from an old wound. (What do you need?) I need to open the box. (Can you?) Yes. These are the memories of my baby. The baby I lost. There are also pictures of Sean. I feel sad that Sean will never know her. I am the only one that knows about her. I am the only one that holds these memories. No one else knows she ever existed. Ana begins to cry.

Postlude
This session brought the memories of Ana's abortion and this loss of this baby back into her conscious memory. She shared that she had never actually grieved the loss of this child. Discovering the pregnancy shortly before her wedding she had felt understandably overwhelmed. Ana underwent an abortion just two days before her wedding and did not share this information with anyone. She felt due to the busyness of wedding details and her pattern of not dealing with her feelings, it became easier to push these emotions and memories away.

GIM: Deprivation and its Contribution to Pain in Eating Disorders

Session #15
Induction: Little girl in a chair
Program: Pastorale

Liadov: (What do you notice?) I see her sitting on a bench by the ocean. We are sitting together. A terrible storm is coming and the winds are blowing. I am trying to protect her. She asks if she will be okay. I tell her, "I will take care of you". Now she is playing by the water. (How do you feel as you see her?) I feel scared seeing her by the water. Sean comes and tells her not to play so close to the water. He knows because his mom taught him how to be safe. Sean brings me to her. She wants to see her reflection in the water. She forgets what she looks like. She is crying and the tears run down her face. I ask her why she is crying. She says she couldn't look in the mirror in the bathroom, because she was afraid she would see the bad man. Afraid she will see her body. She can't feel her body; she needs her body to be numb and not to feel what happened. She is sobbing and drowned in tears. She is looking into the water. Sean tells me its okay to tell her the truth. That it can be scary being a kid and that kids don't always understand why people do those things. Sean tells me it's okay to hold her, hug her, and be in the water with her.

Holst: (What's happening now?) I go into the water and get clean. I look behind me and see all the people who love and support me. This group of people grows and they are cheering me on. They tell me its okay to tell the truth. (How does that feel?) I feel a sense of inner peace. I speak my truth and I feel supported. Everyone wants to be protected. I hug the little girl and she blends into me and becomes part of me. (How does that feel?) So peaceful, I am surrounded by her light. I am holding Sean's hand and we walk away together. The water washed away the shame, blame and imperfections. (How does that feel?) I feel a sense of peace I have never felt before. (Allow yourself to take that in.)

Postlude
Ana felt the little girl in this session was the little girl in her or her inner child. Ana felt her son Sean entered her imagery to remind her that she does know how to nurture this little girl/herself, because she has nurtured him. She did not know that she could nurture herself; she needed to be reminded that she could do this and help herself to heal. While she felt she was not protected as a little girl, in this session she discovered that speaking her truth was not only healing, but also a way of protecting herself.

Through the series of BMGIM sessions, Ana processed the traumatic experiences and her feelings surrounding them. While the face of the man that molested her did not emerge in the process and she could not positively identify the perpetrator, she was able to heal those early wounds. Ana completed her stay in residential treatment and then transitioned to outpatient treatment. She continued to work with me for some additional BMGIM sessions. In time, Ana was able to begin to do volunteer work as well as obtain employment. She shared that she felt more engaged as a mother and a wife now that she could take care of herself.

Case of Mary: Moving from Being Disempowered to Empowered

Mary entered treatment at age 57. She struggled with binge eating for years, but had never received treatment. One-year earlier Mary's niece died as a result of complications of bulimia nervosa. She was having difficulty processing her grief and was finding her own struggles with food intensifying. This prompted Mary to begin treatment for her eating disorder. Mary was also diagnosed with major depressive disorder and generalized anxiety disorder.

Mary was married and had an adult daughter. She described her childhood as challenging, as she often felt like an orphan. Her mother battled schizophrenia her whole life, often going untreated or going off her medication. She described her dad as loving, but often working long hours. Mary had four siblings all much older and established in their lives by the time she was born. She reported often feeling unsafe in life and felt this was due to never knowing how her mom might be doing on any given day. She recalled one episode of coming home from school to find her mother talking to the stove.

Mary shared that she often felt unsafe in the outside world and this often resulted in her staying home and in isolation. She found that she would often use food to soothing herself when she felt anxious, afraid, depressed, and angry. Mary felt unable to process and work through her grief surrounding the death of her niece and she wanted to explore the use of BMGIM to address these feelings.

The session excerpts below provide an overview of Mary's therapeutic process and the feelings and memories that surfaced. She began to make connections between her feelings of grief and loss that related to other experiences in her life. She also began to discover how this related to her relationship with food and her body.

GIM: Deprivation and its Contribution to Pain in Eating Disorders

Session #3
Induction: A box holding something you want to let go of
Program: Relationships

Chopin: (What do you notice?) I feel a sense of exclusion. I often feel excluded. I can feel it in the box. I carry this around with me. I have turned this into that I am not wanted. The truth was I was not wanted by Gladys (Mary's mother). It doesn't mean I am not wanted by anyone. I do want to let go of this. All I could ever see is that I wasn't wanted. If I keep holding onto this box, I stay trapped with it.

Rachmaninoff: I don't think that is what I want anymore. (How do you feel as you hold this?) Angry. (Where do you feel it in your body?) I feel tension and anger in my shoulders and neck. I feel hunched and tense. I don't know how to let this go.

Respighi: The only way I have known how to be is to withdraw. That was safer. This just leaves me feeling unwanted. I don't want to stay stuck with this. (How does it feel to be stuck?) I feel angry and lonely. I want my path to be different. I don't feel wanted anywhere. I have to stop assuming I am not wanted. There are places I belong (Yes, there are places where you belong).

Postlude
Mary recognized that she believed as a child she was not wanted. She often heard these very words from her mother. She was realizing that this message was internalized and this became a truth in her life. When she felt depressed she tended to isolate and this reinforced her belief that she was unwanted. This was the pattern when she felt anxious, angry, or overwhelmed. She was now exploring the possibility that feeling not wanted by her mother was tied into her mother's chronic mental health issues and did not have to be her truth.

Session #4
Induction: Standing in front of a door
Program: Emotional Expression I

Brahms: (What do you notice?) Behind this door is my family. Gladys is there too. (How do you feel as you stand there?) I am fearful and nervous. I don't want to go there. She was so unpredictable. I want to open the door but it will feel overwhelming. It always felt like a landmine, an explosion. I was always afraid. (How do you feel now?) I am afraid and angry. (Where do you feel that in your body?) I feel it in my stomach. It feels upset and unsettled. She would scream at me, yelling, "I hate you!" I would shiver and feel overwhelmed. (Do you feel that in your body?) Yes, I need to protect my stomach.

Brahms: It is really hard to feel my stomach, my gut with all those feelings. It feels like too much to be able to show. How do I feel these feelings without just becoming a pool of nothing? (Do you feel any strength in your body?) I feel it in my head. Strength feels like being planted. (Mary begins to stretch her body) (Stretch and take in that strength.) My dad was as solid as a bowl of jelly. He wasn't strong; he counted on me to be. (Mary continues to stretch) (Take in strength). I can feel it in my legs now. (Let yourself take that in)

Brahms: (How do you feel now?) I feel at peace. (Where do you feel it in your body?) I feel it in my stomach. The music also gives me peace. (Let yourself take in that peace.)

Postlude
Mary was able to connect with some of the emotions that were overwhelming to her. She recognized she never learned how to express or process these feelings. She only knew how to retreat and isolate. In the imagery, when she could stay with the emotions in her body she was able to discover how to find her strength. She felt empowered as she found the strength within. She also noticed that in finding her strength and feeling empowered, she was able to let go of her anger and fear.

Session #5
Induction: Prior to the imagery portion of the session, Mary created a mandala that represented her fear. The image of this mandala was the image utilized at the start of the session.
Program: Creativity I

Sibelius: (What is happening?) I see lightening bolts. They are flying around. I am standing on rings, like the rings of Saturn. The lightening bolts are all around me. I can duck and the lightening bolts don't hit me. (How does that feel?) I am surprised. I never thought I could just duck. I don't have to be the target. I can also use a shield to protect myself. (What do you notice?) I can choose. I don't have to stand there and be a deer in the headlights. There are ways for me to protect myself. (You can protect yourself.) Maybe I can even catch a lightening bolt. (You can catch one). I caught a bolt and place it on my side. (How do you feel?) I feel powerful.

GIM: Deprivation and its Contribution to Pain in Eating Disorders

Vaughn-Williams: I am radiating with the thunderbolt at my side. I look and feel likeWonder Woman. (Wonder Woman.) I need time to learn how to harness this power. It is possible for it to become a part of me. I feel strength in my legs. Before I was able to hold the thunderbolt I felt heavy and bloated.

Delius: (What is happening now?) I am standing with a thunderbolt in each hand. I can put them down and still feel strong and flexible. I hold this power. (Let yourself continue to feel that power.)

Postlude
Mary discovered that she did hold her power and strength and was surprised at this discovery. Following this session, she continued to hold the image of Wonder Woman and the lightening bolts as empowering and healing images. When she struggled or found herself reverting back to old behaviors she would remind herself of her image and continue to reconnect with her power.

This session allowed her to also build strength needed to continue processing her feelings surrounding grief and loss. She found that she was not as afraid of her emotions after this session. She began to explore her feelings in greater depth and allow herself to express those emotions and even cry. She also began to feel more empowered about feeling safe in the world. As a result she became more involved socially, and while it wasn't always easy, she did begin to accept invitations to spend time with friends.

Conclusion

Eating disorders are classified under mental health diagnoses and while this does require addressing the psychological issues, this is only one aspect of disorders. Individuals living with an eating disorder also experience physiological issues as a result of the disorder. These physiological symptoms will vary in severity depending upon how long the individual has been living with the eating disorder and the frequency and intensity of symptom use. It should be noted that severe symptom use can lead to a variety of medical issues.

Psychological issues are often what is underlying and fostering symptom use. The experiences or emotions that the patient is unable to process often serve as impetus for symptom use. As these emotions and experiences become more difficult to ignore, symptom use intensifies. This leads to more serious medical implications and complications for patients.

The BMGIM is a mind-body, music psychotherapy approach utilized to address underlying feelings, memories, and experiences. The case illustrations previously in the chapter, demonstrate how the BMGIM fostered exploration of the psychological and physiological issues. From facing fear of the unknown and choosing a different path, confronting perfectionism, exploring symptoms, working through trauma, and facing underlying emotions of anger, shame, grief, and sadness become achievable tasks.

The music and imagery sessions allowed patients to face their feelings and experiences and discover what they needed to heal. Through this process they found ways to let go of emotions and experiences that kept them stuck in the past. They discovered the eating disorder was only a dead end and they needed to choose another direction for themselves. They felt and tolerated emotions they had long avoided and became empowered. They found it is possible to live life differently and that they could step into life without the eating disorder.

The BMGIM is an in-depth method that lends itself to addressing the complex nature of an eating disorder. This method allows the client to address the issues underlying the eating disorder or the struggle with symptoms. While these case illustrations are anecdotal evidence, they provide a rationale for further exploration and research regarding the BMGIM in eating disorder treatment.

References

1. Collins ME. Body figure perceptions and preferences among pre-adolescent children. International Journal of Eating Disorders, 1991; 199-208.
2. Smolak L. National Eating Disorders Association/Next Door Neighbors Puppet Guide Book. 1996.
3. Neumark-Sztainer D. I'm, Like, SO Fat! New York: The Guilford Press. 2005; 5.
4. Crowther JH, Wolf EM, & Sherwood N. Epidemiology of bulimia nervosa. In M Crowther, DL. Tennenbaum. SE. Hobfoll, & MAP Stephens (Eds.). The Etiology of Bulimia Nervosa: The Individual and Familial Context. Washington, D.C.: Taylor & Francis. 1992: 1-26.
5. Fairburn, CG, Hay, PJ, & Welch, SL. Binge eating and bulimia nervosa: Distribution and determinants. In C.G. Fairburn & G.T. Wilson, (Eds.), Binge Eating: Nature, Assessment, and Treatment. New York: Guilford. 1993; 123-143.
6. Gordon RA. Anorexia and Bulimia: Anatomy of a Social Epidemic. New York: Blackwell; 1990.
7. Hoek HW. The distribution of eating disorders. In K.D. Brownell &

8. C.G. Fairburn (Eds.) Eating Disorders and Obesity: A Comprehensive Handbook. New York: Guilford. 1995; 207-211.
8. Hoek HW & van Hoeken D. Review of the prevalence and incidence of eating disorders. International Journal of Eating Disorders, 2003; 383-396.
9. Shisslak CM, Crago M, & Estes LS. The spectrum of eating disturbances. International Journal of Eating Disorders, 11995; 8 (3), 209-219.
10. Sullivan P. Mortality rates of mental health disorders. American Journal of Psychiatry, Vol. 152 (7), July 1995, p. 1073-1074.
11. Crow, SJ, Peterson, CB, Swanson, SA, Raymond, et al. Increased mortality in bulimia nervosa and other eating disorders. American Journal of Psychiatry; 2009 166, 1342-1346.
12. National Institutes of Health. Research Funding. Retrieved June 7, 2012, from http://www.nih.gov/news/fundingresearchareas.htm
13. American Psychological Association: Diagnostic and Statistical Manual of Mental Disorders, Fourth Edition, Test Revision. Washington, DC, American Psychiatric Association. 2000.
14. Walker LO, & Avant KC. Strategies for Theory Construction in Nursing, 3rd ed. Norwalk, CT: Appleton & Lange; 1995.
15. Pirraglia PA, Hampton JM, Rosen AB, Witt WP. Psychological distress and trends in healthcare expenditures and outpatient healthcare. American Journal of Managed Care. 2011 May;17(5):319-28
16. Ridner, S. Psychological distress: concept analysis. Journal of Advanced Nursing, 2004; 45(5), 536–545.
17. Massee´ R. Qualitative and quantitative analyses of psycho- logical distress: methodological complementarity and ontological incommensurability. Qualitative Health Research. 2000; 10, 411–423.
18. Bulik C. Anxiety, depression, and eating disorders. In C. G. Fairburn and K. D. Brownell (Eds.), Eating disorders and obesity: A comprehensive handbook. New York: Guilford; 2002: 193-198.
19. Kaye W, Bulik C, Thornton L, Barbarich N, and Masters K, Cormorbidity of anxiety disorders with anorexia and bulimia nervosa. American Journal of Psychiatry, 2004; 161(12), 2215-2221.
20. Hudson J, Hiripi E, Pope H, & Kessler R. The Prevalence and Correlates of Eating Disorders in the National Comorbidity Survey Replication. Biological Psychiatry, 2007; 61, 348-358.
21. Abbate-Daga G, Gramaglia C, Amianto, F, Marzola, E. & Fassino, S. Attachment Insecurity, Personality, and Body Dissatisfaction in Eating Disorders. Journal of Nervous Mental Disease, 2010; 198(7), 520-524.

22. Illing V, Tasca G, Balfour L, & Bissada H. Attachment Insecurity Predicts Eating Disorder Symptoms and Treatment Outcomes in a Clinical Sample of Women. Journal of Nervous and Mental Disorders, 2010; 198(9), 653-659.
23. Oldershaw A, Dejong H, Hambrook D, Tchanturia K, Treasure J, & Schmidt U, (2012). Emotional Processing Following Recovery from Anorexia Nervosa. European Eating Disorder Review, 2012; 10, 1170-1181.
24. Hambrook D, Oldershaw A, Rimes K, et al. Emotional dysregulation and emotional process in eating disorder patients. British Journal of Clinical Psychology, 2011; (3)3, 310-325.
25. Harrison A, Sullivan S, Tchanturia K, & Treasure J. Emotion recognition and regulation in anorexia nervosa. Clinical Psychology & Psychotherapy, 2009; 16(4), 348-356.
26. Fox R. & Power M. Eating disorders and multi-level models of emotion: An integrated model. Clinical Psychology & Psychotherapy, 2009; 16(4), 240-267.
27. Pomeroy,C. Assessment of medical status and physical factors. In K. Thompson (Ed.) Handbook of eating disorders and obesity. New York: Guilford Press. 2004; 81-111.
28. Pomeroy C. & Mitchell J. Medical complications of anorexia nervosa and bulimia nervosa. In C. Fairburn & K. Brownell (Eds.), Eating disorders and obesity: A comprehensive handbook (2nd ed.) New York: Guilford Press. 2002; 278-329.
29. Addolorate G, Taronto C, Capristo E, & Babarrini G. A case marked cerebellar atrophy in a woman with anorexia nervosa and a review of the literature. International Journal of Eating Disorders, 1998; 24 ,443-447.
30. Mitchell J, Pomeroy C, & Adson, D. Managing medical complications. In D. Garner & P. Garfinkel (Eds.), Handbook of treatment for eating disorders. New York: Guilford Press. 1997; 167-187.
31. Bonny HL. Guided imagery and music (GIM): Mirror of consciousness. In L. Summer (Ed.), Music consciousness: The evolution of guided imagery and music. Gilsum, NH: Barcelona Publishers. 2002a; 93-102
32. Goldberg FS. The Bonny Method of Guided Imagery and Music. In T Wigram B Saperston, & R West (Eds.), The art and science of music therapy: A handbook. Switzerland: Hardwood Academic Publishers. 1995; 112-128.
33. Ventre M. The individual form of the Bonny Method of Guided Imagery and Music (BMGIM). In KE Bruscia & DE Grocke (Eds.), Guided imagery and music: The Bonny method and beyond.

Gilsum, NH: Barcelona Publishers. 2002; 29-35.

34. Bonny HL. & Pahnke W. The use of music in psychedelic (LSD) psychotherapy. Journal of Music Therapy, 1972; 9, 64-87.

35. Heiderscheit A. The Effects of the Bonny Method of Guided Imagery and Music (GIM) on Adults in Chemical Dependency Treatment: Sense of Coherence, Salivary Immunoglobulin A and Interpersonal Problems. Unpublished Dissertation, University of Minnesota, Minneapolis, MN. 2005.

36. Heiderscheit A. Discovery and recovery through music: An overview of music therapy with adults in eating disorder treatment. . In Brooke, S. (Ed.). The Creative Arts Therapies and Eating Disorders. Springfield, IL., Charles C. Thomas Publisher. 2008; 122-141.

37. Heiderscheit A. Qualitative Analysis of Imagery Themes and Client Perceived Benefits of the Bonny Method of Guided Imagery and Music (BMGIM) with Eating Disordered Clients Concurrent session presented at the IX International Music Medicine Symposium at Augsburg College in Minneapolis, MN. 2011.

38. Heiderscheit A. Presentation at the Annual Music & Medicine Pain Symposium at Beth Israel Medical Center and the Louis Armstrong Center for Music Medicine, entitled, GIM: Deprivation and its contribution to pain. 2012.

39. Swanson SA, Crow SJ, LeGrange D, Swendsen J, Merikangas KR. Prevalence and correlates of eating disorders in adolescents: results from the National Comorbidity Survey Replication Adolescent Supplement. Archives of General Psychiatry. 2011.

Music and Medicine: Integrative Models in the Treatment of Pain

CHAPTER 21

Music Therapy and HIV/AIDS Related Pain

John F. Mondanaro MA, LCAT, MT-BC, CCLS
Christine Vaskas MS, MT-BC

"Music is the concern of all, not of a privileged elite, and if musicality represents an asset, it is not the prerogative of a chosen few, but an endowment of man to man."

Victor Zuckerkandl, Musicologist

Introduction

At this writing, there is no cure for HIV/AIDS. Thirty years after the first recognized symptoms of Acquired Immunodeficiency Syndrome (AIDS) appeared, treatment-planning focuses on controlling the Human Immunodeficiency Virus (HIV) but as of yet not curing it. HIV/AIDS have collectively and profoundly impacted the world not only because of the disease's unprecedented statistics over a relatively short period of time but because its story has sustained social and political centrality. The rapid trajectory of the disease created immediate public demand for not only education and awareness about the disease itself, but for a cure that could bring halt to what was deemed initially as a homosexual disease and later as an indiscriminate one. Achieving pandemic status early on, the quest to surmount HIV/AIDS's has provided the impetus for tremendous positive change from enlightened human rights activism and fair employment practice to perhaps the most poignant to the cause, the acceleration of pharmacological trials by the Food and Drug Administration (FDA).[1] The latter occurred in part as a response to the accelerated interest in alternative treatments due to what was perceived by the growing AIDS community as a lack of governmental response to the epidemic.

While the effectiveness of continued research and development of medications has in fact allowed many infected individuals to live longer lives, such success may run the risk of translating to younger generations as a sort of false optimism. Coupled with the developmentally based propensity of adolescents to view themselves as invincible and to indulge in high-risk behaviors, this lethal combination has contributed to astounding statistics on HIV diagnoses between the ages of 13 and 29 in the United States alone.

An estimated 8,294 individuals in this age group were diagnosed with HIV infection in 2009, with seventy-five percent of these cases occurring in those aged 20 to 24, the peak of sexual and social activity.[2,3] In spite of the statistics that define the impact of AIDS/HIV worldwide and the ongoing educational campaigns, this current trend toward high-risk behaviors seems eerily familiar to the beginning of the epidemic. Successful pharmacological management of the disease may for many individuals relegate the reality that there still is no cure. Adolescents and young adults only partially synthesizing the facts may be apt to make irresponsible and life-impacting choices about sexual safety and other high-risk activities.

The social and political history of HIV and AIDS is significant when discussing the importance of psychotherapeutic support for those living with the virus because of its indelible impact. Survivors from the earliest generation of those infected with the virus to the youth of today who seem to be repeating the same recognizable cycles of behavior live with the reality of incomprehensible loss within a remarkably retrievable past. While the disease is central to this discussion, the history of treatment is also full of compelling controversy.

Pain from HIV/AIDS

The myriad of pain experiences reported by patients living with HIV/AIDS can be understood through the organization of symptoms into three main syndromes identified as Somatic Pain, Visceral Pain, and Neuropathic Pain.[4] While all three have genesis in the virus itself, there may be recognizable types of pain ascribable to the effects of the various medications that are used in treatment as well. A brief description of these areas will be offered to elucidate the range of possibilities and complexity of pain experienced by those living with the disease.

1) Somatic pain manifesting in the skin may ensue from Kaposi's sarcoma, neoplastic infiltration of the skin, and lymphedema. Additionally, various forms of arthritis including Reiter's syndrome and psoriatic arthritis, as well as joint and muscle swelling can cause great discomfort. 2) Visceral Pain Syndrome inclusive of chronic throat pain caused by persistent infections of the oropharyngeal region; various forms of chest pain caused by pneumonia, pleuritus, esophagitis; abdominal pain caused by colitis, hepatitis, pancreatitis; and opportunistic bacterial, parasitic, and viral infections that can result in chronic diarrhea, are among the myriad of conditions that can manifest throughout the trajectory of the illness.[4] 3) Neuropathic Pain from myelopathy, or degeneration of the spinal column, and abnormal cell production resulting in neoplasms may contribute to the patient's experience as well. Headaches, which can occur frequently from

exacerbation of existing conditions to meningitis, and again opportunistic bacterial infections may also be considerable factors.[4]

The pain experience reported by patents living with HIV/AIDS can have tremendous impact on an individual's ability to activate inner resources connected to healthy coping and quality of life. To this end, access to the psychoemotional and/or spiritual resources that may be critical to an individual may well be served by non-pharmacologic therapies such as music therapy that can provide both a space for reflection and reconciliation, and may serve as a recluse from burdensome thought and the verbal processes.

Treatment: Past and Present

The earliest trend toward alternative medicines is understandable in retrospect given the gap that ensued from a lack of a standard treatment during the first five years of the epidemic.[1] The rise and fall in popularity of alternative treatment reflected the changing themes of the first two decades of the epidemic, and empowered the community with a roguish spirit that prevailed as individuals infected with the virus found certain hope, which provided a sense of control. From the easily attained antioxidants (such as Vitamin C and Beta-carotene), Chinese herbs, and Tumeric to the various compounds that received expedited trial by the FDA, there came into greater recognition the need for substantiation and quality control guidance, thus the eventual establishment of the Alternative Medicine Office at the National Institutes of Health.[1]

The increased recognition of this movement challenged care providers to become aware of the alternative treatments being utilized by their patients and to adapt an approach that was supportive and informed rather than dismissive. Acknowledgement, encouragement, monitoring, and referring their patients toward viable alternative treatments, while staying abreast of the evolving standardized treatments redefined the clinical practice of the 1990s.[1] This standard of care has continued to evolve into the twenty-first century with the heightened value on integrative care.

The continued development of antiretroviral drugs and protease inhibitors from the mid-1990s to present day has contributed to longer survival rates as the progression of HIV in the body can be effectively slowed. Current anti-HIV drugs block the virus in specific ways. Non-nucleoside reverse transcriptase inhibitors (NNRTls), Nucleoside reverse transcriptase inhibitors (NRTIs), Proteses inhibitors (PIs), Entry or fusion inhibitors, and Integrase inhibitors, all function to stave off the progression of HIV by directly disabling or indirectly disempowering the virus through deprivation and blocking cell access or growth.[5]

Another notable but puzzling impact of the remarkable progress in pharmacological treatment is the decrease in the number of infected individuals participating in social support programs and community-based resource centers. While better medications have allowed both infected individuals to live longer and infected mothers to give birth to virus free infants, resources available to survivors are at the same time diminishing. Contributing to this shift is a general lack of interest in support services shown by teens and young adults. Common to other chronic conditions that are effectively managed, individuals diagnosed with HIV are more prone to normalization outside of the diagnosis rather than being identified solely within the group.[3]

As the need for support programs diminishes, so does the availability of funding, which results in the restructuring if not dismantling completely of existing programs. Those most profoundly impacted by this combination of impetuses are the survivors of the epidemic's initial onslaught. For many of these individuals, peer and familial support systems directly impacted by the early years of the disease have been rendered negligible. The importance of institutionally based support-programs, made available to the homeless and underprivileged in the past decades is undeniable. For survivors of the original onslaught of the disease, psychosocial support remains important given the degree of loss, isolation, betrayal, abandonment, and guilt they have sustained.[6]

Confidentiality and Ethics

The stigmatization that may occur with any chronic condition is perhaps intensified with HIV and AIDS, because of the social aspects ascribed to the virus. Great consideration has been given to protecting the rights to privacy of any individual pursuing HIV testing, with only subtle variation from state to state. The Illinois AIDS Confidentiality Act[7] and New York State's Public Health Law, Article 27-F_ENREF_124,[8] stand as pillars of such policy, where testing for HIV status is achievable only by consent of the individual being tested. Strict observation of this practice is maintained from state to state, with deviation occurring only circumstantially as follows: 1) required Comprehensive Newborn Screening; 2) self administering with an FDA-approved home testing kit; 3) when needed to obtain, process, or use human body parts; 4) tracking disease trends, and 5) screening for employment in federal programs that require HIV testing such as the U.S. Armed Forces, Job Corps, and federal correctional facilities.[8]

The individual consenting to be tested for HIV receives required information and education about the HIV virus that causes AIDS; the importance of testing as the only course to learning status; significance in pregnancy; the availability of anonymous and confidential testing; and State law's protection against discrimination and adherence to confidentiality and disclosure policy. Person's testing positive are also asked to cooperate with partner notification, which is also handled confidentially. Additional counseling and education are mandatorily provided at the time when test results are given, addressing how to emotionally cope with results; discrimination issues; the importance of intermittent testing; and safe practice against HIV infection.

When results are positive, the sharing of information bidirectionally is emphasized and in some cases mandated such as referral information for medical and psychoemotional care and psychoeducation on preventing further exposure to the virus. Additionally offered is education about the importance of cooperating with professionals in their effort of contacting partners who may have been exposed to the virus, which can be done anonymously if requested.[7,8]

Finally, New York State law maintains that HIV-related information can only be disclosed when the individual has signed an approved HIV release form. Some of the exceptions to the rule include disclosure to members of the individual's treatment team; medical disclosure by a provider to an insurance company; medical personnel coordinating care for a patient who is incarcerated; parents or guardians of a minor individuals only when disclosure is necessary to provide timely care; individuals who need to be notified that they may have been exposed to the virus; and public health officials for the purpose of tracking disease trends.[8]

HIV status as a matter of confidentiality has provided impetus for the building of community, yet even within the HIV/AIDS community and in the context of healthcare where support services can enhance medical care, the issues of trust and confidentiality can impede the efforts to provide programming. While individual counseling more readily ensures the level of confidentiality asserted by state law, group work that offers potentially invaluable peer support can be more challenging to bring into fruition. In spite of the tremendous benefits of altruism and universality among peers relating to one another in a group forum,[9] issues of trust can impede the fostering of group cohesion until enough time can be given to establish consistency and continuity. The following section discusses the provision of support services through a grant-based program at Beth Israel Medical Center known as the Peter Kruger Clinic.

Outpatient Services for HIV/AIDS Treatment through The Peter Krueger Clinic at Beth Israel Medical Center

Beth Israel Medical Center (BIMC) in New York City has been dedicated to optimal HIV/AIDS care for over twenty-five years. The Peter Krueger Clinic (PKC) at BIMC, founded in 1981[10] provides comprehensive outpatient care for patients living with HIV/AIDS. Each patient coming into the clinic receives a primary care team that includes a physician and registered nurse. The clinic also provides other specialty services such as dermatology, gynecology, dentistry, social work, music therapy, and pain management. In the clinic, there is a strong focus on the emotional and life style factors that are associated with this diagnosis, such as stress management, diet, substance abuse and management of high-risk behaviors. The treatment adherence program is also a way for patients to gain support, understand their treatment, manage their side effects and communicate successfully with providers. All of these resources prove to be an essential aspect of the overall care provided to patients receiving care from the clinic. Two constructs within The Peter Kruger Clinic that will be discussed in this chapter are the Peter Kruger Pediatric Clinic and The Women's Project.

The Peter Kruger Pediatric Clinic

The pediatric unit within the Peter Kruger Clinic not only provides crucial medical care, but also has acted as a supportive community for many of the patients and their families. Unlike other illnesses, it is not infrequent that family members may be infected with HIV at the same time, which can add to the stress of poverty, trauma, substance abuse and other social stigmas.[11] The pediatric unit at the clinic provides the long-term medical and psychosocial support necessary for patients and family members to cope with their illness. The Louis and Lucille Armstrong Music Therapy Program has been a vital aspect of the care provided for over twenty years, contributing to the psychosocial well being of patients through the provision of procedural support when needed and ongoing emotional support. The latter point is especially important as the social stigma that is associated with this diagnosis may result in isolation, depression, and related emotional pain.

An individual music therapy session may occur before, during or after a treatment, which can help calm the child and aid medical staff working with the patient.[12] Whenever the session occurs, goals and objectives are dependent on the specific needs of each child. If music therapy is involved prior to the medical treatment, goals may focus on the expression of anxiety or uncertainty that the child is facing. Whether a child is being treated outpatient or on the inpatient unit of a hospital, medical intervention can be a scary and unfamiliar experience. Anxiety that occurs anticipatorily of a treatment can be expressed through songwriting, improvisation and singing. This may also help to normalize the environment and provide grounding or predictability. Having the time and space to express these feelings may lessen some of the burden felt by the patient, which can reinforce existing coping skills during the actual treatment.

During treatment, such as a blood draw, music therapy may be utilized as a forum for procedural support. If the child is fearful of treatment, music therapy may be used as a point of refocusing away from the procedure.[13] Additionally, providing clarification of medical procedures may introduce psychoeducational interventions, which can further build trust between the child, therapist, parent and medical staff.

When a music therapist introduces music as a unique form of auditory stimuli during a procedure, it serves to help the child focus on something other than the treatment and pain. Although refocusing does not stop the child from experiencing pain, it aids in coping with the pain more effectively.[14] Singing a favorite song while the child plays a hand drum or other small instrument may enable the staff to complete the procedure efficaciously while the child still has a sense of control in the space.[15] A favorite song is also a way to acknowledge the child's self-worth which can provide a gateway to communication.[16] Parents can also participate in the singing of favorite songs, which helps to support their child and gives them a sense of empowerment as well. If a child is very aware of their surroundings and their level of anxiety is heightened, a music therapist may use clarification in order to voice the child's fears in the moment. Singing songs about what is going on during a procedure can act as an alter ego and provide value to their feelings. It may also help resolve tension or hesitations that emerge.

When a treatment is over, the child may feel emotionally drained and restless. Music therapy can be used post-procedurally as a reconstitution technique or as a forum for closure and cathartic release so that the child can transition from the hospital with less tension and/or anxiety. Creating a song about what the treatment was like is another way for the child to organize his/her feelings and sensory impressions while acknowledging that they endured a difficult treatment. This is a way for the child to identify personal strengths, which leads to increased self-esteem and mastery. The use of lullaby or song of kin[17] may be another way to center the child and bring a sense of calm. This in turn eases the transition from treatment to the outside world.[18]

It is important to acknowledge that some children receiving care are unaware that they have HIV due to the family's desire to protect them from the social stigmas associated with HIV and AIDS. Such conspiracy of silence can manifest in confusion and uncertainty, especially for younger children. When this is the case, feelings are often intensified before a treatment because the child is unsure of what is about to happen. The dynamics that prevail during these scenarios may pose challenges to all involved including the medical staff. The communication between staff and child can become strained, resulting in the child's increasing detachment from the space.

Improvisational music therapy provides the child with valuable opportunities to gain mastery within an experience laden with uncertainty, through choice making and creative expression. The music that is created during an improvisation may focus on ameliorating the child's anxiety or uncertainty through the provision of a sacred space that is immanently less threatening. Reinforcing the child's sense of control, whether through instrument choice, chosen direction within an improvisation, or recreation of songs from preferred genres or artists can positively reduce stress and provide needed support to immune functioning.[19]

Case Vignette: Kera

Kera a thirteen year-old girl, diagnosed with HIV at birth, had been receiving routine physical examinations annually as part of her care. During one particular visit, she immediately entered the music room and began to emote about her treatment anxiety. During the music therapy session, she told the therapist that she was "scared" to have blood taken and "didn't feel like" seeing the doctor. She also expressed her need to "chill-out" before she was asked "too many questions." After the therapist talked to Kera about other current events in her life (school, family life), her favorite song, "Someone like You" by Adel was played. As time went on, she increased her volume and eventually began to sing the song on her own. Soon, she was singing with strong emotion that was reflected in her powerful vocal tone and animated facial expressions. When the song was over, she took a deep breath in and sat back in her chair. As the therapist and Kera discussed the meaning of the song and how she felt singing it, Kera presented as relaxed and secure in her space. She stated that although it was a "sad" song, she felt that it relayed a positive message and provided hope. The meaning of hope was discussed further as Kera related it to her life. During this session the music acted as a window into some of Kera's emotions and feelings that she had not expressed prior. The session concluded with her report of feeling as though she had "released bad feelings" and of being able to proceed with her medical treatment in a positive frame of mind.

The Annual Peter Kruger Arts Fest

The culmination of the pediatric music therapy program is The Annual Peter Kruger Creative Arts Festival, which provides a group experience for children and young adults living with HIV/AIDS. During this event, children have been encouraged to participate in music and dance performances or share their artwork in an art gallery before the show. This event provides the young children and adolescents with a supportive community where they can express themselves while relating to others.[20]

Additional benefits of such positive group experiences include proven reduction of high-risk behaviors for adolescents and positive influence on decision making regarding peer pressure.[21]

Preparation for the festival has provided as rich an experience as the festival itself, as some patients have sessions with each other to rehearse a dance or musical number. During these sessions, themes about challenges and isolation often arise as the patients share their experiences with each other. Significant songs usually derive from these moments, evoking shared feelings about growing up with HIV. After the themes are explored, the patients are able to bring a sense of closure to the experience when they perform the song. Due to the longevity of the arts festival, many patients have formed strong bonds with one another, and with the staff who also perform alongside patients to contribute to a healthy community spirit. The festival offers not only normalization and a heightened sense of community, but also important validation as families celebrate the accomplishments of the children and adolescents involved.

Due to the fact that the Art Festival has been held annually, some patients have been a part of the event for several years. As they work with the music therapist throughout the year on individual goals, they are able to work toward a completed project that gives them self-esteem and empowerment. Together with the music therapist, a patient may create a song about their experiences living with HIV and then present it at the Art Festival.

Case Vignette: James
James is a 19 year-old singer songwriter who has performed his music in the Arts Fest since its inception. Born HIV positive, James' songwriting as a creative outlet has allowed him to process his experience safely within the structure of song. The forum provided in music therapy sessions offers much needed opportunity for James to share his feelings about both living with HIV, and of how the pain from losing his mother to AIDS has made him "stronger."

Each year James performs several songs that reflect his dreams, interests, and life experiences as a young man. While HIV is the shared context of each performer, the opportunity to shine through the diagnosis for an evening is afforded to all. For James, like many others, hope and altruism abound within the positive atmosphere that is created during this meaningful community event.

Music and Medicine: Integrative Models in the Treatment of Pain

The Women's Project

The Women's Project at the Peter Kruger Clinic was formed in 1996 as a support service that would focus on the unique experience of women living with HIV/AIDS.[1,10] The grant-funded program is available to women living with HIV/AIDS, and who have had a history of substance abuse or who are currently using. After each woman meets with a licensed social worker, they decide on an individualized plan with goals that are related to their physical and emotional health. From there, they are encouraged to participate in one of the groups offered by the Women's Project.

A music therapist runs the music therapy group, with support from one of the social workers on staff. Many of the women who attend the music therapy group have been a part of the Women's Project for three or more years and are familiar with the objectives of music therapy within a group setting. Due to recent program changes and shifts in funding referenced earlier, the Women's Group changed to Project S.h.a.r.e., which has been opened to include men as well. It also focuses on individuals who are currently using methadone and other substances, or who are sober for two years or less. The group vignette presented will focus on the work before and during this transition.

Creating, expressing and sharing in a group setting can offer a sense of grounding, insight and commonality for adults who are experiencing the same side effects from HIV/AIDS. The use of music therapy in a group setting can contribute to process oriented goals, which may motivate patients while reinforcing proactive behaviors. Due to the fact that individuals are attracted to others who they perceive as having similar experiences,[22] a group may act as a second family for some individuals. The social connectedness that is experienced in a group session may aid patients with HIV/AIDS to become aware of factors such as isolation and depression. Therefore, the social support that is provided in a group setting may validate the importance of feeling loved, appreciated and understood.[22]

Due to the fact that HIV/AIDS is still stigmatized in today's society, the issue of privacy remains paramount and is a particularly delicate area to work through within a group. Before any other goals can be addressed and explored, it is essential to build a foundation of trust while developing norms in order for members to feel as though they can express themselves freely in a safe and secure space. Yalom[23] describes group process in terms of self-generating, like a positive self-reinforcing loop that moves from trust, self-disclosure, empathy, and acceptance back to trust once again. This process is vital for group members to become aware of themselves and others while moving toward group cohesion. Although trust within a group is something that continuously grows and develops over time, there are music therapy techniques that may provide a basis for sharing.

Having each member share one of their favorite songs is one way for group members to reveal something about themselves in a conscious and unconscious manner. A favorite song is a window to a person's "outside" world and may display many past and present themes.[24] Although there are many ways to present these favorite songs in a group, the use of Song Sensitation, developed by Joanne Loewy,[25] is a way for group members to gain insight into each other's feelings while discovering common themes within the group. Song Sensitation begins with a relaxation technique that centers on deep breathing and settling into the space. Once the group members are relaxed and centered, the recording of a favorite song from one of the group members is played through a CD player or iPod. It is important to note that the exact recording that the group member requested is played because that particular version may be of significant meaning to the individual. The therapist may also suggest that the group focus on the group member who brought in the song as they listen to the recording. After the group listens to it one time, the therapist hands out the lyrics to the song and encourages the group to underline words or lines that they feel remind them of the one group member as the listen for a second time. Once this is complete, the group analyzes the lyrics and music and discusses why they feel it reminds them of the group member. The group member who brought in the song also shares his or her feelings and states its significant meaning to them. From this vantage point, the group then has the opportunity to create the song communally. The member who brought in the song is empowered to orchestrate how the song should sound, assigning musical roles to each member. This experience can be useful in terms of building trust and getting to know group members in a more meaningful way. The exploration of feelings can also bring emphasis to universal themes, which may invite members to share more about themselves and move toward deeper self-expression.

The identification and expression of feelings, particularly as it pertains to the stage of acceptance to the diagnosis, is an important goal that is addressed within a group setting. Do the group members feel extreme anger? Do they feel hopeless? Are they at a point of acceptance? These questions can be explored through music in a variety of ways. Literature has shown that improvisation may be one of the most useful ways to evoke emotions that are usually difficult to express.[26]

Through improvisation, group members may release their physical and emotional pain while receiving the support and validation that they desire. For a group session, each group member may begin with a verbal "check-in." During this time, they may share feelings that are on the surface, such as how their week has been or any physical pain they may be feeling. After some time, the music therapist guides the group into an improvisation based on their current energy state and emotions. As the music develops, changes in the musical qualities such as texture, dynamics, form, rhythm and harmony may be a deeper expression of the emotions that the patients are experiencing. This is also a time when group roles become more apparent and group cohesion develops. Is one group member imitating another? Is one member playing a different rhythm than the group? There are many different factors that may arise during this time, which can affect the group dynamics. When the musical improvisation is complete, the group is then able to process their feelings further. Some group members might share how they felt in the music and any emotions that came forth. These feelings can either be negative or positive, and conflicts and resolutions may be explored as well. In turn, a full circle of communication is able to flourish and members may share their emotions while relating to each other in a more meaningful way.[27]

Songwriting and lyric substitution may also address self-expression while increasing self-esteem and decreasing feelings of isolation. Group songwriting provides a way for patients to put their ideas into aesthetic form and reflect on their experiences. Sharing in this way also opens doors for validation and support as relationships continue to develop and grow.[28] This process may also enable the group to move toward the goal of altruism.[23] Related themes and experiences may arise from this experience, which may improve individual self-esteem as well as acceptance for each other. Themes such as physical pain, medication use, substance abuse, trust, love and isolation are just a few topics that can be a focus in a song. Through songwriting and lyric substitution, there can be a movement from illness to an aesthetic creation that holds beauty and meaning.[28]

Providing relaxation and release is an important goal within a group as well. Many symptoms of depression and other psychological factors may overlap with symptoms of the HIV infection and HIV medication side effects,[28] therefore the emotional and physical pain that occurs with this illness cannot be separated. Interventions such as drumming have shown to boost immune responses and influence the psychological processes.[29] When group members collectively release through drumming, a sense of wellbeing as well as altered states of consciousness become possible. Other interventions such as guided music meditation and visualization may also bring the group to a collective altered state while retrieving emotions that can be connected to physical pain.

Although the group process takes time and full awareness and dedication from everyone involved, music therapy techniques can be utilized to achieve group goals and develop a sense of safety within the space. Music may also act as an organic transition from themes, conflicts and changes within the group as members are given opportunities to express themselves creatively, which may in turn create an environment of unconditional participation, engagement, and safety.

Group Vignette
Miranda, 51, was one of the members who attended music therapy consistently. She reported HIV transmission from a blood transfusion during a C-section with one of her four children about twenty-five years ago. Miranda has a history of psychiatric diagnosis and is currently on Perphenazine for schizophrenia and Gabapention for neuropathic nerve disruption. Although she reported being addicted to cocaine in the early 1980's, she has been sober for thirty years. At the time of her participation in the music therapy group, she was living with her fiancé but reported that she felt "unsure" of this relationship due to her fiancé's occasional drug use. After a few months in the group, she decided to leave her fiancé and move into a shelter in order to maintain her sobriety and independence. Many of Miranda's conflicts with this decision came up for her within music improvisations and song choices. Due to her sobriety, Miranda graduated from the program and began to attend groups that focused on long-term care.

Another active member in the music therapy group was Lora. She is 53 years old and reports HIV/HCV transmission from risk factors such as substance abuse and heterosexual transmission. Lora has been sober since the early 1990's and due to the fact that she was on methadone, she remained in the music therapy group. During the group, Lora would often talk about her twenty year-old son, reporting that he was her "main priority". She frequently spoke about how she wanted to "protect him" and keep him "safe." Much of the work for Lora centered on the exploration of the meaning of "safety" in her life through verbal and music processing. Disclosure was also important to Lora as she did not share her HIV status to many people in her life and felt that the group was a way for her to receive the support she desired.

Like Lora, Sarah was another group member on methadone due to her history with substance abuse. She is 50 years old and reported transmission through heterosexual contact and/or IV drug use. Since 2009, Sarah has been heroin and cocaine free and reports a history of marijuana use as well. The issue of disclosure was an important commonality between all women, as Sarah's close family members and teenage son were unaware of her HIV status. She often reported the group as her "second family" and a place where she felt "safe" to express herself.

Jessica, 48, reported HIV transmission through heterosexual intercourse in the 1980's. Due to her past employment as a nurse, Jessica frequently expressed her frustration about knowing "too much" about what the infection was doing to her body. Over the course of her treatment, she developed a resistance to multiple medications, which led to depression and anxiety. Her disappointments and anger were often addressed within the music therapy group.

Although each woman had their own story to tell and different life experiences, there were similar themes that surfaced during our work. Relationships and disclosure seemed to be a common issue that the women could all relate to. They also shared experiences with medications and the difficulty about living with HIV in today's society. The physical side effects from the HIV infection and medications such as fatigue, breathing difficulty and body aches were also discussed and explored through the music.

The establishment of trust was critical to the space that would allow for sharing of their experiences with diagnosis, treatment, coping, and substance abuse. The initial goals during the beginning stages were the establishment of trust and development of self-expression. It was initially clear that there was much hesitation to share in both a verbal and musical manner. After presenting the concept of non-verbal expression through improvisation, most of the women did not participate and shared little information about their lives. They would usually pick up an instrument for a few seconds and then put it down before talking about what they did over the weekend or how the weather was looking for the week. The tendency toward surface dialogue was a normal reaction in terms of the group's process. My respect of the group's pace and each member's boundaries allowed the progression toward more meaningful expression to occur gradually.

Establishing trust and gaining insight on each individual occurred through an intervention focused on their favorite songs. This query seemed to break the ice and allow the women to share something about themselves and their outside world. Through Song Sensitation[24] and lyric analysis, the group members began to explore and discuss each other's songs. An example of this was through Lora's favorite song, "Ben" by Michael Jackson. As the women listened to "Ben", they were encouraged to think about Lora and why this song might be meaningful to her. After listening and creating the song together, each woman shared their feelings in relation to Lora and Lora shared why this song was significant to her. Themes about love and taking care of others arose through this process and Lora began to talk about how "Ben" reminded her of her son. She expressed with deep emotion that she wants to "protect him" and that no matter where he goes in life, Lora will always be there for him. This was a chance for the women to share common feelings about children and loved ones in their lives. Further discussion on the meaning of feeling "protected" and why this was so important to them evolved.

As each woman shared her favorite song and the meaning behind it, introducing other techniques such as mandala drawing became indicated as a means to expanding the possibilities for deepened process. Following the group's sequence of listening to a song and creating it live, the members were encouraged to draw what they were feeling in the moment. Through this experience, the women began to share more about their lives in terms of their frustrations and anxieties.

Listening and playing the song "All You Need is Love" by The Beatles, allowed Jessica access to her feeling of being "alone", and the anxiety it caused. After creating a drawing that fused bright colors with dark colors, she reported feeling hopeless at times and didn't know how to see past her pain. Some group members such as Miranda and Sarah shared similar feelings as they supported and validated Jessica's expression. As the group continued to talk about this feeling, they began to discover more similar themes between themselves, and one group member pointed out that there was "hope" in this process because life "has good moments too." At the end of the session, Jessica reported feeling more "stable" in terms of her emotions and expressed appreciation to the group for their support. The drawings from the women's favorite songs were eventually made into a quilt that was featured in the Arts Festival that spring. This was an opportunity for the women to be acknowledged and celebrated.

As the process evolved and the women began to share more about their lives, improvisation became a norm that occurred at the beginning of every session. After expressing themselves during a verbal check-in, there would follow a transition into a music improvisation that reflected the energy of the group members. Although the beginning of this process was met with resistance and hesitation, the women slowly became more expressive and courageous in their musical development. This was evident in their interaction with each other and willingness to try new things. During this time, the women also began to speak about the side effects from HIV and the HIV related medication. Lora and Jessica would frequently talk about their difficulty in breathing and the aches and pains in their bodies. This would be met with extreme frustration and feelings of loss of control. At times like this, music would be used for relaxation and/or release. Depending on the extent of their pain or fatigue, live music would be rendered to support meditation or release through active drumming. Such intervention would usually begin with a deep relaxation followed by an improvisation with a guided meditation. When the meditation ended, the members would create music as a group that reflected the experience. During times like this, many members reported feeling as though they were "floating" or they "left the room." Miranda especially enjoyed this experience and stated that she could "stay there for hours."

Drumming circles within the group proved to be another way for the women to release their physical and emotional pain. At times, the dynamics and pulsation of the drums from each member created a heightened group energy that captured their emotions and brought the group to a natural, free flow. Through this process, the concept of "unloading" came up quite often and many of the women expressed how it felt to be able to do this within the group. The women were encouraged to visualize a suitcase that they could unpack each week. Miranda spoke about how this concept made a profound difference in her life: "The music takes a weight off [of me]. I use to carry a load of weight [but] I learned how to dump it. Once I dump it, it stays here and I can go on."

Emotional release also came in the form of lyric substitution. Once trust in the space and the therapist was established, the women were encouraged to incorporate their words into a popular Eminem song titled, "I'm Not Afraid." The following excerpt was created by Sarah:

> *"I'm not ashamed to tell everyone of my past.*
> *Come with me.*
> *Walk together through good or bad.*
> *We stand together."*

This seemed to be one of many pivotal points in the group's process, as the women not only began to create their own words, but they began to sing them as well. After each group member created their lyrics, the group would participate in a vocal call and response in order to validate and acknowledge the words and feeling of each person.

In late March of 2012, the previously mentioned program changes were instituted, simultaneous to some group members graduating to groups that focused on long-term goal care. Perhaps the most significant change to the group was the extending of participation to men. Considering the psychosocial history of some of the women and the sixteen-year history of the group itself, the changes elicited feelings of frustration, loss, and for some the reactivation of themes of betrayal and abandonment. Lora expressed that she felt "uncomfortable" expressing her feelings in front of men because "they aren't as sensitive as women." Other members felt that this would change the atmosphere of the group and would prohibit members from attending. As time elapsed, fewer core group members attended each week and the frequency of attendance in those remaining also decreased.

Lora continued to attend group however, and appeared to extract meaning from the sessions even when she was the only one in attendance.

This would be charted as an individual session and we would focus on goals and objectives that pertained to her specifically. This individual time with Lora, allowed for rich process that focused on her relationships, pain from HIV medication side effects, and her feelings of isolation. She spoke about the group quite often and expressed her desire to see some of the other members with whom she had bonded. This was also a time when Lora began to express herself more in the music. An example of this was through a song she wrote titled, "Laid Back." In the song she spoke about taking time to settle and relax. The lyrics are:

> *"Get your thoughts together; this is the way life is.*
> *You will find it a lot easier.*
> *Get your thoughts together, life ain't so bad.*
> *You will survive."*

When she began this process, she stated that she had some doubts in herself because she didn't think she could write. Through discussion and improvisation, the song was slowly created, which gave her a sense of ownership for something that was meaningful to her.

Although the changes within the group presented some challenges, the overall process illustrates the importance of support and community with this diagnosis. The music acted as a stimulus for awareness, insight into themes, and the learning of new coping skills.[27] The trust that was built enabled the women to experiment within the music and share intimate details about their lives. As many of the women stated, the group acted as a second family where they felt free to express their anxieties in a safe space that was free from judgment and built from trust and understanding.

Inpatient Music Therapy with HIV/AIDS

Individual casework occurring on an inpatient unit may involve assessment and treatment of not only HIV related symptoms, but a host of co-morbidities that develop when immune functioning is compromised. HIV/AIDS may exist simultaneously with various types of cancer as well as acute and chronic conditions, such as renal disease, respiratory difficulty, gastro-intestinal bowel irritation, and stress-related difficulties with sleep,[30,31] all of which can be exacerbated during hospitalization.

Music therapy as an integrative intervention with both pediatric and adult populations can function well in the treatment of pain,[22,32-34] by offering relaxation focused interventions that assist with release of stress and anxiety that may be existentially based.[9] Thorough assessment, and the establishment of trust can facilitate a foundation upon which meaningful process can occur. At a juncture when a patient's most harbored fears are activated, such therapeutic presence and ability to bear witness can be dignifying. The provision of rich here-and-now experiences through live music for someone who is living with profound loss, and in some cases Post Traumatic Stress Disorder (PTSD),[6,35] can be transforming of the care and perceptions of the care being rendered. Additionally, music therapy facilitated improvisation, or singing of meaningful music identified as significant by the patient can support important reflection and cathartic release of long-held conflict around living with the diagnosis of HIV/AIDS.[35,36]

Children in particular are faced with a variety of emotional and psychosocial distresses. Due to the fact that diagnosis usually occurs at birth, time of disclosure and education about treatment are delicate subjects that family members and health care providers delineate. Other factors such as loss of a parent or guardian, social stigmas, depression, isolation, physical pain and bullying may affect the child's general well-being. Bedside music therapy provides children with a way to explore issues related to their illness in a safe space while offering the support they need to ensure developmental continuance. Providing choices in a music therapy session, such as which instrument to play or what songs to sing, enables the child to gain the control that they are missing due to their illness.

Children are also able to successfully relate to the treatment and medical environment when they have opportunities to express themselves freely in a positive way.[12] A few examples of music therapy applications that may be used to address the emotional, social and physical states are: songwriting, song choice, singing, analysis and discussion of lyrics, improvisation, and playing of instruments.[26] These techniques can provide children and adults for that matter, with opportunities for expression and reinforcement of coping through increased control of their surroundings. In turn, music therapy facilitates the integration of treatment in both physiological and psycho-emotional domains.

The following case vignettes are culminating of the many themes addressed in this chapter, and provide examples of how music therapy can enter rather late in an individual's trajectory of the disease, and still create meaning and aesthetic sensibility to the experience of living with illness.

Case Vignette: Jayden
Jayden was born in July of 2003 in Senegal. At three years old, he moved to the United States with his biological father who eventually took residency in New York City. In the winter of 2011, when Jayden was nine years old, his mother and younger sister came to the United States to live with Jayden and his father. During this time, Jayden began attending a private school where he excelled academically. In the spring of 2012, Jayden was admitted to the

hospital for complaints of respiratory distress and a high fever. During this admission, Jayden was diagnosed with the AIDS virus. A psychosocial history was taken, which divulged that Jayden's mother was HIV positive and that the infection had been transmitted to Jayden during pregnancy. Jayden's father and younger sister both tested negative. Jayden's mother reported to social work, that Jayden's father was physically abusive to herself and her children, and that he had eventually left their home taking residency in a shelter. Further information about the family was unobtainable due to the mother's reluctance to share information that might result in deportation. During Jayden's hospitalizations, it was unclear as to how much Jayden knew about his diagnosis.

Jayden was first referred to music therapy in April of 2012 by one of the in-patient nurses in order to facilitate expression and manage coping. It was felt that throughout Jayden's inpatient and outpatient care, music therapy sessions could provide a needed forum for emotional support, relaxation, self-expression, and playful respite from the hospital milieu. Additionally I would be able to continuously assess Jayden's understanding of his diagnosis and its impact on his emotional state and capacity to cope. The initial session with Jayden in his hospital room also included both of his parents who were present at the bedside.

During the first improvisation, the dynamics within the family began to arise, which lent a better understanding as to how Jayden was coping in the hospital and in his outside world as well. As Jayden's father identified himself as a musician, he would often take the leadership role during the music sessions and would instruct Jayden in how to play certain instruments. It was noted that Jayden would quickly follow his father and become the supporter in the music. Eventually, as a therapeutic relationship with Jayden and his family developed, I suggested to Jayden's father that it was important that Jayden be able to make choices for himself, especially because his choices were limited within the hospital setting. The valuing of Jayden's voice in the space was also modeled within the music by giving Jayden solos and first choice on musical qualities such as rhythm or dynamics. Over time, these roles within the improvisations altered and Jayden began to take the initiative in the leadership role. His father was also supportive while still being able to express his own emotions in a positive and nurturing way. Although Jayden's mother was encouraged to participate in the music as well, she usually chose not to join the sessions.

During music therapy sessions, Jayden presented as a kind, gentle and soft-spoken young boy. He appeared receptive to music and sometimes moved to a deep meditative state while playing an instrument such as the drum or xylophone. During the initial session, he shared his enjoyment of Michael Jackson's music, and reported his favorite song as "Beat It." As soon as the opening chord of the song was played, his energy changed and he began to express himself in an energetic and emotional manner. As a small drum lay in his lap and he held a mallet in his hand, he would beat on the drum in a powerful swift motion as he sang "beat it!" His voice began to gain power and eagerness as he increased his volume and built anticipation in the music. Although he was often soft spoken, this song provided the opportunity to release his emotions and express his inner voice fully. The significance of the song's lyrics to Jayden's personal experience was compelling to imagine, as the song gained importance during the sessions to the point of becoming an opening ritual.

> *You wanna make it through, better do what can*
> *So beat it, (Beat it) Just Beat it (Beat it) No one wants to be defeated*
> *Showin' how funky strong is your fight*
> *It doesn't' matter who's wrong or right*
> *Just Beat it*

Mutually singing and sharing the song facilitated the building of a trust and important therapeutic bond through which further expression and release could occur.

Jayden was discharged from the hospital in late April, but returned several weeks later where he was admitted to the intensive care unit for thrush, and other viral components. During this hospitalization, familiar and comforting music was used for relaxation. He appeared very weak and fragile as he spoke about the pain he felt in his throat and chest. He was also having difficulty sleeping and eating. Familiar and comforting music was used for relaxation during this time and by modifying the meter and dynamics of his favorite songs he was able to fall asleep and feel more at peace in his environment.

During these final sessions, we also continued to explore his emotions through the use of lyric substitution. Once the thrush was clear, he was able to sing again and become more interactive in the music. By using "The Lazy Song" by Bruno Mars, Jayden incorporated his own lyrics to the familiar tune. In the chorus of "The Lazy Song," the lyrics are: "Today I don't feel like doing anything, I just want to lay in my bed." After exploring the song for some time, and asking Jayden what he didn't want to do, he softly said, "I don't want to go home." He shared this in the safety of the therapeutic relationship that had been established, and understandably when no other family members were in the room. Although he never expressed the reasons for why he didn't want to go home, he resolved some of his feelings within the music as he sang about what he did want to do. This session in particular provided insight into the potential degree of emotional stressors that were impeding his ability to cope optimally.

My last session with Jayden, focused on the use of music as a forum for release and expression. During an improvisation, he released through drumming and sang at certain times as well in spite of increasing respiratory difficulty. He did not sing "Beat It" at this time. Many of his other favorite songs were played, while new songs were also created. Following much-enlivened play, Jayden determined the end of the session, and expressed his needs freely requesting music to which he could fall asleep. Later that evening, Jayden died.

For Jayden, music was a bridge to his inner voice and emotional expression. Although it remained uncertain as to whether he knew about the extent of his diagnosis, he was aware of his surroundings and expressed his emotional and physical pain openly through the music. His gentle nature and enduring sprit were able to shine as he created, explored and expressed.

Case Vignette: Maria
Maria was 57 when she was referred to music therapy from The Department of Palliative Care. Having a thirty year history of living with HIV, Maria been diagnosed with Non-Small Cell Lung Cancer (NSCLC) with metastases to the liver. Music therapy was introduced and following Maria's expressed receptiveness, the initial assessment commenced. Maria reported having been a member of the Women's Group for many years before here condition had worsened to the point of it being "too hard to get there". Her references to the group and her friends she had made while attending were positive. At the time of the assessment, Maria described physical pain that she could not easily discern from her fatigue and her general sense of restlessness. Further process elucidated that Maria was under an excessive amount of emotional duress pertaining to the future of her 10 year-old grandson, Xavier. The child had been in Maria's care since birth when her daughter had relinquished her role as primary caregiver in order to finish her education in a trade school.

Maria spoke proudly about her care of Xavier, enthusiastically sharing that he would often hide her cigarettes from her in an effort to protect her from harm. When asked about Xavier's understanding of her current situation, Maria reported that he "knows about the HIV, but not the cancer… he'd be so upset if he knew I had lung cancer". She also expressed concern that he might be sensing something is wrong, because he had recently been acting out and "getting in trouble at school". Expressing this truth caused Maria to emote and further express that she didn't know if he could understand how sick she was. I inquired if Maria would like support in helping Xavier understand the basic facts of her illness in the spirit of inclusion. I further explained that such effort might restore authentic sharing between them.

My offering to create a customized, psychoedcational text, in storybook format (beginning, middle, end), was aimed at providing Xavier a tangible and familiar form by which to gain mastery at a complicated and confusing time. Developmentally appropriate language presented in text form was interwoven with opportunities for creative expression such as drawing, coloring, and stickers, to invite both verbal and nonverbal process. Xavier's choice to read through the book at his own pace, and to do this alone or with family, provided him a unique form of empowerment. Ultimately, I felt that facilitating Xavier's organization of the facts surrounding Maria's illness and treatment was a first step in truly supporting Maria.

On another level, the creation and introduction of the book for the purpose of Xavier's emotional support provided an impetus for his mother's reconciliation with Maria if it was desired. Maria had stated at various times how much she would enjoy a reunion with her daughter, if only for Xavier's sake. Eventually Xavier's mother did participate in a music therapy session in which she, Maria and I read through the book and discussed how Xavier would be best served. Reconciling past differences in the service of Xavier's well being provided the common ground for acceptance and forgiveness as it pertained to their personal history of conflict. In general, this preliminary work seemed to allow Maria a sense of peace across various aspects of the family dynamics to which she had been investing much energy to manage. Whether or not the past history of conflict between Maria and her daughter was completely resolved is unknown, but I do believe the course of Maria's coping with her illness was positively marked by the renewed hope for family unity.

Once a therapeutic alliance was forged with Maria to address these concerns, she was more emotionally available to attend to her own experience with physical pain and discomfort. She seemed to reach a certain acceptance that she was not going to get better, and this shift allowed her to focus on optimizing her experience of life. Music supported breath work was introduced to assist Maria with a form of release that was within her control to achieve. Visualization was introduced as well and it was discovered that nature themes, in particular the beach and seascape, were significant to her. One particular vision Maria would repeatedly conjure was her footsteps in the sand that would be washed away by gentle waves as she strolled into a sunset. The image seemed metaphoric to Maria's wish to leave her grandson and friends in a place of beauty, with only warm memories of her after she was gone.

Music Therapy and HIV/AIDS Related Pain

Music therapy remained present in Maria's care through several transitions from hospital to home, and eventually to the hospice unit where she died five months later. The sessions deepened throughout Maria's care, with interludes of music focusing not on internal resourcing through visualization, but on externalizing her love of family and people with a heightened sense of altruistic focus. These sessions seemed to call her vividly into the life she was immanently leaving, as she would request to sing encores of the 1969 pop hit by Jackie De Shannon, "Put a Little Love in Your Heart".

"Put A Little Love In Your Heart"
(Jackie DeShannon, Jimmy Holiday and Randy Myers)

Think of your fellow man lend him a helping hand
Put a little love in your heart
You see it's getting oh please don't hesitate
Put a little love in your heart
And the world will be a better place (2x)
For you and me You just wait and see
Another day goes by, still the children cry
Put a little love in your heart
If you want the world to know, we won't let hatred grow
Put a little love in your heart
And the world will be a better place (2x)
For you and me you just wait and see
Take a good look around and if you're looking down
Put a little love in your heart
I hope when you decide, kindness will be your guide
Put a little love in your heart
And the world will be a better place (2x)
For you and me just wait and see

Case Vignette: Robert
Robert was 47 when he was referred to music therapy. The discussion of his case during interdisciplinary rounds identified him as a "gentle" man, somewhat isolated, and living with AIDS. The virus was presenting as "classically as the first misunderstood cases in the early 1980s" (Family Medicine Interdisciplinary Rounds, January 13, 2009). Having been stable and well-managed with medication since testing positive for HIV twelve years earlier, Robert was currently being hospitalized frequently for reasons ranging from respiratory distress to severe dysphagia (difficulty swallow-

ing). One medical resident stated it simply, "Robert's body is steadily failing him, and all we can really do is keep him comfortable."

The initial session with Robert focused on bearing witness to his narrative of the sequence of events that had led to his current hospitalization. He spoke with a level of reserve, which seemed to reflect a general lack of trust in others. He appeared stoic in his denial of any pain or discomfort "at the moment", and reported having a good support system of "many friends". His parents and siblings were also supportive, but lived out of state. He was an artist, enjoying a lengthy design career in the theater, and loved "traveling and good food". He had traveled to Spain recently, and was hoping to return, and was also looking forward to getting back to his work, as he was "tired of being in and out of the hospital".

Following Robert's discourse, music therapy was explained as a service for which he had been referred, and that if he was receptive, the therapy could offer various possibilities that might make sense to him in his care. Music therapy in tension release, and for visualization with breath work were explained as a few such possibilities. His response was noncommittal as he stated that he didn't "really need anything, and didn't want to play anything himself", but "listening to music would be okay". He invited the use of guitar because the sound reminded him of Spain, but added that he did not like singing. He offered no qualification for this latter point, but it seemed possible that the use of voice in singing was perhaps too intimate for an initial session.

In our first session, Robert was invited to close his eyes (if he were so inclined), and to focus on deep, steady breathing, which was supported on the guitar. An improvisation over a Spanish chord progression was rendered for approximately fifteen minutes, during which a visiting friend entered the room. Robert invited him in, and made an introduction of the therapist, "he's going to be playing music for me while I'm here". The pride with which he had introduced the music therapy was belied by his earlier affect. Inviting his friend to contribute to the music by playing the Remo ocean drum was an opportunity to extend the session and to impart more understanding of the myriad of possibilities with which music therapy could enhance Robert's care. His friend accepted the invitation and another improvisation developed. At the session's conclusion, Robert expressed his gratitude, stating, "I really enjoyed this…it reminded me of this place I ate at in Barcelona". In retrospect, Robert had attended to the music as if he actually were attending a concert; hands clasped and poised on his lap in enjoyment, and facially displaying calm appreciation for the space that was being defined by the music.

The sessions that ensued from this first meeting became more layered in sound as various other instruments were introduced to him. He enjoyed the Native American flute, as well as an Asian pipe chime, and Mediterranean lyre, which had also been introduced in the course of several sessions. Over time it became clear that the improvisations were providing Robert with much needed interludes of recluse from the aural cacophony of the busy unit upon which he was residing. During our sessions, Robert would experience imagery that he felt was spiritually healing, and it became very clear that his ability to connect to his failing body in this context offered him a sense of purposeful control. It was easy to understand the depth of Robert's connection to our sessions, as they offered him a familiar context of aesthetic structure and sensibility. This was a man whose professional and personal life had been richly immersed in the creation and contemplation of beauty respectively. His endurance, more and more frequently, of extended bouts with the sterility of a hospital environment, had greatly impacted his self-esteem, as well as his emotional and psychological outlook.

Amidst the musical aspects of the therapeutic relationship, trust was also growing as Robert began to more comfortably share his fears and greatest sources of stress. During one particular session, the focus shifted from the provision of music to advocacy on his behalf to have his possessions retrieved from his prior residence. This was a pivotal shift in his perception of the therapeutic relationship that had evolved, and he became even more receptive to the role of music therapy as a helping profession. A minor task in and of itself was monumental to Robert, as he had been ineffective at making such arrangements himself.

At another juncture in his care, he was being advised to receive a gastric feeding tube, because his increasing dysphagia was hindering his ability to take in adequate nutrition. Robert's demeanor changed dramatically and he shared that the experience of eating and drinking was essential to his definition of life, and that he would fight the placement of a tube. His effective self-advocacy allowed him to stave off this intervention, and eventually he regained his strength to the degree of being able to tolerate solids again. He spoke proudly of his success three weeks before he died.

Two and a half months into the work with Robert marked the beginning of his rapid decline. The improvisations had become more richly layered with the acoustic instruments underscored with synthesizer string settings and slow electronic grooves that Robert would select from a bank of sounds presented to him. His music journeying and imagery during sessions was providing him with interludes of deep relaxation marked frequently by semi-incoherent verbalizations from his dreamlike states. He would emerge from these sessions with statements such as: "The music was so beautiful, I felt like I was flying with angels", and "I saw such beauty when I heard the flute".

The last day that Robert was lucid was perhaps the most horrific for him. He had gone into respiratory distress early in the morning, and began to hemorrhage from various orifices on his head and body. To support Robert's request for "anything to help me deal with this", the therapist intermittently throughout the day provided music that had over the months become *Robert's* music. He had also been placed on oxygen, which helped during his anxiety attacks that were occurring with increased frequency. One of Robert's friends was present during these hours, holding his hand, while taking occasional leave to make telephone calls to other friends upon Robert's request. Robert would look up from time to time, and express gratitude for the "beautiful music". Through his fear, Robert continued to ask his caregivers when they would enter the room, how they were doing, and if they were okay? He never stopped thanking them for their care.

Robert lost consciousness by late afternoon, and was transferred to the medical intensive care unit (MICU). There he was placed on support, for several weeks before being moved to a hospice unit where he died early one morning. During these final weeks, music therapy was provided in the form of a 'soundbath', an intervention so named as such by this therapist because the clinical intention was to bathe the patient in improvised music ensuing from the therapists synthesis of environmental stimuli, the patient's clinical presentation, the patient's expressed preferences when lucid, and the aesthetic sense of the therapist himself. Such intervention offered Robert in his unconscious state, not only comfort, but a point of reference to the here-and-now. Additionally, music therapy sessions offered a rich context of support to the many friends who took turns holding vigil at his bedside. It is not certain that he heard the music that was being created for him, but I believed that as long as he was breathing, he deserved to receive beauty from the music that had ensued from his aesthetic choices over the last several months.

Conclusion

The course of HIV/AIDS treatment has evolved to be not so unlike that of other chronic conditions in terms of both psychosocial and psychoemotional goals. The success of symptom management resulting in better prognosis for those living with the virus has led to greater emphasis on quality of life for these individuals. A palliative approach to care brings focus to identifying strengths, resilience, and both internal and external resources for coping with the myriad of pain responses.

Music therapy as a modality that functions in the treatment of both physical and emotional symptoms stands apart from other psychoemotional interventions because of its unique capacity to address patient needs cross-culturally and at both verbal and nonverbal levels. These qualities engendered in the case vignettes, play ephemera to a greater overriding theme of perseverance of the human spirit. Music therapy provides the context for this experience, but it is the therapist's role in supporting the strength and vitality of each patient that reflects the philosophy of the Louis & Lucille Armstrong Music Therapy Program, where live music actively ensuing from the therapeutic relationship is that phenomenon that ultimately calls one into life.

References

1. Sande MA, Volberding P. The Medical Management of AIDS. 6th ed. Philadelphia, PA: W.B. Saunders Company; 1996.
2. Suris JC, Michaud PA, Akre C, Sawyer SM. Health risk behaviors in adolescents with chronic conditions. Pediatrics. Nov 2008;122(5):e1113-1118.
3. CDC. HIV among Youth. 2012. http://www.cdc.gov/hiv/youth/. Accessed 5/18/2012.
4. Portenoy RK. Contemporary Diagnosis and Management of Pain in Oncologic and AIDS Patients. 3rd ed. Newtown, PA: Handbooks in Health Care Co.; 2001.
5. HIV/AIDS: Treatment and Drugs. 2012; http://mayoclinic.com. Accessed 5/18.2012
6. Barskova T, Oesterreich R. Post-traumatic growth in people living with a serious medical condition and its relations to physical and mental health: a systematic review. Disability and rehabilitation. 2009;31(21):1709-1733.
7. Chicago ALCo. HIV and Confidentiality. 2009:1-16. Accessed 7/9/2012.
8. Health NYSDo. New York State Confidentiality Law and HIV: Questions and Answers. 2012; http://www.health.ny.gov/diseases/aids/facts/helpful resources/confidentiality law.htm. Accessed 7/9, 2012.
9. Sumpter J, Ryan C, Homes-Smith S. HIV/AIDS. Mind body and soul. Nursing times. Jun 9-15 1993;89(23):42-45.
10. Center TPK. The Peter Kruger Center/ AIDS Services. In: Center BIM, ed. New York, NY: Peter Kruger Center; 1987.
11. Davey M, Duncan T, Foster JM, Milton K. Keeping the family in focus at an HIV/AIDS pediatric clinic. Families, Systems, & Health. 2008;26(3):350-355.
12. Avers L, Mather A, Kamat D. Music therapy in pediatrics. Clinical pediatrics. 2007;46:575-579.

13. Turry A. The use of clinical improvisation to alleviate procedural distress in young children. In: Loewy JV, ed. Music therapy and pediatric pain. Cherry Hill, NJ: Jeffrey Books; 1997:89-96.
14. Whitehead-Pleaux AM, Zebrowski N, Baryza M, Sheridan R. Exploring the effects of music on pediatric pain: Phase 1. Journal of music therapy. 2007;3:217-241.
15. Loewy JV, MacGregor B, Richards K, Rodriguez J. Music therapy pediatric pain management: Assessing and attending to the sounds of hurt, fear, and anxiety. In: Loewy JV, ed. Music therapy and pediatric pain. Cherry Hill, NJ: Jeffrey Books; 1997:45-56.
16. Boxill EH. Music therapy for the developmentally disabled. Bethesda, MD: Aspen System Corporation; 1985.
17. Loewy J, Hallan C, Friedman E, Martinez C. Sleep/sedation in children undergoing EEG testing: A comparison of chloral hydrate and music therapy. Journal of PeriAnesthesia Nursing. 2005;20(5):323-331.
18. Loewy J, Stewart K. The use of lullabies as a transient motif in ending life. In: Dileo C, Loewy JV, eds. Music Therapy at the End of Life. Cherry Hill, NJ: Jeffrey Books; 2004.
19. Crowe B. Music and soul making: Toward a new theory of music therapy. Lanham, MD: Scarecrow Press; 2004.
20. Boneh G, Jaganath D. Performance as a component of HIV/AIDS education: Process and Collaboration for Empowerment and Discussion. American journal of public health. Mar 2011;101(3):455-464.
21. Stephens T, Braithwaite LR, Taylor ES. Model for using hip-hop music for small group HIV/AIDS prevention counseling with African American adolescents and young adults. Patient education and counseling. 1998;35:127-137.
22. Farber WE. Existentially informed HIV-related psychotherapy. Psychotherapy:Theory, Research, Practice, Training. 2009;46(3):336-349.
23. Yalom I. The Theory and Practice of Group Psychotherapy. New York, NY: Basic Books; 2005.
24. Loewy JV. Caring for the Caregiver: The Use of Music and Music Therapy in Grief and Trauma. Silver Spring, MD: AMTA; 2002.
25. Loewy JV. Song sensitation: How fragile we are. In: Loewy JV, Hara-Frisch A, eds. Caring for the caregiver: The use of music and music therapy in grief and trauma. Silver Spring, MD: Aerican Music Therapy Association; 2002.
26. Knapp C, Madden V, Wamg H, Curtis C, Sloyer P, Shenkman E. Music therapy in an integrated pediatric palliative care program.

American Journal of Hospice & Palliative Medicine. 2009;26(6):449-455.

27. Borczon R. Music therapy: Group vignettes. Gilsum, NH.: Barcelona Publishers; 1997.
28. Cordobes T. Group songwriting as a method for developing group cohesion for HIV-seropositive adult patients with depression. Journal of music therapy. 1997;1:46-67.
29. Bittman BB, Berk SL, Felton LD, et al. Composite effects of group drumming music therapy on modulation of neuroendicrine-immune parameters in normal subjects. Alternative Therapies. 2001;7(1):38-48.
30. Vosvick M, Gore-Felton C, Ashton E, et al. Sleep disturbances among HIV-positive adults: the role of pain, stress, and social support. Journal of psychosomatic research. Nov 2004;57(5):459-463.
31. Vosvick M, Koopman C, Gore-Felton C, Thoresen C, Krumboltz J, Spiegel D. Relationship of functional quality of life to strategies for coping with the stress of living with HIV/AIDS. Psychosomatics. Jan-Feb 2003;44(1):51-58.
32. Jam S, Imani AH, Foroughi M, SeyedAlinaghi S, Koochak HE, Mohraz M. The effects of mindfulness-based stress reduction (MBSR) program in Iranian HIV/AIDS patients: a pilot study. Acta medica Iranica. Mar-Apr 2010;48(2):101-106.
33. Niazi AK, Niazi SK. Mindfulness-based stress reduction: a non-pharmacological approach for chronic illnesses. North American journal of medical sciences. Jan 2011;3(1):20-23.
34. Rokach A. Terminal illness and coping with loneliness. The Journal of psychology. May 2000;134(3):283-296.
35. Smith MY, Egert J, Winkel G, Jacobson J. The impact of PTSD on pain experience in persons with HIV/AIDS. Pain. Jul 2002;98(1-2):9-17.
36. Rotheram-Borus MJ. Variations in perceived pain associated with emotional distress and social identity in AIDS. AIDS patient care and STDs. Dec 2000;14(12):659-665.

CHAPTER 22

Music-Mediated Strategies for the Integrative Management of Pain in End of Life Care

Robert E. Krout EdD, MT-BC

*From a hurt comes a healing, from an end comes a start
From the dark comes revealing, a growing light in our hearts,
thanks to you*
Song lyrics from "Thanks to You" by Robert E. Krout

Introduction

Pain as a care plan problem is prevalent among patients with cancer and other serious medical conditions.[1] This may be especially true with patients in end of life care, where pain is a common concern and symptom.[2] With these patients, pain is also often associated with insufficient prescribing of targeted medical treatments.[3] In addition, a major challenge for the health care professional is that patients with cancer and other serious illnesses often report more than one painful condition simultaneously.[4] As such, non-medical interventions such as music therapy may also be helpful in pain management.[5] In addition, music therapy may help address the patient's pain in an integrated manner. This is because music therapy as used in end-of-life care is designed to improve the patient's overall quality of life. This includes helping to relieve physical symptoms such as pain, while also addressing the patient's psychological, social, and spiritual needs.[6]

The focus of this chapter is the concept and practice of integrative music therapy in pain management and remediation with patients at the end of life. This integrative approach as I describe it brings together four aspects and dimensions – an integrated treatment team, integrated facets and domains of patient pain, treating the patient in the integrated psychosocial context of their family and loved ones, and incorporating an integrated music therapy treatment approach. These four aspects will first be discussed, followed by five brief case examples, which illustrate various music-mediated strategies for the integrative management of pain in end of life care. A summary and discussion concludes the chapter.

Music and Medicine: Integrative Models in the Treatment of Pain

The Integrated Treatment Team Approach

In end of life care, an integrated team approach allows the music therapist to complement other traditional medical and psycho-social-spiritual treatment modalities, and also to address various facets and factors, which may contribute to the reduction and palliation of the patient's perceived pain. In addition to physicians, nurses, nursing aides, pharmacists, and more traditional therapies, other treatment team disciplines may include various adjunctive therapies, dietary and nutrition specialists, spiritual support providers, and others.

The terms interdisciplinary, multidisciplinary, and transdisciplinary are often used to describe such a treatment team. Another concept, that of a synerdisciplinary team approach refers to music therapists embedded in the treatment team and working directly alongside team members in patient/family care.[7] This takes advantage of not only the various modalities within the team, but of the dynamic ways in which clinicians from those modalities can work together with the patient in real time. Thus, in complementing and enhancing medical techniques, the music therapist works as a vital member of an integrated treatment team to meet the pain-related needs of the patient.

Integrated Facets and Domains of Patient Pain

The second integrative dimension is the multifaceted nature of pain. Pain has many components,[8] and music therapy can address a variety of pain sources and symptoms.[9] Many physiological factors may influence a patient's pain response, including inflammation, muscle guarding, exacerbation due to stress, neural sensitization, and altered levels of neurotransmitters.[8] In addition, social, emotional, spiritual, and other stressors can exacerbate physiological stressors.[5] Music may provide a comforting presence, reduce anxiety, and facilitate relaxation and release. The interactions between a patient and family/friends at the end of life can also exacerbate patient pain when discord in present – e.g. a family/caregiver's desire for the needed amount of pain medicine in disagreement with a patient's desired level of pain control. Long-standing family discord (e.g. divorce &/or separation, step-families, "black sheep" of the family, etc.) can overflow when the patient/family relations are stressed due to the terminal illness/prognosis. Music therapy experiences can help ameliorate that discord and redirect energy towards providing psychosocial release and comfort for the patient.[5]

Music Meditated Strategies for Pain in End of Life Care

Treating the Patient in the Psychosocial Context of their Family and Loved Ones

The third integrative dimension is meeting the needs of the patient's family and loved ones (in addition to those of the patient) at the time of a music therapy visit and during a music therapy session. For example, when the psychosocial and spiritual needs of the family are addressed, the patient and family can interact in a more meaningful manner. This may continue even as the patient, in the case of hospice care, declines and ultimately dies. During this difficult time, family members often are faced with the challenge of expressing their feelings to the patient and to each other. In addition, the patient may not able to overtly communicate with or respond to family members due to their advanced disease process or the sedating effects of medications. In this case, family members may feel frustrated when the patient may not be able to look at or speak with them, or even to hold or squeeze their hands. The patient's physical appearance may also be disturbing to the family, as the patient may have noticeably deteriorated since a previous visit. In addition, sounds of congested breathing, apnea, or observed restlessness or agitation may he troubling to the family.

The active expression of feelings of grief and anguish by loved ones during this difficult time may be considered to be both normal and healthy.[10] For example, when family members visit a patient, the music therapist has a unique opportunity to engage them and create a meaningful experience for them with the patient. As each patient's and family's situation is unique, the music therapist can provide individualized interventions based on these needs at the time of the session. Music therapy may involve passive or active participation by the family.[5] As one example, the selecting, singing, or listening to familiar or favorite songs of the patient and family may stimulate discussion relating to life memories, reminiscence, and life review. Family members may request a specific song, listen to or sing with the therapist, and then reflect on the significance of that song to them and the patient. The music may elicit an emotional response that can then allow for the sharing of feelings and emotions. These feelings can then be validated, normalized, and explored by the therapist. For families with a strong religious base, the resourcing of hymns or other sacred songs may create an environment in which the sharing of feelings and faith may result in increased spiritual strength for both the patient and caregiver.

An Integrated Music Therapy Treatment Approach

The fourth dimension is an integrated music therapy approach. Using an integrated treatment model allows the music therapist to incorporate various documented and evidence based-procedures in an approach best suited to the changing needs of the patient during each session. The music used during a session can include live or recorded original, folk, contemporary or popular, jazz, classical, spiritual, and many other styles. The music can also function in a number of ways during the therapeutic process. The first consideration is maintaining the physical comfort of the patient. In addition to facilitating pain control, it can help provide physical and emotional comfort and assist in relaxation, as well as reduce anxiety. By facilitating the physical comfort and relaxation of the patient, perceived pain may be reduced.[11-14] The clinician may in part take advantage of the unique ways in which music is processed by, and in turn may positively affect the central and peripheral nervous systems, including engagement of the parasympathetic nervous system to help reduce stress and pain perception.

Music may also positively affect the endocrine system via efferent pathways and circuits. At a basic level, it is difficult for the brain and central nervous system (CNS) to simultaneously attend to multiple stimuli from the peripheral nervous system (PNS). In addition, proposed mechanisms such as the Gate Control Theory of Pain Perception, one stimulus such as music moving from the PNS to the CNS may block another stimulus such as peripheral pain.[15] Also important in lowering pain perceptions are limbic/emotional responses to music.[16] Cortical and cognitive responses to music can include music elicited fantasy, thought, and imagery. In addition, there may be a thalamic response in which musical rhythms entrain rhythmic movements within the body.[17]

The music therapist may make also use of the Iso-Moodic principle and the process of entrainment.[18,19] Entrainment is the synchronizing of internal rhythms to external stimuli, often through the manipulation of rhythm and tempo.[20] The therapist may first match structural elements (tempo, rhythm, melody, harmony, texture, etc.) of the music to existing patient levels of patient activity, mood, or physiology (breath/pulse/etc.). The music can then be altered to guide these levels/processes in desired directions. This may result in reduced pulse rate, respiration, and other measures, which may help the patient reduce their level of perceived pain. The music therapist may incorporate various techniques such as song choice, active or passive listening, lyric discussion and analysis, instrument playing and improvisation, and songwriting to address and help reduce psychosocial stress and distress within the family unit.[21] This may in turn allow the patient to experience more comfort and less pain.

Following are five brief case examples, which illustrate some of the above concepts. Pseudonyms have been used for all patients, and informed consent was obtained by the patient or family members.

Music Meditated Strategies for Pain in End of Life Care

Clinical Work

The Case of Mr. S
The first case I would like to describe is that of Mr. S.[22] Mr. S was a 49 year-old man with a slow growing and only recently diagnosed brain tumor. Surgery and radiation therapy were only partially successful in removing/shrinking the tumor, and he was referred for hospice services. Mr. S was placed in a nursing facility, where he remained for four months until he died. Because of the slow growing glioblastoma, Mr. S had gradually evidenced negative personality changes in the years leading up to his diagnosis. As such, he was divorced and estranged from his wife. There had been no children, and his ex-wife never did respond to requests from him to reconcile. Mr. S attempted to maintain his independence and sense of control in the nursing home, which became more and more difficult for him. The hospice social worker initiated a referral for music therapy services to address issues of emotional pain, anxiety, anticipatory mourning, and spiritual distress. I initially used song choice and lyric analysis with Mr. S to begin to explore issues important to him and to provide comfort. Mr. S enjoyed hymns, and requested specific selections that we would sing together and then discuss. He shared that he wished he could be reconciled with his ex-wife, with whom he used to go to church, and self-identified this as a source of emotional pain for him. He had attended church only sporadically since his divorce.

As Mr. S continued to decline physically, he also became more emotionally distraught. However, our music therapy sessions appeared to support Mr. S in his appropriate expression of feelings and emotions, as well as his adaptation to and coping with his worsening health and abilities. Although Mr. S had a number of different hymns that he requested during sessions, one that he often requested to end a session was "How Great Thou Art". During this hymn he would sing with me, often closing his eyes and raising his hands as if in praise. During my final four visits, Mr. S became unable to verbally express his thoughts clearly. He began repeating the phrases "Warm hand on my shoulder", "Hot fire in my heart", "Jesus, You are near", "I cried Your name", "Your embrace", "You are my hope", and "Your Godly fire". He would speak and sing these words at various times during the hymn. Because these phrases seemed significant to him, and because he was unable to discuss the meaning of the words with me due to his altered mental state, I used these phrases to re-write the lyrics of "How Great Thou Art". I also re-wrote the title of the hymn to "A Warm Hand on My Shoulder, Hot Fire in My Heart". As such, the hymn truly became that of Mr. S. The original and revised lyrics to the first verse and refrain of the hymn are below.

"How Great Thou Art"
Original title and lyrics
(Swedish folk song. Lyrics based on a Swedish poem written by Carl Gustav Boberg in 1885

O Lord my God! When I in awesome wonder
Consider all the worlds Thy hands have made.
I see the stars, I hear the rolling thunder,
Thy power throughout the universe displayed.

Then sings my soul, my Saviour God, to Thee;
How great Thou art, how great Thou art!
Then sings my soul, my Saviour God, to Thee:
How great Thou art, how great Thou art

"A Warm Hand on My Shoulder, Hot Fire in My Heart"
Adapted title and lyrics

The pain is gone, your right hand on my shoulder
A wife's embrace, I feel your spirit near
Securing me unto your earthly kingdom
Your Godly fire, dear Jesus you are here
I cried Your name, Your warm hand on my shoulder
You are my hope, the pain is gone
I cried Your name, I cried Your holy name
You heal the pain with a hot fire in my heart

During the final session, during which Mr. S was non-responsive, I sang the revised hymn for him at a tempo which matched his observed deep and slow breathing. I told him that the hymn was a gift from all of us at hospice and from those who cared about him at the present time and who had cared about him in the past, including his wife. At the conclusion of my singing, Mr. S opened his eyes and said "You're Robert, you're my music therapist". These were apparently the last words he spoke, and he died several hours after I left.

In summary, although Mr. S was unable to reconcile with his wife, our use and exploration of hymns in the music therapy sessions appeared to give him strength, support, and possibly hope. Mr. S appeared to me, and the treatment team, to be more at peace and not exhibiting the same level of emotional or spiritual pain as before music therapy was begun with him. Music therapy may have helped him feel re-connected with positive memories of his wife, and to be more emotionally at peace.

The Case of Ms. R
The second case is that of Ms. R.,[23] a 40-year old woman who was widowed and had four children. Ms. R was diagnosed with HIV/AIDS, which she reportedly contracted from her husband. Ms. R reported that her late husband had lied to her about his HIV status and transmitted the virus to her before his death. Her husband had also died under the care of the hospice organization where both I, and a music therapy intern under my supervision worked. This intern provided music therapy services to Ms. R, and will be referred to as the therapist.

Upon referral to music therapy (at time of admission to hospice), the care plan identified the following problem and goal areas: to facilitate anticipatory grieving; support her emotional needs, reduce spiritual distress, reduce pain, minimize extra pyramidal side effects of pain medications, and provide the patient a peaceful death with dignity. The spiritual needs assessment identified Ms. R as a Baptist whose faith was important to her, and noted that she found comfort in prayer and rituals. Ms. R had several placements during her hospice care, including home, the hospice in-patient acute care unit, and the skilled nursing facility where she eventually died.

The therapist reported that during her initial music therapy visit, Ms. R requested spiritual music, and that she preferred to listen to the therapist sing and play. Ms. R would reportedly lay back in her bed, close her eyes, and listen to the familiar hymns she had requested. As pain was a problem in her care plan, the hymns were played and sung to help her relax, and she was able to fall asleep when listening to her favorite spiritual songs. This suggested that these songs may have provided Ms. R some physical and/or emotional release from pain.

As a rapport between the therapist and patient developed, Ms. R became a more active participant in the music therapy sessions. She appeared to use the spiritual songs to send messages to others, e.g. "I like that song for you, I like it for me, I like it for the whole world", gain comfort and reassurance, e.g. "It is soothing me already", and recapture positive spiritual feelings, e.g. "Singing songs and thinking about Jesus makes me rejoice". She appeared to the therapist to be connecting to the meaning of the hymns via her careful attention to the words and her own selecting of phrases to continue singing or discussing. She also appeared to be connecting to the entire ambiance of the music, and Ms. R commented several times about the "soothing" quality of the music.

One hymn in particular, "God Will Take Care of You," was one Ms. R had requested in multiple sessions. At one point when the song was over, Ms. R said softly to the therapist, "I'm afraid that God won't take care of me." When encouraged to elaborate, Ms. R shared that she was afraid that God wouldn't take care of her because she hadn't forgiven her husband for transmitting the HIV to her. Ms. R and the therapist discussed the difference between forgiving and forgetting, and Ms. R made a number of positive and negative statements about her relationship with God. After exploring these issues, she asked the therapist to play "God Will Take Care of You" again. During the music, Ms. R closed her eyes and began to smile. When the song was over, Ms. J asked to hear it a third time, and a peaceful smile spread across her face as she lay and listened to the words that seemed so meaningful to her:

"God Will Take Care of You"
Text by Civilla D. Martin, music by W. Stillman Martin 1904

Be not dismayed what e'er be tide,
God will take care of you
Beneath His wings of love abide,
God will take care of youGod will take care of you,
through every day, o'er all the way
He will take care of you, God will take care of you.

In her final music therapy session, Ms. R initiated the closing of the session, asking the therapist to pray with her. She offered a prayer that was full of praise for God and thanks for her life. Her prayer appeared to mirror some of the thoughts and feelings embodied and expressed in the hymns sung and discussed during the sessions. Ms. R died at the skilled nursing facility four days later.

In summary, a number of fears and concerns, as well as feelings of anger and helplessness, were expressed by Ms. R in the music therapy sessions. It appeared that the hymns played and discussed were effective not only in facilitating the expression of those feelings, but also in offering validation, support, and reassurance. These in turn may have helped the patient in reducing her perception of emotional, spiritual, and physical pain.

The Case of Ms. J
The third case is that of Ms. J.,[22] a 60- year-old woman dying from mesothelioma. She was receiving music therapy services provided by a graduate music therapy student I was supervising at a local hospice in-patient facility. This graduate student was a credentialed music therapist. The sources of pain were many in Ms. J's life, as she had a childhood history of abuse, as well as spousal abuse. She was referred to music therapy with high levels of distress and acting out, with some observed delusional and obsessive symptoms. Physical and emotional pain, spiritual distress, and isolation were identified as initial problem areas for Ms. J. The psychosocial assess-

ment shared by the social worker indicated that the patient had significant abandonment and grief issues. These appeared to be exacerbated by the fact that her only daughter had recently moved overseas. The treatment team felt that addressing these psychosocial issues could potentially help Ms. J. in her overall pain control.

The initial goal targeted by the treatment team and music therapist was to establish a therapeutic relationship with this woman who appeared to feel so alone in the world. Using song choice as an initial intervention, the therapist offered popular songs for Ms. J. to select and listen to. The therapist played and sang these, and was able to share and use these songs as entry points for talking about Ms. J.'s present situation and various aspects of her history. It appeared to the therapist that aspects of Ms. J's difficult life story were dominating her thoughts and exacerbating her emotional pain. However, Ms. J. began to appear very philosophical about her terminal diagnosis and hospice placement being in effect a new stage in her life. When asked by the therapist what she most wanted in life at this time, she said, with tears in her eyes, "1 want peace and happiness', and she asked the therapist to play "something spiritual". Asking Ms. J. to close her eyes and imagine herself at peace, the music therapist sang the African-American spiritual Peace like a River, substituting Ms. J.'s words. The original and revised lyrics are below.

"Peace like a River"
African-American Spiritual Hymn
Original Lyrics – Verse 1

I've got peace like a river, I've got peace like a river,
I've got peace like a river in my soul.
I've got peace like a river, I've got peace like a river,
I've got peace like a river in my soul.

Revised Lyrics

I want peace and happiness, I want peace and happiness
I want peace and happiness today
I want peace and happiness, I want peace and happiness
I want peace and happiness all my life

The music therapist reported that Ms. J appeared to relax while listening to her play and sing this hymn with which she related so strongly. Through the ongoing relationship with the therapist, Ms. J. explored aspects of meaning and purpose in her own life, allowing the music to go beyond what her life had been to date. Ms. J. had shared that she had no formal religious affiliation, but that she strongly believed in an afterlife.

The final song she requested the therapist to sing for her during the last music therapy session was the Welsh folk song "All Through the Night". Ms. J. shared with the therapist that the final words of the song seemed to sum up her life journey to a point of closure. She and Ms. J. reflected on those words - "Though our hearts be wrapped in sorrow, from the hope of dawn we borrow promise of a glad tomorrow all through the night'. Ms. J. died the following day, reportedly at peace and with no complaints of pain, abandonment, or distress. It appeared that the music and shared experiences with the therapist, who had become a trusted ally for her, had created a safe space in which to experience the final passage of her life.

The Case of Ms. P
Our fourth case is that of Ms. P, a 37-year-old woman with ovarian cancer who was in an acute care unit of a hospice organization. I learned of her admission to the unit during the daily morning treatment team "huddle", or mini-treatment team staff meeting during which time new admissions were discussed and referrals for treatment services made. Ms. P was referred for music therapy to address her impending death and the anticipatory grieving and spiritual distress on the part of her family.

Immediately before meeting with Ms. P and her family, I had been visiting with another patient in his room on the unit. As I provided live songs as comfort and support for the other patient, Ms. P's aunt and brother stopped outside the room to listen (the door to the room was closed). When I exited the room they asked if I would see Ms. P. They both appeared somewhat distraught, and the brother shared that "We are worried that she is dying and there is nothing we can do to help her". They had both travelled across the country to visit, as Ms. P did not have family in the immediate area.

Upon entering the room, I observed Ms. P reclining in bed. Her eyes were partly open and her breathing appeared and sounded shallow. Ms. P seemed to be minimally responsive and not able to communicate with her family members, and impending death had been noted on her care plan. She did not appear to me to be in physical pain or distress. Ms. P's brother stated "She can't hear us, she's almost gone." I told them that Ms. P might be able to hear us even though she could not speak. I addressed Ms. P directly, telling her "My name is Robert. I'm a music therapist and you are with us here at hospice. You are very safe and your family is here with you. We will keep you comfortable. I am going to sing some songs to help you relax. Just listen to the music. It is a gift from your family to you and it is a privilege to visit with you". I then asked Ms. P's aunt and brother what type of music she enjoyed. Both replied "hymns and gospel." Ms. P's aunt asked to hear "Amazing Grace and "anything else you

Music Meditated Strategies for Pain in End of Life Care

like." I began with "Amazing Grace," I then continued to play a medley of spiritual songs, including "Michael, Row the Boat Ashore," "He's Got the Whole World in His Hands," ."This Little Light of Mine," and "Kumbaya " During "Amazing Grace", both family members listened. As I continued to sing, Ms. P's aunt began to sing with me (I had provided copies of the words), and Ms. P's brother then sat next to the patient with his hand resting lightly on her shoulder.

Incorporating both the Iso-Principle and the principle of entrainment, I began the songs at a moderate tempo to match the observed rate of the patient's breathing and apparent stress level of Ms. P's family members in the room. I then slowed the pace for following songs and also lowered the volume of the voice and guitar playing. "Kumbaya", as the final song, was thus sung in a gentle and tender manner. The final words of the song were "Oh Lord, come by here," the translation of the song title from Angolan to English. Both Ms. P's aunt and brother appeared to appropriately express feelings and emotions during the session, crying quietly at several points. They also appeared more calm and relaxed as the session progressed.

After concluding the music, I stayed with the patient and family to provide support and to thank them for traveling across the country to visit. I also explored and reinforced the importance of their own support systems while validating their feelings of impending loss. Ms. P's and brother thanked me several times for visiting, saying that the music helped them interact with Ms. P in a meaningful manner. Ms. P died later that night. In summary, Ms. P's ant and brother had offered a cue that music was meaningful to them and to the patient by stopping in the unit to listen as I provided music for another patient. They had also shared that they were in emotional pain and felt helpless in the current situation. In the room, their interaction with the patient and me shifted from passive (listening) to active (singing with me). Both family members also shared with me that the music helped them say goodbye to their loved one. This sharing from the family was significant for me, as my goal had been to help the family by reducing their emotional pain at this difficult time.[10]

The Case of Ms. G
The final case is that of Ms. G. Also a patient in an acute care unit of a hospice organization, she was a 78-year old woman with a terminal diagnosis of dementia. As with Ms. P, I learned of Ms. G's admission to the unit during the daily morning treatment team "huddle". Ms. P was referred for music therapy to address her impending death and anticipatory grieving on the part of her family. At the request of the family, I had provided some music for her and several of her adult children the previous day. Although Ms. G had presented as minimally responsive during this initial session, the family requested that I return

again.

During my second visit, Ms. G again presented as minimally responsive, but appeared to be comfortable, and not evidencing terminal distress or agitation. There were several family members in the room with her. One adult daughter shared "The hardest part is not being able to say goodbye". Apparently, this was due to the dementia and patient's physical decline which prevented Ms. G from responding to, or overtly interact with, her family.

As I was speaking to the family to gauge their needs at that time, one daughter asked me to play and sing the Bette Midler song "Wind Beneath My Wings." We briefly spoke about the meaning of the song, and she shared that "Beaches" had been a favorite movie of both hers and the patient. The movie had been released when the patient was younger and still fully healthy. She also shared with me that the patient had "always been there" for the family, and that they wished they could do more now or at least say goodbye in a meaningful manner. I validated and reinforced this sentiment for the family, noting that this was a time that the family was able to "be there" for their loved one, and that Ms. G might know that they were there to say goodbye, even if Ms. G was not able to express that due to her decline. We next briefly explored the theme of the song and movie (support of a loved one during a long terminal illness), with the support metaphor being the wind beneath the wings. I also addressed the patient directly stating, "This is a song of love and support from your family. It is a gift they would like to share with you now."

During the singing, family members focused their eyes and attention on the patient. Two daughters, one on each side of Ms. G's bed, held her hands. Several family members cried lightly and grasped tissues to dry their eyes. Throughout the song, the patient appeared comfortable but did not appear to respond to the music in an overt manner. After the song ended, a period of silence and stillness filled the room, and no one spoke for about 30 seconds. This silence was not uncomfortable for me, nor did it appear uncomfortable to the family members, who now appeared at peace and not distraught. Although it could not be measured quantitatively, the stillness felt like to me like it was comforting for all persons in the room. I waited until a family member spoke before I spoke, to avoid intruding upon the family's moment. A son then expressed sincere thanks to me for helping to provide comfort for his mother and bring the family together at a difficult and painful time. Ms. G died the next day.[10]

Conclusion

As discussed in the introduction, an integrative approach to address patient pain may bring together four aspects and dimensions – an integrated treatment team, integrated facets of patient pain, meeting the needs of the family in an integrated way, and an integrated music therapy treatment approach. An integrated approach allows both the music therapist and the entire treatment team to design a treatment package designed that addresses the holistic and dynamic nature of the physical, psychosocial, and spiritual needs of the patient. Each of the five case examples described illustrated aspects of these integrated approaches, and for each of these patients and their families, their end of life journeys were made more meaningful in part by music therapy. Table 1 illustrates how the needs of each of the five patients were met in this integrated manner.

	Mr. S	Ms. R	Ms. J	Ms. P	Ms. G
Integrated Treatment Team	X	X	X	X	X
Patient Pain	X	X	X		
Family Context				X	X
Music Therapy	X	X	X	X	X

As can be seen in the table, three of the four integrated approaches were present in all five cases, and all four integrated aspects were present in two cases. In addition, while family members were not present during sessions with the patients in the first three cases, the sessions did address family dynamics, which had been central to their life stories.

In conclusion, as a music therapist who had the privilege of working with these five patients and their families, I truly appreciated the opportunity to work in such an integrative manner. As such, I recommend that all music therapists working in the area of pain management consider incorporating an integrative approach to their work whenever possible.

References

1. Kuru T; Yeldan I; Zengin A; Kostanoglu A; Tekeoglu A; Akbaba YA; Tarakci D. Prevalence and aetiology of neuropathic pain in cancer patients: The prevalence of pain and different pain treatments in adults. J Turk Soc Algology. January 2012;23:22-27.
2. Steindal SA; Bredal IS; Sørbye LW; Lerdal A. Pain control at the end of life: a comparative study of hospitalized cancer and non-cancer patients. Scand J Caring Sci. Dec, 2011; 25: 771-9.

3. Bennett MI; Rayment C; Hjermstad M; Aass N; Caraceni A; Kaasa S. Prevalence and aetiology of neuropathic pain in cancer patients: A systematic review. Pain. February 2012;153:359-65.
4. Davis JA; Robinson RL; Le TK; Xie J. Incidence and impact of pain conditions and comorbid illnesses. J Pain Res.2011;4:331-45.
5. Krout RE. Hospice and palliative music therapy.: A continuum of creative caring. In American Music Therapy Association, ed. Effectiveness of music therapy procedures: Documentation of research and clinical practice - 3rd edition. Silver Spring, MD: American Music Therapy Association; 2000: 323-411.
6. Bradt J, Dileo C. Music therapy for end-of-life care. Cochrane Database of Systematic Reviews 2010, Issue 1. Art. No.: CD007169. DOI: 10.1002/14651858.CD007169.pub2
7. Krout RE. A synerdisciplinary music therapy treatment team approach for hospice and palliative care. Aust J Mus Ther. 2004;15:33-45.
8. National Institutes of Health. NIH pain information page. Available at http://health.nih.gov/topic/pain. Accessed January 26, 2012.
9. Loewy, JV: Spingte, R. Music soothes the savage breast. Mus Med. 2011;3: 69-71.
10. Krout RE. Music therapy with imminently dying hospice patients and their families: Facilitating release near the time of death. Am J Hos Pal Care. 2003;20: 129-34.
11. Krout, R. The effects of single-session music therapy interventions on the observed and self-reported levels of pain control, physical comfort, and relaxation of hospice patients. Am J Hos Pal Care. 2001:18; 383-90.
12. Krout, R. E. Therapist-composed music and song in end of life care. In Dileo, C, Loewy, J, eds. Music therapy at the end of life. Cherry Hill, NJ: Jeffery Publishers; 2005:129-40.
13. Miller, EB. Bio-Guided Music Therapy. London: Jessica Kingsley; 2011.
14. Krout, R. Music listening to facilitate relaxation and promote wellness: Integrated aspects of our neurophysiological responses to music. Arts Psych. 2007;34: 134-41.
15. Melzack R, Wall PD. Pain mechanism: a new theory. Science. 1965; 150: 971-79.
16. Bernatzky, G, Presch, M, Anderson, M, Panksepp, J. Emotional foundations of music as a non-pharmacological pain management tool in modern medicine. Neurosci Biobehav Rev. 2011;35: 1989-99.

17. Altschuler, I. A psychiatrist's experience with music as a therapeutic agent. In: Schullian, D, ed. Music and Medicine. New York: Books for Libraries Press; 1948.
18. Taylor, DB. Biomedical Foundations of Music as Therapy. 2nd ed. Eau Claire: Barton Publications; 2010.
19. Rider, M. The Rhythmic Language of Health and Disease. St. Louis: MMB Music, 1997.
20. DiMaio, L. Music therapy entrainment: A humanistic music therapist's perspective of using music therapy entrainment with hospice clients experiencing pain. Mus Ther Persp. 2010; 28: 106-15.
21. Groen, KM. Pain assessment and management in end of life care: A survey of assessment and treatment practices of hospice music therapy and nursing professionals. J Music Ther. 2007;44: 90-112.
22. Hepburn, M., & Krout, R. E. (2004). Meaning, purpose, transcendence and hope – music therapy and spirituality in end of life hospice care. New Zeal J Mus Ther. 2004; 2: 58-82.
23. Tanguay, C. Will god take care of me? A case study addressing spirituality and hope through music therapy in the hospice setting with a woman with AIDS. Unpublished paper; 2001.

Music and Medicine: Integrative Models in the Treatment of Pain

SECTION IV

MULTICULTURAL PERSPECTIVES

CHAPTER 23

Culturally Informed Music Psychotherapy: Using Latin American Music and Repertoire in the Treatment of Pain and Anxiety Experienced by Individuals Receiving Chemotherapy

Jillian Hicks MA, MT-BC
Erik Baumann Cornejo MMT
Natalia Garrido MMT

Gracias a la vida que me ha dado tanto
Me ha dado la risa y me ha dado el llanto,
Así yo distingo dicha de quebranto
Los dos materiales que forman mi canto
Y el canto de ustedes que es el mismo canto
Y el canto de todos que es mi propio canto[*]
Violeta Parra

Introduction

The need for integrative, individualized care for the treatment of pain has become apparent in the international health community.[2] In the United States, a report by the Institute of Medicine showed,[3] that the emotional, cognitive, and physical complications of chronic pain affect approximately 116 million Americans. Pain as a valuable indicator informs us that something is happening to our body that requires special attention. However, if the pain persists beyond the point of providing beneficial information, it may become a separate disease.[3(p3)] This "disease of pain" has physiological, psychological, social, and spiritual components. If the pain becomes

---

[*] "Thanks to life that has given me so much, It´s given me laugh and cry. That's how I distinguish joy from sadness, to be broken.the two materials, which form my song and your song which is the same songnd everybody´s song, which is my own song."

chronic, the nervous system changes becoming progressively worse as the pain cycle deepens and remains.[3(p3)] As anxiety can significantly affect a person's perception of pain and create anticipatory nausea and vomiting, it is critical to address it in order to successfully treat cancer related pain.[4] A study shows[5] that patients who reported having cancer related pain were also found to have higher scores for mood disturbance, tension, depression, anger, fatigue, and confusion which were linked to longer durations of pain. In another study,[6] fear of nausea, vomiting, infection, hair loss, and weight loss were the most frequent worries in those at the beginning of treatment. Research supports a strong correlation between pain and mood; they are inter-related.

There are many specific factors involved with cancer related pain. According to written communication with oncology nurse practitioner, Eugenie Spiguel, N.P. (April 2012), some of the common physiological cancer related side effects include: fatigue (most common complaint), sleep disturbances,[7] alopecia (hair loss), nausea and vomiting, mucositis (mouth sores), myelosupression (decrease white and red blood cells as well as platelets), peripheral neuropathy (numbness of fingers, hands, toes, feet, and sometimes legs), diarrhea or constipation, discoloration and breaking of the nails and skin, skin rashes, allergic reactions, and infusion reactions. Alopecia can also cause chronic nasal drip due to lack of nose hair and ingrown eyelashes. Nausea may induce lack of appetite and weight loss. Mucositis can also manifest as painful sores in rectum and anus. Myelosupression may cause a wide variety of complications. It may cause long-lasting fatigue and dyspnea (difficulty breathing), tendency to have recurrent infections or mild bleeding but can also induce life-threatening complications. When peripheral neuropathy becomes advanced, it causes difficulty with fine motor skills and may cause people to trip, fall, or drop things. The chemotherapy drugs and/or anti-nausea medications commonly prescribed can cause severe constipation. All of these side effects are likely to have adverse psychological implications.[8]

The psychological components of cancer diagnosis and long-term effects[9] are subjective and every individual person experiences the stressors related to diagnosis, acceptance (or non-acceptance) of diagnosis, treatment, and recovery or end-of-life differently. Each person has his/her own history, culture, and set of tools for dealing with adverse conditions. However, there are some common psychological issues that may arise such as worrying thoughts about being a burden on care-givers,[10-12] increased anxiety and/or depression,[13] feelings of panic and isolation, existential crisis, the emotional impact of the financial burden of illness, and identity issues (becoming a patient). Additionally contributing to the psychological stress of a patient are changes in his or her role within family unit and/or work environment, struggles with independence vs. dependence, strain on relationships, and the trauma of facing life threatening illness.[14] Patients who had surgery for breast cancer or colo-rectal cancer may have additional factor for depression because of drastic changes in their body image. Caregivers of these patients may also suffer from depression, which can in turn negatively impact the quality of life experienced by cancer patients.[15]

The pain and anxiety associated with cancer manifests itself differently for each individual.[3(p133)] Therefore, one has to tailor the care to each individual patient. Each individual comes with a unique identity that is the result of one's life experience, coping skills, individual culture, family dynamics, past traumas, resilience level, and belief systems. The need for psychological support and inner resourcing is great, because the changes surrounding cancer diagnosis affect every aspect of a person's life. Screening patients who are newly diagnosed can help identify patients in need, and best direct supportive care services.[16]

A Cultural and Preferred Music Therapy Approach to the Treatment of Pain and Anxiety

The physical aspects of pain and its psychological components are totally intertwined. In fact pain associated with advanced cancer is multifaceted and complex, and is influenced by physiological, psychological, social, and spiritual phenomena.[17] We must treat all aspects of a person, because of the inextricable connection between the mind and the body.[18] Growing research supports the use of music therapy as a treatment for all aspects of cancer-induced pain and anxiety.[19-24] The purpose of music therapy intervention is to provide a forum for cancer patients to reconnect to their healthy and intact inner components. Music therapists provide support for the person to build and enhance their resilience and the coping skills needed to reduce pain and anxiety.

Music therapy intervention has been found to relieve pain, nausea, and lessen stress, anxiety, and depression in patients with cancer.[25] The treatment of pain is a team issue and may be best addressed by integrating all those involved in the patient's care including the medical and supportive staff, family and caregivers, and most importantly, the patient. In her chapter about pain and music therapy,[18(p59)] Kwan identifies six themes for successful treatment of a patient in distress: trust, presence ("being with"), caring, physical empathy, sympathetic resonance and empowerment. All of these themes can be utilized by music therapists providing thorough care to oncology patients.

When one approaches an oncology (or any) patient, it is imperative to be aware of the individual's cultural identity. This is especially critical when considering culturally influenced beliefs about pain and differing terminology used to describe pain.[26] Music is one of the things that help to define cultures. It is inextricably linked with identity.[27] Humans have different musical preferences, which are associated with memories, culture, life experiences, identity, family, friends, and emotions. This "music identity" develops over the course of a lifetime. By using music that is personally meaningful to the patient, the music therapist is able to tap into the patient's "music identity" leading to a deeper level of connection within the therapeutic relationship. The music is a way to enter into the patient's cultural life script, potentially unlocking personal beliefs about pain. Both therapist and patient can the use this information in order to build suitable mechanisms for coping with pain.

Cultural Considerations: Pain and Anxiety in Latin American Oncology Patients

There is a kaleidoscope of various cultural identities attempting to blend into the everchanging social landscape of life in the United States. People move to the US for a multitude of reasons, ranging from economic freedom, employment, and refuge from violence and/or war. Specifically, the Latin American sub-group in the US has accounted for a large percentage of the population. According to a recent census, Latin Americans represented the second largest ethnic group with 29.1% of the extremely diverse population of New York City. Non-Hispanic whites were the largest group with 33%. If we take into consideration the whole country, the Latin American population corresponds to 16%. Between 2000 and 2010, the increase in the Latin American population was responsible for more than half of the total population growth of the United States.

A study which focused on cultural factors involved in the care of Hispanic patients with cancer related pain[29] demonstrated that pain may not be outwardly spoken about or shown due to: stoic responses, belief in folk and nondrug remedies, and language barriers leading to noncompliant pharmacological intervention. Healthcare providers must never assume a patient is not in pain simply because they do not outwardly express it. Latin American communities commonly place great importance on family and religion. These two items have been related to overall quality of life.[30] For Latina breast cancer survivors, religion/spirituality was found to be strongly linked with quality of life and higher levels of functional well being.[31]

Spirituality plays a predominant role in Mexico, the Caribbean, Central American, and South American countries as well as for Latin Americans living in foreign countries. In this culture, spirituality is commonly a part of the everyday life and serves as a foundation of strength in coping with life's struggles.[33] Spirituality was found[32] to be the most common coping mechanism in Latina, African American, and Asian American women who had survived breast cancer. Within the domain of spirituality, there are a variety of perspectives among these countries. The majority of the population identify themselves as Catholic (around 83%), or Christian, Protestant or Evangelical.[28,33,34] The spirituality is intertwined with cultural values[33] and is also a large contributing factor to social identity.[35] A study of breast cancer survivors reports,[36] African Americans, Hispanics, and those who self-identified as Christians, were more likely than other groups to feel comforted by God.

The coping mechanism associated with spirituality itself has been found to be associated with several positive outcomes such as less distress and better quality of life regardless of perceived life threat.[37] Spiritual well-being has been significantly associated with an ability of people with cancer to continue to enjoy life despite high levels of pain or fatigue and has been found to be inversely related to depression.[37] Due to the importance of spirituality in the Latin American culture, these findings may be significant in addressing the challenging needs of oncology patients.

Because spirituality plays a major role in Latin America, and has been identified as a primary coping mechanism for so many, music therapists may chose to focus on this inner resource in the care of oncology patients. Each individual country has its own culture, and within every person is a unique cultural identity. This cultural approach to treatment is the lens through which one can practice music therapy. Music therapists support the patient's expression of what is personally true and meaningful. Individualized assessment allows for the provision of treatment that is culturally sensitive and specific to the patient's cultural identity.

Music Therapy Intervention: Latin American Music

There are a variety of ways one can utilize culture as a resource for therapeutic interventions.[38] The music psychotherapy approach to pain treatment is done through building a supportive environment. In this trusting realm, pain and anxiety treatment is addressed and processed. Music is a unique and effective way to access all aspects of the nuanced cultures of patients undergoing chemotherapy treatment and their caregivers. Through culturally informed music psychotherapy intervention, music therapists can best meet the needs of patients.

The following section discusses some of the relevant attributes of Latin American music and its link to the culture. The concept of Latin American music represents the musical movement that originated after the Spanish, French, Portuguese and Italian colonization in America. Latin

American music includes: the sounds of mambo, samba, salsa, mariachi, tango, Celia Cruz, Agustín Lara, Mercedes Sosa, Joao Gilberto, bongos, congas, maracas, charango; ideological power, expressive melodies, and romantic moods. The modern concept of Latin American music excludes Native American cultural traditions, however rhythms and harmonies from these cultures are incorporated into the music.[39]

Alejo Carpentier wrote, "Latin American Music exploded into existence rather than evolved in coherent and measured patterns. Its beauty and strength lay in its non-classical forms."[40] It is a complex concept because the genre's name encompasses a multitude of styles originating from different countries and eras. There are twenty-three countries including Spain, where Spanish is the primary language spoken. Each country has a multitude of styles that contribute to the genre termed, Latin American music. The music of Brazil is also considered within the Latin American tradition although the primary language of the country is Portuguese. Latin American music is born from the fusion of traditional rhythms and harmonies indigenous to each country. Strong influences are found from the African rhythms of the slaves transported to South and Central America and the traditional music of Spain. Throughout the nineteenth and twentieth centuries Latin American music has been styled by Spanish, European classical, and North American folk music such as jazz and R&B.

Ed Morales referred to Latin American music as an essential part of Latino identity, meanwhile non-Latino are drawn to it for its strange complexity and its expressive possibilities.[1(p12)] Features that differentiate Latin American music from other music styles are syncopated rhythms, the use of the clave in 5- over two measures (rhythmic structure), and the African "question-answer" percussion sections. Of course, these three features are a generalized and simplified way of distinguishing Latin American music. For instance, there are a multitude of differences between the music from Cuba to Mexico. Sometimes music styles are classified by their country of origin such as the tango from the slums of Buenos Aires and the samba as a true symbol of Brazil. However, various parts of Latin America produced different kinds of music that are identified beyond political borders. The music of the Caribbean, Central America, and South America are all uniquely different.[1(p12)]

The contexts in which Latin American music is inseparable include religious practices, activities, leisure, the life cycle,[40(p53)] and social-political situations. When music therapists use Latin American music in their work, they need to be aware of the turbulent history of Latin America that is reflected in songs considered within the protest genre. The traditions of the troubadour and politically committed songwriters have a long history in Latin America and are established genres of contemporary Latin American music. When using this kind of music, one must be careful as intense associative memories and difficult feelings may arise.

There are echoes of Latin American music in the music of the United States of America. The Latin American tradition came before jazz was born in New Orleans. In fact, Jelly Roll Morton developed the New Orleans piano style that he called, "The Latin Tinge", which influenced the development of jazz in America. Additionally, the ragtime style of Scott Joplin contains echoes of Afro-Cuban styles.[1(p16)] To this discussion, King (2004) contributes:

> The vitality of Latin American music and its extraordinary capacity for transformation, its ability to respond to new social and political circumstances, and to incorporate new traditions and forms. They have resulted in its distinctive sounds, the unique voices of many communities, hybrid of many sources, which have not only been heard around the world and have affected music worldwide, but which continue to adapt, to change and surprise us.[39(p256)]

Clinical Work

The following vignettes and case studies illustrate the use of culturally informed music therapy techniques in the care of physiological, psychological, emotional, social, and spiritual needs of Latin American oncology patients. Music therapists from the Louis Armstrong Department of Music therapy conducted all therapy sessions. The music therapy department is a part of the integrative approach to health care at Beth Israel Medical Center and the Cancer Center at St. Luke's Roosevelt Hospital in New York City. Addressing the mind, body, and spirit of a person is at the forefront of the work at these medical institutions.

Acute Interventions Thematic of Spirituality

Portrayed here are examples of how spiritual Spanish music can be used in music therapy interventions. They are meant to provide a clear perspective on the role of spirituality in Latin American culture and spiritual Latin American music. In the first vignette, music therapy is used as a way of creating a calmer, relaxed state in a patient undergoing a medical procedure. The second vignette involves a woman having difficulty connecting to her experience with illness and treatment. The work demonstrates the clinical importance of identifying clear goals and creating opportunities for success in reclaiming inner resources for coping. In both vignettes, the same song is utilized in different contexts. The third vignette depicts a newly diagnosed oncology patient and the work of connecting to positive feelings about her faith as a way of identifying and activating effective coping mechanisms to process feelings surrounding diagnosis.

"Victoria"
Procedural Support: Accessing Coping Mechanisms within Spirituality
Victoria, a seventy year-old female from Puerto Rico, was undergoing chemotherapy for breast cancer. She arrived in the outpatient infusion suite for her sixth cycle of treatment, accompanied by a friend from her church. We had worked together twice before, and in these initial sessions, had identified themes that were recurrent for her. The most important theme was that she was facing a similar illness as the one to which she had lost her husband twelve years prior. She was born and raised as a Catholic, but after losing her husband she had found a new relationship with her spirituality and was attending an Evangelical Latin American church. She identified her faith as her primary coping mechanism. On the day of the third music therapy session, Victoria was experiencing problems with the placement of an intravenous (I.V.) line for the chemotherapy. She became increasingly tense and nervous. As these psychological and physiological factors increased, so did the pain in her arm (reported by her). I asked Victoria if she wanted music therapy while she waited for the nurse's return to attempt placement on her other arm. Victoria agreed, and I began by asking her how she was feeling while improvising around a chord progression based on a Christian song called "Pescador de Hombres." I played the guitar chords C, G and F while simultaneously playing the ocean disc. Victoria and her friend both held egg-shakers as I matched the tempo of my guitar strumming to her respiration. Within the intervention, I specifically entrained the Remo ocean drum to her exhalation. The music progressively relaxed and deepened her breathing. Her posture changed and she looked calmer.

Shortly after we began our improvisation, Victoria's nurse returned to make another attempt at placing the I.V. This time it was successful. Victoria continued listening to the music during the procedure and after the I.V. was placed, she affirmed to the therapist that the music made her feel, "calmed and relaxed".

Victoria spoke about the importance of faith in her everyday life. She expressed wanting to play "Pescador de Hombres" together. As we played this song, Victoria sang while her friend joined in playing the egg-shakers and singing. When the song was finished Victoria expressed how this song made her feel, "happy." It reminded her of the first time she felt God in her whole body while attending church, and what an incredible experience it had been. Her whole body responded to this song with a similar relaxed posture and she expressed no longer feeling tense.

"Juana"
Setting Personal Goals in Musical Prayer
Juana, a 56 year-old female from Ecuador, was undergoing chemotherapy for breast cancer treatment. Her entire family relocated to New York in the late 90's. During assessment, Juana spoke about being a very active person and was anxious about the possible side effects chemotherapy might have on her. She worried how it would affect her everyday life. Prior to receiving chemotherapy, Juana had experienced difficulties with her stomach, which had affected her appetite. Juana identified herself as Catholic and described her religion as giving her great strength. Juana was a very strong willed, independent woman and would frequently avoid the subject of how she was doing by saying, "Things are the same," or "It's all so-so." She was afraid of chemotherapy and did not want to think too much on how it was actually affecting her.

Throughout our work together, Juana asked to play a variety of boleros and music from her country. We finished nearly every session by playing "Pescador de hombres" and improvising lyrics on the verse. The first time we did this, after singing the chorus for the second time, I began playing the verse and asked Juana if she felt like putting her own words into the song. Almost immediately Juana began praying to God. She began declaring all the things she wanted to achieve before her next treatment and asked God for strength to be able to do them. Recurrent themes involved her appetite and energy level. After every verse, we sang the original chorus together. The setting of goals in the form of musical prayer was a useful tool in helping her obtain a clear perspective on her feelings and needs. She was able to notice that her response to the chemotherapy treatment was more positive than what she had imagined it would be.

"Beatriz"
Expression and Acceptance through Spiritual Musicing
Beatriz, an eighty-three year-old female from Mexico, diagnosed with breast cancer, came with her husband to the United States almost thirty years ago. One of her daughters, Ana, lives in the USA, while the other two remain in Mexico. Beatriz was referred to music therapy in order to help her cope with her new diagnosis. Her situation was complicated by the fact that her daughter, Ana, had just finished treatment for breast cancer. At the time of the music therapy assessment, Beatriz mentioned feeling "grey" and "not able to find out what my feelings are." She was confused, and when we spoke about her illness and personal experience, she was very often unable

to find words to finish the sentences. According to her daughter, Beatriz had always taken care of everyone: her husband's diabetes, Ana's cancer, and the rest of her family. It was very difficult for her to be in the role of the one needing care. She and I began working on a session "warm-up" (as developed by Dr. Joanne Loewy) using a bolero song she remembered her father playing for the family when she was a kid.

After Beatriz experienced the music, she tried to explain how she felt. I noticed her becoming increasingly tense as she recognized that she could not complete her sentences. All she could elaborate was that she felt "grey." I began playing some chords (uneven guitar chord progressions that did not contain much repetition) while she narrated her experience. I asked her if she could recall a place that had made her feel calm. She mentioned a particular church she used to attend. As I asked her to narrate what this place looked like, I switched to a steady, rhythmic chord progression between C and F, entraining it to her respiration. We continued working on the image of this place until she was able to find a particular item within it. It was a painting, which she used to stare at while sinking into her thoughts and prayers. It had given her much peace. As we went deeper into her associations with this painting, she closed her eyes and sank into thoughts of this image. I asked her what this painting would say to her if it could tell her something. She whispered, "Be calmed...Be calmed...It will be all right." The moment following this visualization was the first time Beatriz was able to calm her thoughts and process her diagnosis.

It is possible to see the differences of how people relate to their own spirituality in all three vignettes. It is important to be aware of these differences and pay attention to how the individual person relates to his or her own spirituality.

Pain Management:
Re-experiencing the Past to Explore the Present

"Carlos"
The following case reflects the use of music therapy pain management techniques while involving Latin American music. Carlos, a fifty-five year-old, Puerto Rican male who moved to NYC as a teenager, was admitted to the hospital for a gastrointestinal cancer. He was referred to music therapy primarily because of high pain levels, and secondarily for psychological support. At the time of the first session, Carlos mentioned that he was in such great pain that he had not been able to sleep more than two hours in the last three days. When I asked him to rate his pain on the Wong-Baker Faces Scale,[41] he rated it between 9 and 10 (10 highest level of pain), and located the pain on the right side of his chest and rib cage. When asked about his

Latin American Music and Repertoire with Pain and Chemotherapy

musical preferences, Carlos told me he preferred salsa. He looked very tired and said he was, "willing to try anything" that could help him manage the pain.

I offered him an ocean-drum and told him that he could play if he wanted to. I began playing a slow tempo *son* (one of the rhythmic roots of salsa) on a Dm, F, Gm and A chord progression based on the song "Chan-Chan" by Buenavista Social Club. Immediately Carlos began exploring the sounds of the Remo ocean drum, changing the intensity from strong short expression to long softer ones. Meanwhile I let the way he played the Ocean-drum set the rhythm for the improvisation. I reflected the intensity of the "waves" with the guitar. Carlos' expression changed to a look of concentration. I asked him if this music made him think about any place, and he responded that he immediately thought about his hometown in Puerto Rico, a small fishing town by the ocean. He described a beachside landscape. I asked him to think about the colors of that place, the way the sand felt on his feet, and to think about the smells. Carlos described the place and I asked him if he remembered how the ocean felt. Carlos began to narrate how he and his friends used to swim on the ocean and how they used to play on that beach. As the music continued reflecting what Carlos was playing on the ocean-drum, his posture began to change. He became more relaxed and continued narrating several scenes from his childhood including playing with his friends and helping his mother with some of the house tasks. He mentioned several times how happy he had been, and how neither he nor his friends had had anything to worry about. He described how they had grown up in a very dangerous neighborhood but that they had learned how to be happy. By the time the music finished Carlos mentioned feeling almost no pain at all and rated it at a level 2 out of 10 on the Visual Analong Scale (VAS). He said, "This is the most relaxed I've been since I came to the hospital with this pain."

We spoke about his current life status and his new struggle with cancer. He told me he was trying to recover from years of addiction to heroin. He mentioned that he never wanted to be a bad father or husband, and that he tried not to mix his addiction with his family. Carlos said he lived a very different life when he was not at home, which was something he was tired of. He spoke about his desire to change and of living a less complicated life.

In this case, music therapy addressed Carlos' immediate need for pain management. By providing a musical environment that was familiar to him, he became calm and experienced a significant decrease of his pain. By giving him the opportunity to set the rhythm and intensity of the music, Carlos gained control over his environment where he had previously felt helpless. Exploring his past made it possible for him to look at the present.

He discovered some of his most immediate needs. By providing a music that was closely linked with his identity, Carlos was able to freely associate with some of the core aspects of his *self*. From this place, he was able to express a desire for change. One can only change that which is understood. By recovering one's sense of the *self*, it is possible to strengthen the nucleus of the identity,[42(p176)] a process that the psychoanalyst Bollas defines as "destiny."[42(p176)]

The Use of Mantra Techniques: Processing New Diagnosis

Mantra is a Sanskrit term[43] commonly used to describe Vedic words, which have meter or any Hindu or Buddhist word/syllable that holds spiritual meaning that is repeated for focus. Traditionally it is used in a religious context as a way to meditate on one concept. For the context of this paper, the term is defined as repeating a single word or short phrase in an improvisational musical framework. Mantra provides a simplification of verbal options for expression thereby enhancing the focus, meaning, and depth of a single word or phrase. The possibility for an increase in emotional connection is afforded. Using this technique in my work with Spanish speaking patients has created profound moments of tension release, life review, expression, and inner resourcing. The mantra can begin with the word(s) provided by the patient or with words that I think capture the theme of the mood or what has been processed. My primary language is English and I have what I would consider a novice level of Spanish that enables me to understand some of what is verbally said and a small vocabulary with which to respond.

One of the unique benefits of the music therapy modality is the ability to work outside the verbal scope. I have found that sessions with Spanish speaking people can be highly effective and ethical when I am transparent and present with the patient about the limitations of my language abilities. The therapeutic relationship that develops within the music and sessions primarily happens in a musical context. Music can be used as a tool, which affords expression, connection to emotion, identity, culture, evokes physiological responses such as changes in heart rate, oxygen saturation, respiratory rate, movement, energy, and relaxation. It is abstract, can take over where words fail, and stimulates memories. In a study,[44] fMRI imaging was collected off a human brain while a person played improvised music. The results showed the activated areas of the brain were the same as those, which activate during autobiographical speaking. Here we see a possible rationale for why music improvisation can be such a meaningful, personal experience. This enables people to non-verbally communicate aspects of him/herself that are deeply personal and gives music therapists tools to work on the autobiographical, expressive level with patients outside the directly verbal realm.

The method of using mantra naturally lends space for empathizing and reflecting both lyrically and musically. My authentic presence can be felt in the music. By repeating their contributions back to them, patients are able to hear and experience their strengths enhanced.[45] Many times, people create their own mantras; freely contributing words that are of personal significance. Music goes beyond verbal communication and the depth of the process is significant. Also, working in a creative medium can allow the patients to put their pain, anxiety, and experience into a transformative context. When used non-verbally within the constructs of music, the result of manta can be a powerful catharsis, feeling of support and understanding.

"Silvia"

The following case study illustrates the use of mantra with a patient referred to as Silvia, a forty-nine year-old female diagnosed with right breast cancer. Her maternal Grandmother and Aunt were both diagnosed with cancer. One of her friends told me that both family members had gone into remission. Silvia reported no past traumas. When asked about her current beliefs about chemotherapy treatment, she stated, "Pienso que es bueno porque reduce el cancer" ("I think it is good because it reduces the cancer"). She has three children and is married. The session took place during her first chemotherapy infusion, to which she was accompanied by her husband, sister-in-law, and a family friend. The session was conducted in both Spanish and English, as Silvia was originally from the Dominican Republic where her primary language was Spanish. This effort was important for purposes of inclusion, as Silvia's husband and friend were bilingual as well. An important digression here is to mention that in cases where bilingualism is a factor, the extra burden of translating treatment information can often be placed on the caregiver. Health care providers should approach this issue sensitively and intelligently by enlisting interpreter services which are provided by healthcare institutions in accordance with state law.

As I approached Silvia at the infusion suite at St. Luke's Roosevelt Hospital, I noticed that she was surrounded by family and friends and was holding onto a portable music player. During the initial intake and assessment, she reported being at a stress level of two on the Wong-Baker Faces Scale.[41] She said she felt, "tranquila" and stated the most stressful part of the treatment was the I.V. placement. On a color analysis scale (CAS),[46] Silvia drew marks and described what they meant for her. She was nervous and had hopes and wishes. Her breathing was shallow and controlled. She told me she used music everyday in her life and that Christian music was the most important genre for her. Silvia listened to Christian praise music in

Spanish, which was sung by Latinas. Some of her favorites included Lily Goodman, Nena Leal, Marcela Gandaba, and Isabelle Valdez.

Verbal communication was difficult because of language barriers but we connected with each other by both mutually explaining that we each spoke a tiny bit of the other's language. As we began the session, I quickly realized the need to form clear direction for Silvia and her caregivers. Everyone had a different idea about what we were going to do with the music. I wanted to incorporate their ideas and direction, but also needed to provide direct grounding for them to join together and apply music psychotherapy techniques. I did a "tour of the room" which is a music therapy assessment tool.[47] After demonstrating each instrument, I handed everyone the instrument they acted the most curious about. Silvia chose the Remo ocean drum to begin, but quickly handed it off to me once she felt finished with it. This also occurred with the egg shakers. I was not sure why she did not sustain instrument playing, but it felt as though we had not yet discovered something in which she could express herself. I continued forming the session by moving from the assessment into exploration of her preferred genre, Christian music.

The family friend pulled out an iPad to play her favorite Christian song. Silvia responded to the song selection by rocking back and forth, closing her eyes, and appearing as though she was thoroughly enjoying the music. Knowing that live music creation could potentially reflect Silvia's emotional state and address her need for a deepening of breath, we focused on a single line from the chorus of the song. I asked what it meant and how to say it. The words were "Este tiempo es tuyo," which means, "This time is yours". The song was a about a strong woman. The family seemed pleased that I was trying to speak and understand the Spanish and the meaning of the song. The goal was to create an opportunity for the family to feel culturally and spiritually validated. After listening to the recorded song for a little time, I proposed that we create our own version of the music live with our prospective instruments. I began playing the guitar and singing the single line, "Este tiempo es tuyo" as a type of mantra, meditative theme. Everyone seemed to lighten and smile as they recognized the single line from the song. Collectively we all created the song together contributing unique parts, which fit together. Silvia's sister-in-law played the drum and continued for the duration of the session. She had a clear, steady, defined beat and I got the sense from her music and her disposition that she may have played her role in life and within the family unit similarly to the way she played the drum. Her music fit into the tapestry of music being created without dominating or being submissive: steady, strong, constant.

During the improvisation I periodically interjected an improvised line, "Silvia con su familia, este tiempo es tuyo" ("Silvia, with her family.

This time is yours.") The first time I sang her name, she giggled a little, which I thought may have indicated that she was slightly uncomfortable. The second time I sang her name within the context of the song and mantra, she began crying steadily and with increasing intensity. She sobbed as the song continued.

Afterward, a conversation developed in which different caregiver members spoke about their process around the diagnosis and the fears they had. A common thread that ran throughout the session was that of faith as the centerpiece of everyone's experience and strength. Silvia would interject with an "A-men" every time one of her relatives spoke about something that was important/rang true for her. The discussion became a little disjointed with every family member speaking about something different in little groups and at me. Silvia giggled at her husband and told me that he was her "clown" and that he always made her laugh. I thought I could see sadness, but calm strength in his face. Silvia looked at him at one point and said, "I love you!" in English. Their connection appeared to be deep.

As the discussions came together again, I proposed that we could do a musical improvisation around prayer. I asked what the Spanish word for prayer was ("orar") and motioned with my hands in a prayer pose. Silvia asked if it would mean that she would sing. I assured her that she was welcome to sing, but she could also speak the prayer and we (her husband, sister-in-law, family friend, and I) would provide a musical frame for her words. Her sister-in-law played the drum steadily on the beat. Silvia chose the chords she wanted to use. I gave her choices between major or minor chords. She chose two minor chords, Em and Am, which I strummed back and forth on the guitar in triple meter. The family bent over with their heads bowed. Silvia moved to the end of her infusion chair. She spoke the entire prayer and sobbed through her words expressing deep gratitude to God for her life and all her blessings. In between she'd say "Amen" repeatedly. Her family pulled the curtain over partially so they would have more privacy in the infusion suite. After the prayer was over I sang, "Amen" a few times and visualized the prayer being sent with full intention.

Afterward, Silvia looked me in the eye and said over and over, "Thank you. Thank you. Thank you." There was a moment when I thought the session was coming to a natural end, however the group moved into a spontaneous joyful expression of one of their favorite Christian songs. Everyone sang and played instruments. Silvia's affect changed greatly. I got the sense that she had experienced an intense cathartic release of emotion.

The session contained a full range of emotions including deep, continuous crying, utter joy, and laughter. I think the session was a place of a deep release for all the fears and tensions Silvia had been holding onto. In a post questionnaire in reaction to the music therapy session, she reported being at a stress level of 0 and wrote, "Me siento liberada, mucho mejor" ("I feel free; a lot better"). She wrote that her body felt, "Más fortaleza" ("I feel more strength"). Silvia said the music therapy session benefited her by giving her strength in her soul. In the post color analysis scale, she reported no feelings of nervousness.

When Silvia thanked me for the opportunity for improvised musical prayer, I felt that she had accessed a part of herself that was emotionally connected and experienced tension release. She had an expression on her face that was relieved and relaxed. She looked like she was present in her body: still and steady. Perhaps like the sister-in-law's drumbeat.

The Use of Music Therapy Techniques focusing on Bossa Nova for the Treatment of Anxiety

Joao Gilberto is considered one of the musicians who greatly contributed to the birth of Bossa Nova. There is an anecdote from Gilberto's era when Brazilian artists used to meet at parties. Fellow artists remember him playing the guitar differently than they were accustomed. In addition, he had an almost whispering quality to the melodies he produced with his voice. They say that Gilberto explained how he intended to apply the breathing techniques used by the yogis to sing long melodic phrases.[48]

When I found this wonderful anecdote it made me want to investigate the possible music qualities of Bossa Nova that I could include in music psychotherapy techniques. I discovered the concept of *Saudade*: an intrinsic feature of Bossa Nova. *Saudade* is a Portuguese word, which expresses a feeling closely related to melancholy resulting from nostalgic feelings from something that is distant, temporarily lost, or absent. At the same time, this feeling involves the desire to return and to achieve that, which was lost. It is a dance between the sadness of what is missing and the hope to reach it again. Spanish theologian, Andres Torres Queiruga rejected any interpretation of *Saudade* as static. For Queiruga it displays an intrinsic, dynamic orientation to the roots of existence. He says there is a progression in which you go deeper and intensify in its experience. This explains the tendency of *Saudade* to occupy the whole psychic life of the person experiencing it. The completion coincides directly with the openness inherent in *Saudade* to the Transcendent.[49]

I have incorporated different ways of using Bossa Nova to the music therapy sessions. When I have an encounter with a patient who is in pain or in a state of anxiety I visualize the intervention in three stages:

1) Anxiety, pain. LOSS. *Musically match the situation.*
2) Transition. DESIRE. *Entrain-deep breathing.*

Latin American Music and Repertoire with Pain and Chemotherapy

3) Relaxation. TRANSCENDENCE. *Achieve relaxation and access inner resource.*

In the first stage, I emphasize the rhythmic syncopation of the bossa nova, to connect with the patient's psychological and physiological state: matching the rhythm of their agitation and superficial breathing. When we are perfectly synchronized we move into the transition stage. The rhythmic pattern becomes de-emphasized, leaving sonic space for the melodic pattern produced by the voice. Initially, the vocal melodic phrases are short and become progressively longer to encourage deepening of respiration. I demonstrate the deepening of the breath through exaggerated inhalation followed by lengthening Bossa Nova phrases. When the patient achieves a state of relaxation, the melodies contain maximum duration, deepest breath, and a whispered voice. In this moment, chord variations are minimal and the guitar suspends the sense of defined rhythm.

Anxiety and pain are experienced when there is a loss of health. It is the loss of a state that once existed. Patients are aware of how they used to be. There exists a desire to achieve it again. There is a direct link to the definition of *Saudade* and this same feeling is reflected in Bossa Nova.

"Rosa"
The following case involves the use of Bossa Nova within a music therapy intervention known as Story Song, created by Dr. Joanne Loewy. The technique provides a forum in which the patient creates a story while the music therapist improvises music, which reflects the patient's feelings and experiences pertaining to the themes of the created story. One of the important features of Story Song is to lead your patient to a therapeutic end; a place that is healthy and safe.[50]

Rosa, a 47-year-old female, newly diagnosed with stage III breast cancer, reported only a brief medical history of having undergone knee surgery as a younger adult. She had been born in Puerto Rico, but raised in New York City, and was a single parent of two sons. The oldest of her sons was diagnosed with Down syndrome, and the youngest was attending college outside of New York City. The first day I met Rosa, I was working in the Infusion Suite at St. Luke's Roosevelt Hospital. I had been working with another patient when a nurse approached to inform me that there was a patient in the smallest infusion room crying and experiencing high levels of anxiety. It was her first day of chemotherapy treatment and all the fears had come to her in the form of an emotional avalanche.

During my assessment session with Rosa, she told me her worries were about how the treatment would affect her and if her physical condition would allow her to keep taking care of her oldest son. The most stressful part of the treatment was, "Not being able to resume my typical life," and experiencing hair loss. After several sessions working on procedural support and relaxation, Rosa recounted the feelings she'd had the day she found out about her cancer. She said,

> "When you find that you have cancer, you go through so many stages. "Why me?" "How could this happen?" "My children. My family. "When you are alone at home and you think about the whole journey (She commonly referred to her breast cancer and the healing process as a "journey"), you could sit there and think about the same things for hours. Thinking about...Oh my God! You're gonna die soon, this is what's gonna happen."

After listening to her, I suggested that she could make a journey from her home, her own concept of an ideal place; a place where she could be safe, secure, and calm. The goal of the Story Song was to help her connect with her fears, support her in the moment, and provide her with sensations of movement and transition in order to reinforce her existing strengths. This gave her an internal anchor, which provided an emotional safety net for her to confront and walk through the trauma of cancer diagnosis.

I distributed the instruments around her and invited her to close her eyes while imagining her home. I asked her to remove from her home all the things she did not like or made her feel uncomfortable. I told her it could be an idea, feeling, sensation, decoration, association, or place. I gave her space, in the form of silence, to think and feel about what this might be for her. Rosa began to cry. She opened her eyes and told me the following:

> "When I found out that I have... (She didn't ever use the word, "cancer") I was in this journey: my son went to college. Before he went the conversation was about everything, it was vast, it was important. So now that he left and I'm going through this I don't talk a lot the way I do. I don't converse the way I do."

After her disclosure, Rosa wanted to remove the lack of conversation from her home. I asked her to look at the instruments pick up the one she thought represented this concept. Rosa took the djembe. She picked this instrument, as she explained to me, because, "If you don't play it, it wasn't going to make any sound or noise." She played it for nearly the entire song.

I put her words into an improvised song and enhanced them with a harmonic chord progression found in the Bossa Nova style. I used this music style to lead her story and used the Remo ocean drum to entrain to her breathing pattern. I wanted to give her the sensation of *Saudade;* by addressing something that she missed and connect her at the same time with the desire and ability to achieve it again.

Rosa's Story Song "journey" occurred in a boat. From this boat, she described a blue-green sea similar to the one she remembered as a child in Puerto Rico. She connected with a memory when she was young. Rosa's family used to go to the beach. She liked to swim a lot and did not pay attention to how the conditions of the sea changed every day. Her mother used to tell her "Rosa, watch out because the sea is treacherous." I captured this sentiment by using some chords that represented the feeling of a "treacherous sea".

Finally our boat arrived at an island. Rosa described it as "Beautiful" and "Where the waves come in and out but you cannot hear it. The waves don't make noise." At this point in her imagery, she decided to make a hole and to bury the lack of conversation. She laid down in silence and relaxed. It was the first time that she experienced the sensation of calm after she started, this "Journey." Following Rosa's completion of relaxation, I continued playing the Bossa Nova improvisation, entraining the rhythm with the depth of her breathing; extending the sensations of relaxation that she reached.

Conclusion:
Thoughts for Future Work

The pain experience is influenced by beliefs, culture, and emotional states. It is only through an integrative team approach to treatment, that all aspects of suffering can be addressed. Music therapy has been found to be an effective modality to incorporate into pain treatment plans. It has the potential to reach the psychological, physiological, social, and spiritual needs of patients.

The field of the music therapy naturally extends the reaches of therapeutic work to new depths in appreciating the importance of multicultural perspectives. Still, further research is needed to deepen understanding of cultural identity and the treatment of pain and anxiety through music therapy intervention. As Even Ruud wrote:

> Music therapist must have a musical cultural understanding, a deep respect for the individual or idiosyncratic and sometimes sub-cultural representation of music. If they do not, they reduce themselves to suppliers of a new language or a new model through which the client may rewrite her experiences. This in turn deprives the client of the chance to live

as deeply as possible through her own preverbal experiences of music.[27(p.24)]

References

1. Morales E. *Ritmo Latino: la música latina desde la bossa nova hasta la salsa.* Barcelona: Robinbook; 2006:12-16.
2. Davidhizar R, Giger JN. A review of the literature on care of clients in pain who are culturally diverse. *Int Nurs Rev.* 2004; 51(1):47-55.
3. IOM (Institute of Medicine). Relieving pain in America: A blueprint for transforming prevention, care, education, and research. Washington, D.C.: The Nation Academies Press; 2011.
4. Velikova G, Selby pJ, Snaith PR, et al. The relationship of cancer pain to anxiety. [abstract]. *Psychother Psychosom.* 1995; 63(3-4):181-184. http://www.ncbi.nlm.nih.gov/pubmed/7624464?dopt=Abstract. Accessed July 10, 2012. PMID:7624464.
5. Glover J, Dibble SL, Dodd MJ, Miaskowki C. Mood states of oncology outpatients: Does pain make a difference? *J Pain Symptom Manage.* 1995; 10(2):120-128. http://www.ncbi.nlm.nih.gov/pubmed?term=%5B6%5D%20Glovr%20J%2C%20Dibble%20SL%2C%20Dodd%20MJ%2C%20Miaskowki%20C.%20Mood%20states%20of%20oncology%20outpatients%3A%20Does%20pain%20make%20a%20diffeence%3F%20J%20Pain%20Symptom%20Manage.%201995%3B%2010(2)%3A120-8.%20%20. Accessed July 11, 2012. PMID:7730684.
6. Passik SD, Kirsh KL, Rosenfeld B, McDonald MV, Theobald DE. The changeable nature of patients' fears regarding chemotherapy: Implications for palliative care. *J Symptom Manage.* 2001; 21(2):113-120. http://www.ncbi.nlm.nih.gov/pubmed/11226762. Accessed July 11, 2012. PMID: 11226762.
7. Kwekkeboom KL, Cherwin CH, Lee JW, Wanta B. Mind-body treatments for the pain-fatigue-sleep disturbance symptom cluster in persons with cancer. *J Pain Symptom Manage.* 2010; 39(1):126-38. http://www.ncbi.nlm.nih.gov/pmc/articles/PMC3084527/?tool=pubmed. Accessed July 12, 2012. PMCID:PMC3084527
8. Dhingra L, Shuk E, Grossman B, Strada A, Wald E, Portenoy A, et al. A qualitative study to explore psychological distress and illness burden associated with opioid-induced contipation in cancer patients with advanced disease [abstract published online ahead of print June 25 2012]. *Palliat Med.* 2012.

9. Stein KD, Syrjala KL, Andrykowski M. Physical and psychological long-term and late effects of cancer. *Cancer.* 2008; 112(11 Suppl):2577-2592. http://www.ncbi.nlm.nih.gov/pubmed/18428205. Accessed July 11, 2011. PMID:18428205.

10. Kowal J, Wilson KG, McWilliams LA, Peloquin K, Duong D. Self-perceived burden in chronic pain: Relevance, prevalence, and predictors [abstract published online ahead of print June 13 2012]. *Pain.* 2012. http://www.ncbi.nlm.nih.gov/pubmed/22703692. Accessed July 8, 2012. PMID:22703692.

11. Davis-Ali SH, Chesler MA, Chesney BK. Recognizing cancer as a family disease: Worries and support reported by patients and spouses. *Soc Work Health Care.* 1993; 19(2):45-65. http://www.ncbi.nlm.nih.gov/pubmed/8153845. Accessed July 12, 2012. PMID:8153845.

12. Lambert SD, Jones BL, Girgis A, Lecathelinais C. Distressed partners and caregivers do not recover easily: Adjustment trajectories [abstract published online ahead of print June 28 2012]. *Ann Behav Med.* 2012. http://www.ncbi.nlm.nih.gov/pubmed/22740365. Accessed July 8, 2012. PMID:22740365.

13. Linden W, Vodermaier A, Mackenzie R, Greig D. Anxiety and depression after cancer diagnosis: Prevalence rates by cancer type, gener, and age [abstract published online ahead of print June 20 2012]. *J Affect Disord.* 2012. http://www.ncbi.nlm.nih.gov/pubmed/22727334. Accessed July 8, 2012. PMID:22727334.

14. Bisson JI, Chubb HL, Bennett S, Mason M, Jones D, Kynaston H. The prevalence and predictors of psychological distress in patients with early localized prostate cancer. *BJU Int.* 2002; 90(1):56-61. http://www.ncbi.nlm.nih.gov/pubmed/12081771. Accessed July 8, 2012. PMID:12081771.

15. Heidari Gorji MA, Bouzar Z, Haghashenas M, Kasaeevan AA, Sadeghi MR, Didehdar Ardebil M. Quality of life and depression in caregivers of patients with breast cancer. BMC Res Notes. 2012; 5: 310.

16. Hartl K, Engel J, Herschbach P, Reinecker H, Sommer H, Friese K. Personality traits and psychosocial stress: Quality of life over 2 years following breast cancer diagnosis and psychological impact-

factors. Psycho-Oncology. 2010; 19(2):160-169. http://www.ncbi.nlm.nih.gov/pubmed/19189279. Accessed July 9, 2012. PMID:19189279.

17. Magill L. The use of music therapy to address the suffering in advanced cancer pain. *J Paliat Care*. 2001; 17(3):167-172. http://www.ncbi.nlm.nih.gov/pubmed/11816757. Accessed July 12, 2012. PMID: 11816757.

18. Kwan M. Music therapists' experiences with adults in pain: Implications for clinical practice. *Qualitative Inquiries in Music Therapy*. 2010; 5:43-85. http://www.barcelonapublishers.com/QIMTV5/Kwan(2010)QIMT5(2)43-85.pdf. Accessed July 11, 2012.

19. Igawa-Silva W, Wu S, Harrigan R. Music and cancer pain management [abstract]. *Hawaii Med J*. 2007; 66(11):292-295. http://www.ncbi.nlm.nih.gov/pubmed/18065118. Accessed July 8, 2012. PMID:18065118.

20. Hanser S. Music therapy in adult oncology: research issues [abstract]. *J Soc Integr Oncol*. 2006; 4(2):62-66. http://www.ncbi.nlm.nih.gov/pubmed/19442337. Accessed July 12, 2012. PMID:194422337.

21. Magill L. Role of music therapy in integrative oncology [abstract]. *J Soc Integr Oncol*. 2006; 4(2):79-81. http://www.ncbi.nlm.nih.gov/pubmed/19442341. Accessed July 11, 2012. PMID:19442341.

22. Richardson MM, Babiak-Bazquez Ae, Frenkel MA. Music therapy in a comprehensive cancer center. *J Soc Integr Oncol*. 2008; 6(2):76-81. http://www.ncbi.nlm.nih.gov/pubmed/18544287. Accessed July 12, 2012. PMID:18544287.

23. Ferrer AJ. The effect of live music on decreasing anxiety in patients undergoing chemotherapy treatment [abstract]. *J Music Ther*. 2007; 44(3):242-255. http://www.ncbi.nlm.nih.gov/pubmed/17645387. Accessed July 12, 2012. PMID:17645287.

24. Tan X, Yowler CJ, Super DM, Fratianne RB. The efficacy of music therapy protocols for decreasing pain, anxiety, and muscle tension levels during burn dressing changes: a prospective randomized crossover trial. *J Burn Care Res*. 2010; 31(4):590-597. http://www.ncbi.nlm.nih.gov/pubmed/20498613.Accessed July 13, 2012. PMID:20498613.

25. Mahon EM, Mahon SM. Music therapy: a valuable adjunct in the oncology setting. *Clinical Journal of Oncology Nurings*. 2011;

15(4):353-356. http://www.ncbi.nlm.nih.gov/pubmed/21810567. Accessed July 13, 2012. PMID:21810567.
26. Garro LC. Culture, pain and cancer. *Journal of Palliative Care.* 1990; 6(3):34-44. http://psycnet.apa.org/psycinfo/1991-10306-001. Accessed July 13, 2012.
27. Ruud E. *Music Therapy: Improvisation, Communication, and Culture.* Gilsum, NH: Barcelona Publishers. 1994.
28. Population Reference Bureau (PRB), The Changing Demographics of Roman Catholics. Available at: http://www.prb.org/articles/2005/thechangingdemographicsofromancatholics.aspx Accesed July 15, 2012.
29. Juarez G, Ferrell B, Borneman T. Influence of culture on cancer pain management in Hispanic patients [abstract]. *Cancer Pract.* 1998; 6(5):262-9. http://www.ncbi.nlm.nih.gov/pubmed?term=Juarez%2C%20G.%2C%20Ferrell%2C%20B.%2C%20%26%20Borneman%2C%20T.%20(1998).%20Influence%20of%20culture%20on%20cancer%20pain%20management%20in%20Hispanic%20patients.%20Cancer%20Practice%20Suppl.%206(5)%3A%20262-269. Accessed July 13, 2012. PMID: 9767344.
30. [28] Juarez G, Ferrell B, Borneman T. Perceptions of quality of life in Hispanic patients with cancer. *Cancer Pract.* 1998; 6(6):318-324. doi: 10.1046/j.1523-5394.1998.006006318.x. Accessed July 13, 2012.
31. Wildes KA, Miller AR, de Majors SS, Ramirez AG. The religiosity/spirituality of Latina breast cancer survivors and influence on health-related quality of life [abstract]. *Psychooncology.* 2009; 18(8):831-840. http://www.ncbi.nlm.nih.gov/pubmed/19034922. Accessed July 13, 2012. PMID:19034922.
32. Ashing-Giwa KT, Padilla G, Tejero J, Kraemer J, Wright K, Coscarelli A, et al. Understanding the breast cancer experience of women: a qualitative study of African American, Asian American, Latina and Caucasian cancer survivors [abstract]. *Psychooncology.* 2004; 13(6): 408-428. http://www.ncbi.nlm.nih.gov/pubmed/15188447. Accessed July 13, 2012. PMID:15188447.
33. Campesino M, Schwartz GE. Spirituality Among Latinas/os Implications of Culture in Conceptualization and Measurement. *ANS Adv Nurs Sci.* 2006; 29(1):69-81.
34. Central Intelligence Agency CIA. Field Listing: Religions. Available at:

https://www.cia.gov/library/publications/the-world-factbook/fields/2122.html Accesed July 15, 2012.

35. Baron RA, Byrne D. *Psicología Social*. 8th ed. Madrid: Prentice Hall Iberia;1998.

36. Levine EG, Yoo G, Ewing C, Au A. Ethnicity and spirituality in breast cancer survivors [abstract]. *BioBehavioral Journal of Cancer Survivors* 2007; 1(3):212-25. http://www.ncbi.nlm.nih.gov/pubmed/18648972. Accessed July 11, 2012. PMID:18648972.

37. PDQ Cancer Information Summaries [Internet]. Bethesda (MD): National Cancer Institute (US). [date unknown]. Spirituality in Cancer Care (PDQ). 2003. http://www.ncbi.nlm.nih.gov/books/NBK66000/. Accessed July 11, 2012.

38. Davidhizar R, Giger JN. A Review of the literature on care of clients in pain who are culturally diverse. *Int Nurs Rev.* 2004; 51(1):47-55.

39. King J. *The Cambridge Companion to Modern Latin American Culture*. 8th ed. Cambridge: Cambridge University Press; 2004.

40. Olsen DA, Sheehy DE. *The Garland HandBook of Latin American Music*. vol. 1. 2nd ed. New York: Routledge Taylor & Francis Group; 2008:53.

41. Wong-Baker Faces Pain Rating Scale. Wong-Baker Faces Foundation. 1983. Available at: http://www.wongbakerfaces.org/. Accessed July 14th, 2012.

42. Baumann E, Cornejo D, Vecco P. Escuela de ángeles D1: la danza como alternativa para el crecimiento psíquico. *Transiciones 15: Revista de la Asociación Peruana de Psicoterapia Psicoanalítica de Niños y Adolescentes*. 2010; 15:169-176.

43. Mantra. Collins English Dictionary Complete & Unabridged 10th Edition. http://dictionary.reference.com/browse/mantra. Accessed July 10, 2012.

44. Pochmursky C. *The Musical Brain* [DVD]. Canada: National Geographic; 2009.

45. Austin D. *The theory and practice of vocal psychotherapy: Songs of the self*. London: Jessica Kingsley Publishers; 2008.

46. Loewy J. Tonal Intervallic Synthesis in Medical Music Therapy. In Baker S, Uhlig Eds. *Voicework in Music Therapy: Research and Practice*. London: Jessica Kingsley Publishers; 2011:252-268.

47. Loewy J. Music psychotherapy assessment. *Music Therapy Perspectives*. 2000;18(1):47-58.

48. Castro R. *Bossa Nova. La historia y las historias.* Ed. Madrid:Turner Publicaciones S.L.; 2008:158.
49. Queiruga AT, Piñeiro R. *Nova Aproximación a Unha Filosofía de Saudade: Discruso Lido Na Recepción Pública de 20 de Xuño Do 1980.* Ed. Galicia:Artes Gráficas;1981.
50. Loewy J, Stewart K. Music therapy to help traumatized children and caregivers. In N. Boyd Webb Ed, Mass trauma and violence: Helping families and children cope. New York: Guilford Publications, Inc.; 2004:191-215.
51. Kattari K. Building Pan-Latino Unity in the United States through Music: An Exploration of Commonalities Between Salsa and Reggaeton. *Musicological Explorations.* 2009; 10. http://journals.uvic.ca/index.php/me/article/view/149/181. Accesed July 11, 2012.

Music and Medicine: Integrative Models in the Treatment of Pain

APPENDIX

Basic Latin American Rhythms and Genres

Bossa Nova
Bossa nova is a Spanish music style from Brazil. It is a fusion of samba with elements of jazz. It is played with nylon string guitar, sung in Portuguese, contains syncopated rhythms, long phrases, and incorporates major and minor 7th chords, with extensions typical from jazz. Typically bossa nova is played on the guitar without a pick with the fingers, which alternate between bass with the thumb and the higher strings. The percussion is not considered essential to the style, but is sometimes added by tapping the body of the guitar with a two-bar rhythmic pattern, the first bar offset and the second in time. "The Girl From Ipanema." is typical example of Bossa Nova.

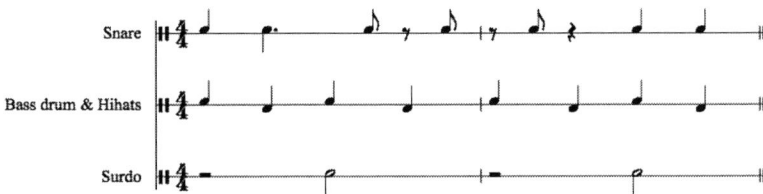

Bolero
Bolero music is slow romantic music, which originated in Spain. It is more popular among the older generations of Latin Americans, and it was widespread through the whole continent. It is played often on acoustic guitars, and bongos. The güiro often plays 8th notes. Famous *Trios* like "Los Panchos" were famous since 1940, and its music can still be heard in some radio stations. *"Bésame Mucho"* is a good example of bolero. Two Basic Bolero rhythm examples:

Bachata
Bachata originates in Dominican Republic, and has influence mostly from bolero, but also from merengue, and son, among others. It is usually played with less instruments than salsa; guitars, güira, bass and bongos the most common. The second guitar, called *segunda* has the task to add syncopation to the music, while the fist guitar plays arpeggiated chords. Themes usually are romantic, but also can be of heartbreak or sadness. *"Me Enamoré"* by Anthony Santos is a good example of how this music souds. Bachata is

music for dancing, and has it's own dance style. Basic bachata rhythmic pattern on bongos and güira:

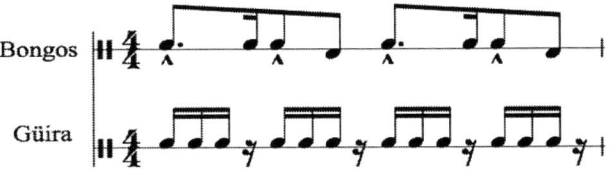

Salsa
Salsa music was originally from Cuba, but was also largely developed in Puerto Rico by Puerto Ricans and Cubans in New York City. It is played by ensembles and it has very complex rhythms. Pianos, trumpets, trombones, bass, guitar, flute, and other instruments play the melodic part of the songs, while the rhythmic section is divided between the bongos, timbales, congas, claves and güiro. One of the key elements is to listen the "Clave". Piano usually plays a rhythm that originated in Cuba, called Montuno, while the Bass plays the Tumbao. Themes can vary from very simple romantic music, to very radical political subjects. Song structures often include a verse and a "call and response" chorus, where the whole orchestra answers to the singer's lyrics. "Son" is a Cuban music genre that influenced many of the elements found in salsa, considered one of its roots. Some of the most popular salsa artist are: Hector Lavoe, Ruben Blades, Fania All-Stars, Eddie Palmieri, Willie Colón and Celia Cruz, among others. "La Vida es un Carnaval" by Celia Cruz is a good example, this song speaks about being happy even through the bad times. Here's an example of the clave, bongo's and the bass "tumbao":

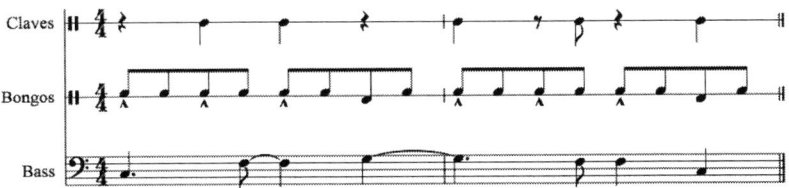

Merengue
Merengue music was originated in the Caribbean, mostly in Dominican Republic, but is popular in nearly every Latin American country. Merengue is often faster than salsa and played by smaller orchestras. Bongo, claves, güira, tambora (drum), trumpet, bass, and guitar are some of the common instruments. Breaks often mark the begging of the chorus, which usually has a call answer form. It is music that people usually dance to, and the themes found in lyrics are usually romantic. However, contemporary artist Juan

Music and Medicine: Integrative Models in the Treatment of Pain

Luis Guerra sings about his Christian spirituality. "Me Enamoro de Ella" by Juan Luis Guerra is a good example of genre:

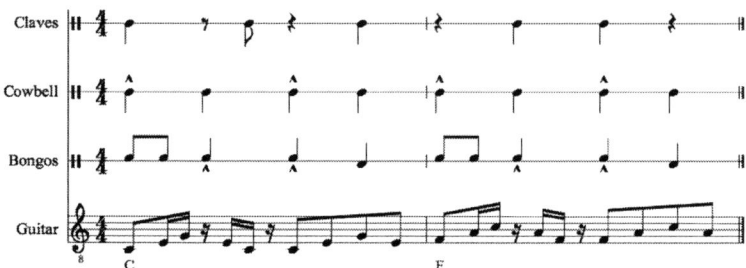

Reggaeton
Reggaeton music is very popular among young Latin Americans.[51] It is the result of many fusions, and also contains influences from hip-hop and rap. This music often uses loops and samples played with the characteristic "Dem Bow" rhythm, which provides an easy structure for lyric improvisation. The structures of this songs are very similar to hip-hop; containing a melodic chorus alternating with rap verses. The themes of this genre commonly speak about sexuality or neighborhood pride and often demonstrate explicit lyrics. Reaggeton rhythm ("Dem Bow") can be played on melodic instruments in a I, II and iii progression such as C, D and Em, using the single low notes for the bass and higher notes for the snare:

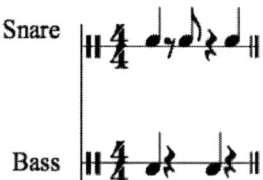

Ranchera
Ranchera is a traditional Mexican music genre, associated often with the mariachis. Originally it was sung by one singer and a guitar, but currently it is commonly played with guitar, vihuela (5 string Mexican guitar), trumpet, violin and guitarrón (as bass). The basic rhythmic figure is a syncopated triplet with a steady bass, and it has influence from bolero, waltz and polka. Even though this genre is associated with the Mexican culture, it is also popular in other countries. Themes are often romantic or patriotic and have melodic vocal parts. Some of the most popular artists are Pedro Infante,

Latin American Music and Repertoire with Pain and Chemotherapy

Javier Solís, Vicente Fernandez, among many others. Mexicans often sing "Las Mañanitas" at birthdays and other celebrations. "Cielito Lindo" is also a popular song and a good example of the genre. Ranchera rhythmic chord progression:

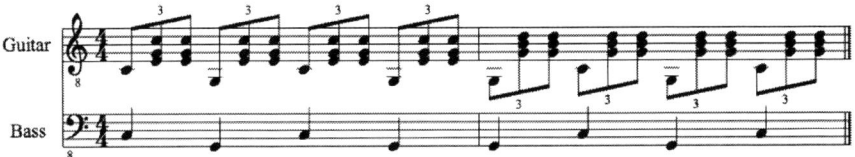

Tango

Tango music is from Argentina and Uruguay. It is the fusion of European influences, like the polka, and the waltz, and some of the traditional Argentinean rhythms. It became a worldwide phenomenon in the 1930's, before that it was originally associated with the lower class of Buenos Aires. Tango has a marked rhythm and intense melodies. It is played usually by a six-piece band, with violin, piano, guitar, flute and bandoneón (concertina like instrument). Carlos Gardel is one of the most famous artists in the genre. "Mi Buenos Aires querido" is a traditional song of the genre. Basic tango rhythm:

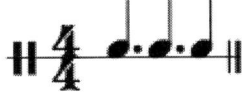

Rumba

Rumba (flamenca) is a music genre from Spain. It's one of the music styles of flamenco. It is played with acoustic guitars and the rhythm is marked by clapping, cajón, and castañuelas. The band know worldwide for playing this kind of music is, The Gipsy Kings. Their song, "volaré" is classic example. The rhythmic guitar can be very complex and rumba players often clap on their guitars. A good chord progression to begin with this rhythm is Am/G/F/E. Rumba rhythm:

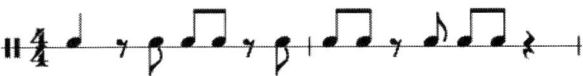

CHAPTER 24

Confronting a Different Great Wall: Using Environmental Music Therapy to Provide Psychoemotional Support for Asian and Asian-American Patients in a Radiation Oncology Waiting Room

Thomas J. Biglin, Jr. MA, MT-BC
Yi-Ying Lin MA, MT-BC

"*Music makes the blood flow, frees the spirit, and inspires a positive mind.*"[1(p162)]
Shi-Ji (Book of Odes)

Introduction

This chapter recounts the reflections of two music therapists on their implementation of Environmental Music Therapy (EMT) during a clinical internship. The context for this work is within a radiation oncology suite serving a demographically heterogeneous population of patients including patients of Asian and Asian-American heritage. EMT involves applying a therapist's clinical intuition to provide music in order to create a healing environment for all within the space. To further clarify the technique of EMT, we thought it best to reference the words of Andrew Rossetti, MMT, MT-BC, the music therapist at Beth Israel who had been our primary mentor and guide in using EMT within this suite:

> *Environmental Music Therapy seeks to create an integrative healing environment by combining the needs and state of patients, caregivers and staff in an interactive soundscape constructed in such a way as to incorporate ambient noise as well as visual and aural clues from those present in a music experience that may reduce stress responses and is conducive to more positive mood states. Given that in this particular music therapy strategy individuals and individual elements are incorporated in the intervention, it may be viewed as a "multi-individual therapy" rather than a "group therapy" concept.*[2(p30)]

Music and Medicine: Integrative Models in the Treatment of Pain

When we would conduct an EMT session in the radiation oncology waiting room at Beth Israel Comprehensive Cancer Care Center – West Campus (BI West), we would consider *everyone* in the room to be a recipient of music therapy, not simply the individual undergoing medical treatment. By no means does this minimize the significance of the physical and psychoemotional pain for each particular patient with cancer receiving treatment. However, the individual's caregivers and other family members, as well as the numerous staff members present—medical doctors, nurse, radiation specialists, social workers, administrators, volunteers, and, yes, music therapists—are all capable of being affected by the environment and therefore have the potential for being aided therapeutically by a conscious adjustment of the room's sonic landscape or *soundscape*.

While there has been a great deal of information about pathology and pathophysiology of pain,[3] we would like to address what we very often worked with in our EMT sessions: namely, psychoemotional pain. Specifically, how people of different cultures may relate to their pain and to our roles as music therapists in helping them with their pain.

In finance, the term *Chinese wall* refers to "the ethical barrier between different divisions of a financial (or other) institution to avoid conflict of interest."[4] While learning to apply EMT to a diverse population, which included people of Chinese descent, two music therapy interns—one Asian, one Caucasian—used music as a therapeutic modality as well as a means of communication to help navigate the cultural and linguistic barriers that sometimes separated us from these recipients of EMT. And, in the process, occasionally, a few bricks in the wall were removed.

Exploration of Asian Culture

In the Chinese culture and in traditional Chinese medicine, the mind, body, spirit, and nature are seen as united and interrelated. Eastern philosophies of Buddhism, Taoism, and traditional Chinese medicine adopt a holistic conceptualization of an individual and his or her environment.[5(p15)]

Holistic View of Mind and Body

From Chinese medicine's perspective, the mind and body are considered inseparable; and pain is mostly related to poor blood/air circulation, which might be induced by emotion. This holistic view has been referenced in several ancient Chinese classics.[1,5,6] More than two thousand years ago, the earliest Chinese medical book *Huang-Di-Nei-Jing*[1(p63)] (黃帝內經) had mentioned that changes of moods are closely related to the organs. Each mood is dominated by a specific organ. "Heart rules happiness; liver dictates anger; spleen dominates thought, lungs control worry; kidneys decide fear."[1(p63)] In addition, Chinese medicine claims that emotions may affect blood flow. Blood flows when breath is flowing, and the directions of breath flow are decided by emotions. "Breath is flowing up when one is angry; going down when one is fearful; disturbing when one is startled; vanishing when one is sad; condensing when one is thinking; and relaxing when one is happy."[1(p69)] Therefore, the priority of healing cancer is increasing happiness and improving the quality of life.[1(p111)]

Similarly, the emphasis on mind-body balance was also mentioned in the Chinese Philosophy Classic *Analects of Confucius*. "In the late spring after new clothes are made, gather a group of adults along with some children to go hiking, bathing in the riverside and enjoying the breeze on the mountain slope, and then singing along on the way home."[6(p6)] One's health can be achieved when the life is not under too much stress and the tension can be released through developing suitable interests.[6(p6)] Therefore, medical treatment cannot be set outside of mind-body care.

Music, Body, and Mind

Among various paths for easing pain and achieving mind-body health, the effect of music was emphasized in the Chinese ancient classics as well. In *Analects of Confucius*, Confucius once listened to the music composed by legendary ruler Shun and was completely captivated by it. The beauty of the music made him forget the taste of food. He said, "I did not think listening to the music could actually make me reach this level of happiness." Another Chinese ancient classic, *Shi-Ji* (Book of Odes) also recorded "Music makes the blood flow, frees the spirit, and inspires a positive mind."[1(p162)] This shows the power of music that makes people forget about physical sensations and promotes the spirit.

In addition, *Huang-Di-Nei-Jing* proposed the concepts of "Penta-tone Therapy." The penta-tone means the five notes in traditional Chinese music. They are gong (宮), shāng (商), jue (角), zhǐ (徵), yǔ (羽). Comparing the five notes to the modern Western scale, it can be approximately interpreted as Do, Re, Mi, Sol, La. The idea of Penta-tone Therapy was based on the Statement of Five Elements (五行), which posits that patients' emotions can be categorized into five elements found in nature: metal represents sadness, wood stands for anger, water reflects despair, fire shows irritability, and earth illustrates isolation. Furthermore, those five notes correspond to the five elements as well: gong for earth, shāng for metal, jue for wood, zhǐ for fire, and yǔ for water. Therefore, in order to maximize the effects of music, selection of music should consider the listener's elemental characteristics in order to create a shift in an existing mood state.[1(pp163-164)]

Music and Medicine: Integrative Models in the Treatment of Pain

Emotional Expression

> The Chinese family came in to the waiting room. We had already seen this Chinese family three times before. The patient was an elderly man, perhaps in his 80s. The first time, there were five additional people accompanying him to the hospital, and the second and the third time we saw the patient, he was with two other different family members. They did not speak in Mandarin so I could not be absolutely sure of their nationality, but they always brought a paper bag with Chinese characters printed on it. Today, the elderly man came with two younger-middle-aged females. Usually while he was waiting, the accompanying family members would be chatting, but this time he did not join the conversation. He just waited quietly. Following the tempo and style that had been established, I strived to make a connection with them by playing the Chinese tune and attempted to make eye contact. However, they seemed to avoid any kind of connection with the whole environment. They did not make eye-contact with anyone in the waiting room, nor respond to the environment or music through their body language. It seemed like they felt more comfortable only being in their "family circle." Thus, I did not try to make further connection with them. We respected them and left space for them to be where they were in the moment. Maybe that was the best way to react with them then– just wait for them until they felt emotionally ready for more interactions. We then continued with the EMT session, playing a new piece.
>
> ~ Extracted from Yi-Ying's log

Patients with cancer often suffer from pain. However, feeling pain does not only relate to physical sensations, it also connects to challenging psychological factors. Sometimes, mild discomfort might be exacerbated due to mental distress. Many traditional Asian and Asian-Americans tend to describe their emotional pain through somatic complaints according to their holistic view of mind and body. This may also include possible shame towards emotional difficulties. Especially for Asian males, expressions of emotions are regarded as immature and demonstrative of out of control behaviors. Common descriptions for depression or feelings of sadness are boredom, discomfort, pain, dizziness, headaches, fatigue, restlessness, disturbances in sleep, and loss of appetite. It is worth noting that when working with Asian or Asian American patients, a direct focus on emotions might elicit negative reactions such as discomfort and shame. Therefore, the therapist should focus more on behaviors than on emotions, and acknowledge the patients' feelings in a more indirect manner.[7 (pp365-366)]

Popular Chinese Folk Songs with a Very Familiar Western Chord Progression

During the course of our EMT sessions, we were able to use a simple I-V-vi-IV-V structure in the key of C to play a very well-known contemporary folk/pop song that would be immediately recognizable to a broad demographic spectrum of Asian patients. Prior to playing the song for the first time with Yi-Ying, Tom had never heard it before. While he did not know the lyrics, and while he did not have any direct cultural relationship with the song, the song was very much a I-V-vi-IV-V structured piece, a chord progression very familiar to Western listeners. Tom was not able to understand any of the words of the song because he did not speak the Chinese language, but all of the chords fit on the fretboard of his guitar. He might not have been able to sing the lyrics with understanding, but he could play the chords and vocalize the melody. Although the song was selected by Yi-Ying to appeal to the Chinese patients who were in the waiting room at that moment, the appeal was not restricted to an Asian sensibility. We posit that, like Tom, the other Western patients in the waiting room could appreciate the melody and the aesthetic and emotional qualities of the song without understanding a single word.

What significance did this have for us as music therapists? And, more importantly, what effect did this have on all the patients in the waiting room? Clearly, while we cannot speak for each individual in the room, music's ability to cut through the difficulties of verbal language is one if its powerful and sublime characteristics. Leveraging music's *wordless communication*—even when involving sung lyrics—can be a powerful therapeutic tool for the music therapist, especially when working with EMT, where there is not necessarily much direct or active verbal engagement with the patients.

This is not to say that music therapists working with EMT do not *talk* with the patients. Nor does this mean that every Asian song will sound consonant or familiar to Western listeners. We know, from experience as music therapists, that there are various pentatonic, microtonal, and other scale patterns that are not familiar to many Westerners. Since our EMT involved a culturally mixed collection of individuals, we as the music therapists wanted and needed to incorporate music that would be effective for this disparate population. One of the sublime lessons Tom learned from his partner, Yi-Ying, occurred during her teaching him and their playing of that popular Chinese tune: Tom could play the music without understanding the words; he could experience an emotional connection to the piece without understanding its cultural significance; and, most importantly for our work in the radiation oncology waiting room, all the people in the room could be provided with music that could help adjust the soundscape of the environment for maximal therapeutic effect.

Sure, Yi-Ying might be able to converse with a particular patient and his/her caregivers if they were able to speak the same Chinese dialect. Just because everybody else in the waiting room, besides Tom, was Chinese did not mean that they could understand what each other was saying. People who only speak Cantonese, for instance, would not be able to easily understand those who spoke only Mandarin, if at all. And vice versa. This, combined with Tom's ability to say only "hello" ("nǐ hǎo") and "thanks" ("xièxie") in Mandarin, meant that he was prevented from engaging in a verbal dialogue with everyone else in the room. Tom was severely limited in his ability to introduce himself, to inquire how others were feeling, to ask for preferred styles of music or even a favorite song. However, the fact that he couldn't make himself understood verbally did not impede our effectiveness as music therapists using EMT. Mostly because of that middle letter, "M." The music was able to cut through the language barriers and establish a common foundation upon which to share ourselves with each other in the here and now. Music allowed us to talk to each other in ways that words couldn't.

While the focus on this chapter may rest upon patients of Asian descent, we included references to the other patients of non-Asian background who were also present, because it is important for the reader to appreciate the rich demographic background of people who comprise the radiation oncology waiting room. EMT, like the patients it treats, does not occur in a vacuum. During this span of time in the waiting room, before and after cancer treatment, patients of various cultures may interact, or at the very least, exist with each other. And so does the music we provide for them with EMT.

The following are some of the Asian musical elements that can be incorporated into EMT sessions with Asian patients:

Asian Scales
Asian music involves pentatonic sounds and emphasizes the variation on melody and rhythm. Different from Western music, Asian music has less emphasis on harmony. During EMT sessions, using various instruments while improvising music around these Asian scales with different rhythm usually offered diverse "flavors" to the atmosphere.

Environmental Music Therapy with Asian and Asian-American Patients

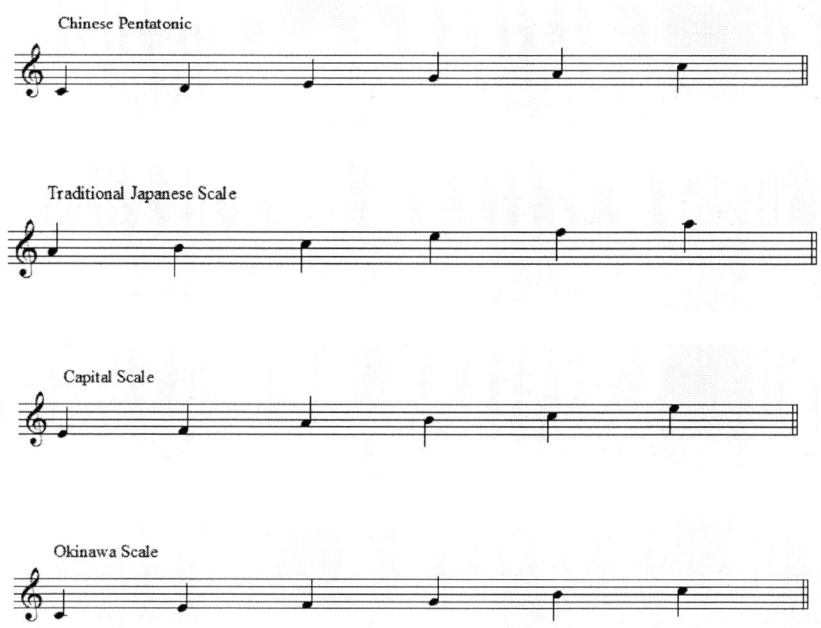

Asian Instruments

The ancient classification for Asian musical instruments was based on the materials called *eight sounds*: metal (金音), stone (石音), earth (土音), leather (革音), silk (絲音), wood (木音), gourd (匏音), and bamboo (竹音). As cultural exchanges became more frequent, instruments from Western culture were adapted to Asian music as well. Current classifications include percussion, wind instruments, plucked instruments, and bowed instruments. Some musical instruments are not strange to Western culture, such as: Chinese violin – *erhu*; bamboo flute – *dizi*; double-reed horn – *suona*; Asian lute – *pipa*, Japan Okinawa *shamisen*, Korean long drum – *taiko*, These Asian musical instruments' tuning can be coordinated with Western temperament. Therefore, applying Asian instruments when performing Western tunes is another feasible way to incorporate different cultures in one environment. While we did not have any native Asian instruments available to use during our EMT session, this would be something for other music therapists to strongly consider putting into practice as another method for helping bridge the Western-Asian cultural divide.

Music and Medicine: Integrative Models in the Treatment of Pain

Asian Tunes

During our EMT sessions we selected several Asian tunes that were most popular. While applying these tunes in EMT, music therapists do not have to stick to the suggested chord progressions written in the scores. Changing the meter, rhythm, styles, major/minor keys, as well as improvising around the themes, are highly recommended.

Chinese folk song *Jasmine Flower (*茉莉花*)*

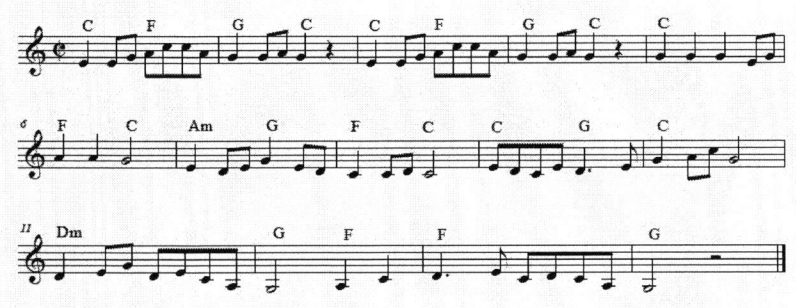

Excerpt from *Night Life in Shanghai (*夜上海*)*
Music by Chen, Ge-Xin; lyrics by Fan, Yan-Qiao; sang by Zhou; Xuan, released in 1946[8]

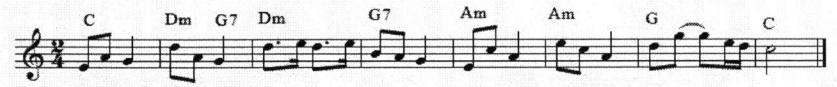

The following three excerpts are cross-generational, cross-nationality Chinese songs found widespread in Asian society, originally sung by the legendary Taiwanese singer Teresa Teng (1953-1995). She was popular in Taiwan, China, Hong Kong, Japan, and in the Chinese community in Southeastern Asia. During the Cold War period, her voice was the only common language able to pass through political barriers among the Chinese community. To this day, there are still many pop singers inspired by her songs who cover her music, thus continuing to spread the music's popularity throughout Asian communities. Since her songs are regarded as classics, they are usually first introduced to the Westerners who are interested in Asian pop music. Therefore, it is easy to evoke resonance from people with different cultural orientations by playing her songs.

Environmental Music Therapy with Asian and Asian-American Patients

Excerpt from *Wishing We Would Last Forever (但願人長久)*
Music by Liang, Hong-Zhi; Lyrics by Su, Shi

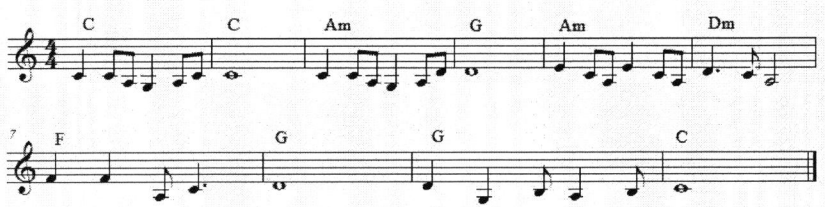

Excerpt from *The Moon Represents My Heart (月亮代表我的心)*
Music by Sun, Yi; lyrics by Weng, Qing-Xi, released in 1973[8]

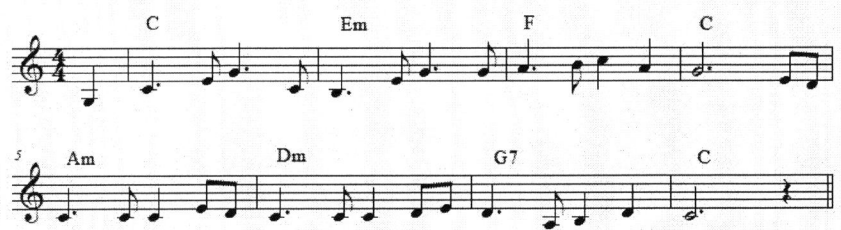

Excerpt from *I Only Care About You (我只在乎你)*
Music by Takashi Miji, lyrics by Shenzhi
In the Japanese version, the song is called 《时の流れに身をまかせ》

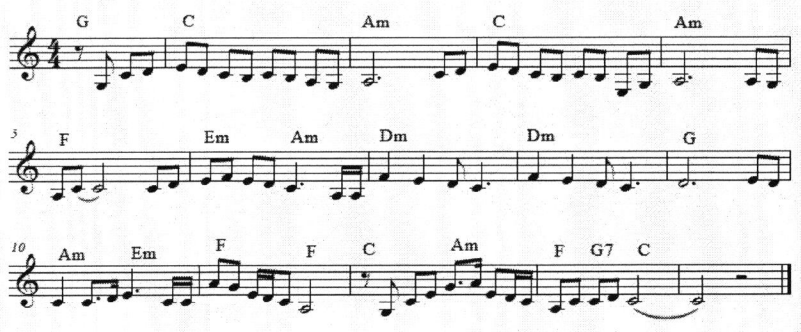

Music and Medicine: Integrative Models in the Treatment of Pain

Excerpts from EMT Sessions

Vignette 1: A Multicultural Focus

Perspectives from a Caucasian Music Therapist
Because of the nature of EMT, where direct verbal interaction isn't the primary focus, we therapists don't usually get to know the patients' names or their medical histories and diagnoses. Also, as previously mentioned, we consider everyone in the radiation treatment waiting room–where we conduct EMT–to be a recipient of music therapy. Whether they are the ones receiving radiation or the caregivers supporting them, everyone in the room contributes to the energy of the room and subsequently is a candidate for the therapeutic treatment we provide through EMT.

We began the first of two 45-minute weekly EMT sessions, as we usually did, with a warm-up song for the room. We liked to use a musical selection to make time to "take the temperature" of the room, and also give ourselves time to allow our clinical intuition to inform us what the various clients in the room may need from our music. This often involved an instrumental improvisation, mostly on an acoustic guitar, played at a moderate tempo and an *mp/mf* dynamic. I tended to play a fingerpicked arpeggiated chord pattern of Cmaj7-Am7-Dsus2-G6 with a legato rhythm and an *mp/mf* dynamic. While there is soothing quality to the melody, the rhythm and the fingerpicking allow for subtle shifts in dynamic and tempo to provide means for *tension and release* to the clients in the room. Yi-Ying would usually play her recorder or her chromatic harmonicas along with my guitar playing. Oftentimes, we took turns with the melody: Yi-Ying with her recorder or harmonicas, I on vocals.

On this day the sessions had two distinct energies, yet each was incredibly profound for us. During the first session, there was an elderly Chinese woman and a young boy around 8-10 years old who we presumed was her grandson in the waiting room. Once we started to play, especially once Yi-Ying started to play a popular Chinese folk song on her recorder and, later on, her harmonicas, both the grandmother and her grandson recognized the tune. They both gave us a smile and a look of recognition. The grandmother even began to sing along to the melody *sotto voce*. As Yi-Ying was playing a second Chinese folk song a Chinese man returned from the radiation rooms. Immediately upon hearing the tunes, he, too, smiled at us and sang along *sotto voce*. We suspected him to be the boy's father and the grandmother's son. Unfortunately, we were not able to confirm this before the family left for the day. It was energizing to be around a multi-generational Chinese family who was experiencing and sharing in familiar music of their homeland as played by Yi-Ying on her harmonicas and recorder. It was great to be able to be a part of this music making: Yi-Ying was able to describe to me the chords (C-Am-F-G) of this popular Chinese song. So while she played the melodies, I was able to provide arpeggiated finger picked and strummed rhythmic patterns on the acoustic guitar.

It was also wonderful to have a patient—"Michael," a pseudonym—actively engage in the music making by singing along with us, even harmonizing to the melodies of our songs. Michael had arrived sometime during the middle of the Chinese music that we were playing and sat down to Yi-Ying's immediate left. Michael, who was not Asian, warmed up rather quickly to the music we were playing. We noticed that Michael had started to tap his foot during one of our more upbeat selections, *Folsom Prison Blues*. In fact, there were a couple of other patients who were also tapping their feet and bobbing their heads in time with the music. Beyond the personal and professional satisfaction of feeling like were doing a "good job," it felt great to see that we were able to effect active responses from the patients in the room to our music. The patients were reacting in their own individual way to the environmental music therapy.

This personalized response to the music was further made manifest by the reaction of the middle-aged Latina during the second session. We had seen other patients during past sessions sometimes tear up and sniffle a bit while listening. One does not forget the primary reason all of these patients are here: they have cancer. But, this was different. While she wasn't wailing or sobbing loudly, this woman was crying more profusely than any other patient we had seen during our sessions to-date. While crying can provide a cathartic, physical benefit to the person, it also can be an emotionally upsetting event for that person and the others in the room—including the staff—who may have a difficult time with the highly personal display in such a public environment. It was also confusing because, being relatively new to EMT at the time, we weren't sure if we should stop playing immediately or continue—albeit respectfully and mindfully of what was unfolding. What happened was that once it was clear that this woman was becoming emotionally overwhelmed, one of the receptionists and a visiting volunteer moved to console her. The song having ended, Yi-Ying also crossed the room and knelt down in front of the woman to see how she was doing. I chose to remain where I was across the room and improvised a tune with similar chords to *Lean On Me*, but slightly more upbeat. I didn't want both of us to completely stop providing music and I didn't want to crowd the crying woman, who was already being attended to by three people. But also, I wanted to maintain a sense of continuity to what we had established thinking that it could provide some musical grounding for the rest of the room. What I was saying, through my guitar playing was, "I acknowledge that you're crying and seem to be upset. While I'm not

Music and Medicine: Integrative Models in the Treatment of Pain

exactly sure what you need at this moment, I would like for you to feel supported by this new music. I also want to let the rest of you sharing the space to know that we are here for you as music therapists and as human beings to offer support the best way we can: through our music and our presence."

At another point toward the end of our session, a middle-aged man of either African-American or perhaps Caribbean descent—"Ted," also a pseudonym—had seemed somewhat emotionally upset during the session but in a quiet, contained way. We had been playing and singing *Amazing Grace*, which was chosen mostly because of what was intuited from this gentleman. Yi-Ying had started off playing her recorder while I finger-picked the chords on my guitar; about midway through the piece I felt that our presence was too strong. I motioned a suggestion to Yi-Ying to cease playing the melody on her recorder. I shifted away from singing the lyrics and we simply hummed the melody with an *mp* dynamic. This just felt better to me because I sensed that this felt better to the gentleman. This is another example of a developing clinical intuition. After the song ended and we were packing up, I overhead the man tell the radiation technician that his father had just died and he was also feeling very apprehensive about the necessity for starting radiation treatment. The following week, this same gentleman approached me during one of our breaks and shared with me how our EMT sessions transformed significantly his time in radiation oncology into a more pleasant experience. He referred to his difficulties from last week and said that the work that we were doing helped him get through the day.

Perspectives from an Asian Music Therapist
When Tom and I went to BI West Radiation Oncology, there were a few people in the waiting area, including a Chinese woman and boy who looked to be a grandmother and grandson. We met the woman the previous week, and she seemed to remember us. She asked the boy to listen to us. When we took out the guitar, recorder, and the harmonica, the boy was visibly excited to see all these instruments and told us that his school also taught students how to play the recorder, but he had not learned it yet. Both the grandmother and the grandson paid attention to our preparation. I heard them speak in some kind of Chinese dialect, so I asked them from what part of China they came, and the grandmother answered, "Shanghai." Thus, I chose to start with the Chinese song *Night Life in Shanghai (夜上海)*. Immediately, the grandmother smiled and hummed along with the music when I played the

melody. I did not finish playing the whole song because I could not recall the chorus part, but the grandmother was still surprised and joyful. Then I picked the other Chinese song that was sung by Teresa Teng, the most famous singer in Chinese society. The grandmother knew this song very well and sang along to the entire piece. The grandmother and grandson applauded in the end of the song, and the other people in the waiting area also looked at us in a friendly manner.

Soon after playing the Chinese song, Tom and I shifted to a warm-up improvisation and then transitioned to other songs. Because of the interactions we had shared with the Chinese family, the other people in the waiting area—all non-Asian—now seemed to be paying more attention to us than had been the case earlier. It was obvious that some patients were really engaged in the music and were enjoying it, tapping their feet and giving us positive verbal feedback to show their appreciation. Some just made friendly, short eye contact with us and smiled, as did some of the staff who passed by frequently. I saw some patients and their families smiling, and hugging each other before leaving the radiation oncology waiting room

One patient—"Michael," a pseudonym—who introduced himself as Filipino, harmonized when Tom and I sang *Blowing in the Wind*. When the song ended, Michael said, "Hallelujah!," which led us to sing the song, *Hallelujah*, by Leonard Cohen. Michael knew the song too, and he harmonized to our vocals again. People applauded at the end of almost every song we sang and played, and Michael took an active role in some of these songs. He even sang the lyrics of *The Boxer* to an instrumental improvisation. This led to another Simon & Garfunkel song, *The Sounds of Silence*. He reported that the music had a therapeutic effect on him. He said he "came into the waiting room feeling heavy" but was now feeling "lighter."

Similar to Michael, the Chinese family who was involved in the beginning of the session now also paid closer attention to our playing. In addition to the first Chinese song I played earlier, I chose two other Chinese tunes and quickly wrote the chord progressions for Tom. I saw the Chinese boy was playing a video game and it gave me an idea to play a Chinese song, *Childhood (童年)* for him. While we played *Childhood*, the boy's father returned from his treatment room humming the tune with a smile on his face. The three of them left soon afterward, all with smiles on their faces.

Such involved participation by patients in the waiting area was unusual for our EMT sessions. In the beginning of the session, the Chinese family paid close attention to us even before we started making any music. The Chinese song provided a cultural connection, and seemed to create for them a warm feeling. However, we did not want to exclude the other people in the waiting area, so we also offered some familiar American pop songs. Interestingly, the Chinese family seemed to be a "role model" for the other people and in a way acted as a "catalyzer" between the therapists and the environment. Many other people in the waiting area showed the same behaviors (i.e., singing along, making eye contact, conversing with us), which seemed to raise the energy of the entire room.

Vignette 2: Negotiating Roles and Services

The radiation oncology waiting room is a milieu that hosts many tiers of caregivers including volunteers who give their time in serving others but who may also be fulfilling their own personal needs. The skill to negotiate the various roles is one that must be built by the music therapist through recognition of and empathy for these various underlying intentions, especially when they may be at cross purposes to the clinical applications of EMT.

Andrew accompanied us to BI West to observe our session and to provide supervision on our work, particularly concerning a recent challenge that had presented itself regarding a Chinese volunteer who had been scheduled simultaneously with EMT session. The volunteer's presence had become problematic during some of our recent sessions due to his talking quite loudly with the Asian patients he was assisting while the rest of the patients were awaiting treatment and taking in the music. We did not know whether or not the volunteer would be present during today's sessions, but during our individual supervision we had been prepared and reassured of the fact that we were an integral part of the care of BI and that, while it is important to team build, we also could take umbrage in the fact that we were providing music psychotherapy to these patients. This was the main point that needed to be explained to the volunteer.

Yi-Ying brought up the fact that in Chinese culture, age matters. This can be a sensitive issue when providing constructive criticism, as it can prove challenging for someone younger to offer this criticism to someone older without seeming disrespectful. Nevertheless, we had been prepared to find the most positive and constructive manner in which to proffer such criticism to the volunteer, if the situation required it. Understanding the important difference between *responding* versus *reacting* to a situation had been imparted throughout our training, and was pertinent to this situation. Reacting comes from an immediate, reflexive place, where you have not processed your interaction. Responding, however, implies that there is a thought process before any answer is provided.

As it turned out, the Chinese volunteer was in the waiting room already talking with a couple of Chinese patients before we began our session. At first, the volunteer's voice volume was not much of a hindrance; there was a lot of commotion going on in the room—patients talking with receptionists, staff joking with each other—so, while this was not the usual volume level in the room (it tends to be less noisy), there was nothing particularly unique about the volunteer's vocal presence, at least not until we started to play and sing Leonard Cohen's *Hallelujah*. It was clear to both of us, that the patients in chairs were captivated by our playing and singing of this song. You could feel the energy, and also see each person's level of engagement. You could almost hear their listening to the song. Then, during one of the quieter verses, as nearly everyone in the room was engaged with us, the volume of the volunteer's voice escalated noticeably. We did not feel that the volunteer was being intentionally intrusive; however, it seemed to us that speaking with a loud voice was part of his culture.

There are sensitive cultural issues here at play—the differences of speech volume between some Eastern and some Western cultures—but, as a member of the caregivers' team, his voice volume was somewhat impeding the therapeutic effect of the work we were doing with the patients. As we were in the middle of the piece, there weren't any realistically viable options: we were not about to stop the work we were doing to verbally address the issue with the volunteer in public.

While we continued singing and playing the song, we contemplated the most opportune time to address this issue. Thankfully, this became moot: at some point after the end of the song, the volunteer, completing his work, arose to leave the waiting room. At this point we could see that Andrew took it upon himself to address the volunteer privately beyond earshot of the waiting room, and those remaining in it. As a consequence of Andrew's intervention, we learned that the volunteer's seeming obliviousness to the therapeutic services being provided by music therapy was also due in part to his own story and motivation in his work. The volunteer had shared that as a cancer survivor himself he was invested in making sure the patients were comfortable.

The conversation elucidated for Andrew that this volunteer was working from a place of personal connection that was laden with unprocessed feelings of his own and much countertransference evoked from the environment. Andrew had skillfully validated the volunteer in the value of his work while also educating him as to the role of music therapists working with both the patients and the sound environment of the waiting area. The approach with this volunteer, encompassing both validation and psychoeducation, was effective and he became much more aware of his voice volume in our subsequent EMT sessions.

Tom learned a great lesson on cultural differences from Yi-Ying. Oftentimes in Asian cultures low talking or whispering in public can imply a serious, somber, or worrisome situation. It can cause those taking part in the conversation to become anxious, concerned that the subject of the conversation contains some horrible, bad news. And, yes, there may be something to the fact that different cultures have different norms for conversational volume.

There was a chronic issue for patients of various ethnicities sharing the waiting room—namely, the differing levels of what would be considered a "normal" acceptable level of volume for a conversation between adjacent conversers. This did, at times, present problems for the various patients in the radiation oncology waiting room.

One time in particular a non-Asian male got up and verbally chastised an Asian family for talking too loudly while the music was playing. As music therapists using EMT, this confrontational situation presented us with an uncomfortable yet necessary opportunity for allowing the patients in the room the freedom to express themselves, but also for encouraging them to engage with each other respectfully. In general, from our clinical observation, Asian patients would sometimes converse at higher volume levels than other patients of different ethnic backgrounds, although we want to stress that this wasn't limited to nor was it a universal occurrence with the Asian patient population with whom we worked.

It is important to remember that these are only our clinical observations. Clearly, this can be a delicate situation to navigate, much less describe. We believe that this subject warrants further study and could provide a wellspring of insights for cultural sensitivity, especially when working with an ethnically diverse population.

On a lighter note, it was something of a revelation for Tom, a Caucasian native New Yorker, when Yi-Ying, a native of Taiwan, was no more able to tell whether a patient was Chinese or of some other Asian background, than she could easily tell whether they could speak Mandarin, Cantonese, or Taiwanese simply by their appearance. This speaks volumes about cultural assumptions and about the subtle but nevertheless insidious problem of making judgments based upon appearances or of thinking that there can be some kind of "one size fits all" approach to working with any ethnic group. Even for music therapists who are part of that group.

Conclusion

"Humans interact with music, both consciously and unconsciously, at behavioral, emotional, and physiological levels."[9 (p96)] The clinically intuitive aspects of EMT require that music therapists working within this modality develop an "inner ear" for listening beyond language to what a patient is communicating. Music, with its capacity for traversing the landscape of language through the creation of a therapeutic soundscape, has the potential for wordless healing. Pain, while very real,[3] is also so very subjective.[10]

Working with a diverse group of individuals, especially a group that involves a variety of cultural dynamics, can provide significant challenges but also opportunities for the music therapists.

There is still much more to learn about working cross-culturally. Being sensitive and aware, and remaining open and flexible to learning and adapting are key qualities that would serve music therapists well. EMT is only one of the many tools available to music therapists in working with pain. While there are significant differences between how Asian and Western patients relate to their pain[1,5-7,11,12] it is imperative, especially when working within an open environment of a radiation oncology waiting room, that music therapists find common ground. Only by learning to appreciate these differences can music therapists create a truly integrative therapeutic soundscape for a diverse population.

References

1. He Y, Yang K. Healing Cancer from Mind: Psychological Key for Cancer Healing. Taipei: Da-Guan Press; 2011.
2. Biglin TJ, Jr. An Integrative Approach to Keeping Creative in Medical Music Psychotherapy. [unpublished master's thesis], New York University; 2012.
3. Portenoy R. Pain Medicine: Best Practices. Music and Medicine: Integrative Models in Pain Medicine Symposium; January 30, 2012; The Louis Armstrong Center for Music and Medicine Beth Israel Medical Center.
4. Chinese Wall. [cited July 7, 2012]; Available from: http://www.investopedia.com/terms/c/chinesewall.asp
5. Edrington J. The Experience of Cancer Pain and Barriers to Cancer Pain Management in a Community Sample of Chinese American Cancer Patients. [unpublished doctoral dissertation], University of California; 2007.
6. Lee C. Twelve Fatal Diseases: Supplements from Chinese and Japanese Doctors. Taipei: Kang-Yin Press; 2011.
7. Sue DW, Sue D. Counseling the Culturally Diverse: Theory and Practice, 5th Edition. Hoboken, NJ: John Wiley & Sons, Inc.; 2007.
8. Encyclopedia of Taiwan. [cited July 15, 2012]; Available from: http://taiwanpedia.culture.tw/web/content?ID=10015
9. Ellis RJ, Koenig J, Thayer JF. Getting to the heart: Autonomic nervous system function in the context of evidence-based music therapy. Music and Medicine. 2012;4(2):90-99.
10. Loewy J. New Frontiers in Pain Treatment: Integrating Key Aspects of Mind and Body in Clinical Practice & Research. Music and

Medicine: Integrative Models in Pain Medicine Symposium; January 31, 2012; The Louis Armstrong Center for Music and Medicine Beth Israel Medical Center.

11. *Asian Family Caregiver Handbook.* New York, NY: Beth Israel Medical Center; 2010.
12. Dileo C. Cultures of Pain: A Meta-Perspective on Decision-Making in Music Therapy Treatment. Music and Medicine: Integrative Models in Pain Medicine Symposium; January 30, 2012; The Louis Armstrong Center for Music and Medicine Beth Israel Medical Center.

APPENDIX A

Asian Culture and Western Medicine[11(p119)]

- Every family works differently. There are some values and beliefs that are important to Asian families that can affect how you relate to the healthcare system.
- Individual rights may not be as important in your culture as they are in Western culture. Some families consider that the interests of the whole family are more important than the individual's interests or concerns.
- Some families prefer that doctors give information to caregivers, instead of to the patient. It is then up to the caregiver whether to pass the information along to the patient.
- In some families, the husband or son may be the decision makers, while the women provide caregiving.
- In some Chinese cultures, the caregiving process reflects some of the Confucian concepts of filial duty. Therefore, children may feel they do not want their parents to be in hospice care or a nursing home because they believe that it is their traditional duty to care for their dying parents.
- It's important to tell the health care team about your values and beliefs so they have a better understanding of how your relative wants to make decisions about medical care and treatment.
- When communicating with a physician, you may feel that it is disrespectful to ask questions, speak directly to the physician, or look at him or her directly in the eye. But in the American medical system, such behavior is a sign that you have heard and understood what the doctor is saying, and that you are being truthful.
- If you do not agree with the doctor about a treatment or test, or if your relative has religious or cultural concerns about a particular procedure, such as having blood drawn, it's important to speak up and tell the doctor or nurse.

Music and Medicine: Integrative Models in the Treatment of Pain

APPENDIX B

Original Text in Chinese Classics

- 《黃帝內經》中指出，情志的改變可以使人發病。古人認為人有五臟化五氣，以喜、怒、悲、憂、恐，為五志；七情則是喜、怒、憂、思、悲、恐、驚。情志的變化和臟腑密切相關，一定的臟腑由一定的情志所主，心主喜、肝主怒、脾主思、肺主憂、腎主恐。正所謂：「暴怒傷肝火上頭，肺病最怕添憂愁，思慮過度傷脾胃，驚恐傷腎尿自流，過喜氣緩心無主，真心劇痛命自休。」

- 《黃帝內經》中已發現：「怒則氣上、恐則氣下、驚則氣亂、悲則氣消、思則氣結、喜則氣緩……」並基於此創立「內情傷志」理論，中醫理論認為「氣行則血行」。

- 《論語・先進篇》子路、曾皙、冉有、公西華侍坐。子曰：「以吾一日長乎爾，毋吾以也。居則曰：『不吾知也！』如或知爾，則何以哉？」子路率爾而對曰：「千乘之國，攝乎大國之間，加之以師旅，因之以饑饉；由也為之，比及三年，可使有勇，且知方也。」夫子哂之。「求！爾何如？」對曰：「方六七十，如五六十，求也為之，比及三年，可使足民。如其禮樂，以俟君子。」「赤！爾何如？」對曰：「非曰能之，願學焉。宗廟之事，如會同，端章甫，願為小相焉。」「點！爾何如？」鼓瑟希，鏗爾，舍瑟而作。對曰：「異乎三子者之撰。」子曰：「何傷乎？亦各言其志也。」曰：「**暮春者，春服既成。冠者五六人，童子六七人，浴乎沂，風乎舞雩，詠而歸。**」夫子喟然歎曰：「吾與點也！」三子者出，曾皙後。曾皙曰：「夫三子者之言何如？」子曰：「亦各言其志也已矣。」曰：「夫子何哂由也？」曰：「為國以禮，其言不讓，是故哂之。」「唯求則非邦也與？」「安見方六七十如五六十而非邦也者？」「唯赤則非邦也與？」「宗廟會同，非諸侯而何？赤也為之小，孰能為之大？」

- 《論語・述而篇》子在齊聞韶，三月不知肉味。曰：「不圖為樂之至於斯也！」

- 《史記》「故音樂者所以動盪血脈，通流精神而和正心也。」

- 《黃帝內經》中「五音療法」，是依據五行學說，運用宮、商、角、徵、羽等不同音調，採取對症下「樂」。不同的音樂曲調，產生不同的效應。《靈樞·陰陽二十五人》中根據五形人的不同特點，與五聲音節對應，土形人選宮音、金形人選商音、木形人選角音、火形人選徵音，水形人選羽音；認為這樣對調整心態有較強的作用。

CHAPTER 25

Journeying through Cultures: Personal Explorations of Indian and Persian Music Traditions in Music Therapy Practice

Soniya K. Brar MA, MM, MT-BC
Oksana Rosenblum MA

> *"Of the many domains of culture, music would perhaps seem to be one of the least necessary; yet we know of no culture that does not have it."*[1]
> Bruno Nettl

Introduction

This chapter looks at multicultural approaches to pain management, specifically from Indian and Persian music traditions. In the first section, Oksana Rosenblum discusses the historical and theoretical context to these traditions, suggesting how melody and rhythm can be used for healing and psychological growth. The dialogue continues, as Soniya K. Brar discusses how Indian musical elements can address pain management in music therapy practice. It is our objective to examine how to connect ancient healing traditions and contemporary music therapy.

Using Classical Indian and Persian Music in Music Therapy

Personal Reflections
Music has always been a mystery for me. As a child, I remember pressing a key on my piano and wondering where the sound wanders - whether it is always heard and is just getting quieter, or whether it disappears at some point but we are still able to hear it in our mind. That was before I knew anything about physics and the wave nature of sound.

While learning piano and solfeggio at the music school in Soviet Ukraine, where great emphasis was placed on the study of theory, I was taught to not question, experiment, or actually "play" with the material. It was much later that I understood the playfulness of music, in a sense Hindu culture talks about the concept of *lila,* the Divine play that brings about creation.

Music and Medicine: Integrative Models in the Treatment of Pain

Intrigued with the psychology of altered states of consciousness, and how they were perceived and worked out within different culture, I became especially interested in the mystical trends of world religions. It was clear to me that music facilitated the passage to the "other reality", yet it did not occur to me that perhaps I could be the facilitator of such passage by accessing my own musical creativity.

A new chapter opened in 2003 when I arrived to the United States, motivated in my decision by the diversity of world music traditions accessible in New York City. I began studying privately the vocal and drumming practices of the Middle East, India, and Balkan and Slavic countries, while reading extensively on the history and theory of these traditions.

I soon realized that classical Indian and classical Persian music were teaching me something about healing. When I started studying those traditions approximately five years ago, I was not prepared for a life-changing experience. I was coming from a different place, different culture, and was working on issues of transition in my life. Little by little, however, I started to feel transformation in my inner world. Singing would bring up strong emotions. I experienced flashbacks from the past, and images full of water, mountains, colors, etc. I felt as one with the universe, transported to a different realm, alive and present. I wanted to sing this music all the time and everywhere I went. There was a strong connection between this kind of music and death – a lot of Persian poetry actually talks about the death of the Lover for the sake of Beloved. In my view, it was about the death of the subject, or Ego.

Music in Healing Practice

In this chapter, my aim is to provide an overview of how Indian and Persian music have been used historically for healing, and give some examples of how one can create a synthesis of Western "scientific" and Eastern, or "intuitive" approaches (obviously, the notions of scientific and intuitive are relevant here only in part, as both traditions contain the opposite to a degree). Also, more specifically, my colleague Soniya and I would like to consider how these music traditions can facilitate pain management.

In a way, the traditional approach has been and continues to be used throughout the Eastern world in daily rituals, be they religious or secular, without people being necessarily aware that they are evoking the healing aspects of music, or perhaps being aware of it in a very general context (for instance, someone reports feeling better after a concert, but the feeling cannot be connected to any specific improvement in well-being). This is what we call therapeutic power of music. Within the western therapeutic approach, the distinction between *music as therapy* and *music in therapy* is being made. While in the first case the music serves as "the primary medium and agent for therapeutic change",[2(p39)] the second one provides opportunity for a person to experience music within a different context, perhaps as a background for a different therapeutic modality.

As early as the 9th century, one can trace in the Arabic world a well-developed doctrine on how to use music for medical purposes. It was based on Aristotle's theory of four humors of the human body. The opinions differed, however. According to Ibn Hindu (d.1019), physicians should have made use of certain music modes when treating ailments. They should have hired musicians to do this work professionally. Ibn Sina, aka Avicenna (d.1037) considered all theories that connected astrology, music and medicine as nonsense. However, in his *Canon on Medicine*, he talks about a certain relationship between music and medicine that combines rhythm, consonances and pulse as indicators of either good health or sickness.[3]

A review of traditional Indian healing methods, including musical ones, has been done by Sumathy Sundar.[4] The author mentions a number of traditions: Vedic chants and hymns, Ayurveda, and nadayoga. According to Sundar, "music therapy practices" use various verses of Vedic texts to enhance attention, improve concentration and help with relaxation. More specifically, pentatonic rāgas have been used for curing diseases, sickness and bad health, hexatonic rāgas to attain beauty, youth and charm, and *sampoorna* rāgas (rāgas with all the notes) for strength, wisdom, wealth, good harvest, prosperity and children.[4(p400)]

In the Indian world, the healing aspects of rāga music go back to Rāga *Chikitsa*, an ancient text in Sanskrit that documents the therapeutic aspects of rāgas (TV Sairam, personal communication, March 23, 2012). However, according to T. V. Sairam, the text of Chikitsa has not survived until present moment in its entirety, and only the fragments are available.

In a diary of 1921, Graf Hermann Keyserling, a philosopher and traveler from Prussia, of aristocratic origin, who was one of the first European philosophers to bring public attention to oriental cultures, pinpoints (as cited in Hamel, 1984) some very important characteristics of Indian music: it has a unity of mood, it is of the same nature that Indian dance is; while listening to it, one feels intensely alive; and generally speaking, this music lies in a different dimension to ours [Western], and it is a dimension of pure intensity. People find themselves trembling, gesturing with their hands, weeping...

According to Hamel, Indian music is based on the prolonged sound of a single note, or of a recurring sequence of notes, which "is more likely to make an exclusively mentally oriented person edgy and irritable".[5] It requires the listener to let go of herself, and to follow patiently the minute developments of melody and rhythm, staying with the same emotion for a long time. While this observation can be challenged by a particular experience of working with various clients, Graf Keiserling's perceptiveness as to the nature of Indian classical music is striking and presents an early example of European reception of that musical tradition.

Historical Background of Indian Music

It is impossible to define what *rāga* is in one term. In short, one can say that in Hindūstāni and Karnatak music, rāga is a melodic mode that consists of particular upward and downward movement, connection between notes, and characteristic phrases. Once part of the same tradition, Hindūstāni or the Northern music system and Karnatak or the Southern one became differentiated by the 12th century. The former came heavily under the influence of Persian and Arabic music under Muslim rule. Hindūstāni music relies more on improvisation, while Karnatak follows more strictly the rules of composition.

Traditionally, rāgas have always been associated with a particular season, time of day, male or female principles, and planets. Based on these extramusical characteristics, there existed a system of treating people with rāga music. It would have been very tempting to reconstruct it; however, according to Suvarnalata Rao, there exist at least two major obstacles: first, we do not know how to relate the rāgas of today to those that are mentioned in treatises of hundreds of years ago. Similarly to the stars that change their position and routes in the sky over the decades and centuries, the rāgas "shift" as well. Secondly, there is a disparity between the traditionally prescribed rasa of a particular rāga and the way it is experienced by listeners.[6] For instance, the solemn mood of rāga Bhairav can be experienced in different ways: while one person perceives it as uplifting and calming, another might be bored, etc.

Indian musicology goes back approximately two thousand years, and so do attempts to analyze the emotional impact of music on a listener. *Rasa* is a term used to describe an aesthetic emotional experience that one undergoes when engaged in perception of any genre of the arts, be it poetry, drama, music, dance, or painting. It entails total identification with the artistic creation. It was first used in the treatise on dramaturgy, *Nātya Shāstra*, ca 3 BC.[7] In this work, rasas were classified into nine categories, or static emotions, and thirty-three transitory ones. One should note that a classificatory approach is an important characteristic of Indian culture, and Indian philosophers have been known for classifying and organizing the knowledge "with endless taxonomic lists that included intricately worked cosmologies covering the remotest corners of theology, philosophy, and natural science".[8(p69)] These nine rasas describe the complexity of human feelings, and for centuries have been represented in chanting, music, literature, and dance. They are:

- *shringara*: love;
- *hasya*: humor;
- *karuna*: compassion;
- *raudra*: anger;
- *vira:* valor;
- *bhayanaka*: fear;
- *vibhatsa*: disgusting;
- *abdhuta*: wonder;
- *shanta:* peace.

Hindūstāni and Karnatak schools
The main characteristics of both Hindūstāni and Karnatak schools that manifest themselves during the performance are the following: the contrast of unmetered with metered, the progression from free rāga improvisation to emphasis on rhythm, and the fusion of traditional composition with improvisation.[7(p74)] Let us look at the structure of Hindūstāni and Karnatak performance.

Hindūstāni Instrumental Music Performance:
- *alāp*: slow, meditative, rhythm-free melodic improvisation that establishes the mood of the rāga;
- *jor*: rhythmic pulsation; tempo increases at the end;
- *gat:* composition - follows with solo variations (*gamakas* or ornaments and *taans*);
- *jhala*: accelerando that ends with culminating virtuoso conclusion.

Karnatak Music Performance:
- *varnam*: a composition presented in medium or slow tempo, with no variation;
- *kirtana*: a composition in praise of Lord Ganesh;
- pre-main rāga, the purpose of which is to prepare the ground for main rāga;
- *rāgam*: includes *aalapana,* an extended vocal improvisation, free of rhythm; followed by the main rāga;
- *tanam*: extension of rāga, plus rhythm;
- *pallavi*: main rāga accompanied by percussion;
- *tani-avartanam*: percussion solos.

Music and Medicine: Integrative Models in the Treatment of Pain

When envisioning the difference between Hindūstāni and Karnatak music in terms of images, I often think of the former as developing horizontally, the latter – vertically. The melodic development in Hindūstāni music is more successive and gradual, if compared to the "jumpy" character of Karnatak. This might have to do with the fact that the ornaments, or gamaka-s, are profuse in Karnatak music. Basically, every pitch is ornamented with a shake of a definite interval.[7(p73)] The potential of using these differences in a music therapy context, such as in offering particular pieces from both traditions to patients, depending on their psychosomatic state is compelling. If paired with imagery exercises, the system will be even more effective for those who are either better able or willing to explore the visual channel of their perception. For instance, the gradual melodic development in Hindūstāni can be envisioned as a long and calm river, while in the Karnatak as a rapid stream of water in the mountains, or a waterfall. The experience of listening and performing in these traditions can be compared to a massage: in Hindūstāni, one is being "caressed" with slow, soft, gradual movements, as opposed to Karnatak, where one is being "pinched" in a rubato style. We need both approaches in different periods of our life, depending on our emotional state – sometimes we need to be supported (*sample: aalap – Rāga Chayanat*), and other times – lightly pushed in order to move forward (*sample: Karnatak - Pallavi*) (see note 1).

From a perspective of pain management, a more mellow and gradual melodic development in Hindūstāni genres seems aptly indicated for patients who suffer physically, as opposed to the invigorating and energizing nature of Karnatak music.

There is no fixed pitch in Indian music, which creates even more freedom to experiment with an individually determined tonic, depending on the range of a patient. Traditional Ayurvedic principles are employed by present day music therapists in their work with patients. In Karnatak vocal therapy, a music therapist establishes a *swara* (note) for every energy center in a human's body. According to Rajam Shanker, a Karnatak music therapist based in Andhra Pradesh, there exist seven *swaras*, which correspond to seven main energy centers, from *Muladhara* to *Sahasrara* chakra. When the note reaches the respective center, the healing vibration is produced. The usage of each note should be calibrated accordingly, in order to "to provide the corrective charge to boost this energy center".[9] Detoxification is a prerequisite of the energy work.

A similar view is developed by Sumathy Sundar, a Hindūstāni music therapist based in Chennai. She combines Ayurvedic principles of the four *doshas* (types of human constitution) with 22 *shruti-s* of Indian music, and then connects those to energy centers, or chakras.[4(p400)] Another traditional philosophy – *nadopasana* – is an integrative method that includes meditation and yoga practice. In her research on nadopasana and cancer patients, Dr. Sundar was able to integrate this traditional healing method in a cancer treatment as a supportive strategy in terms of modern music therapy, in order to find out the effects of music on cancer related pain and state anxiety.[4(p402)]

Generally speaking, Indian music therapists seem to be philosophically attuned and open to traditional methods of healing, such as Ayurveda, yoga, and nadopasana. Among Western music therapists, the clinical approach of quantitative and qualitative methods dominates, although sensitivity toward culturally specific music therapy is an established trend (see, for instance: Kenny C, Stige B. *Contemporary Voices in Music Therapy – Communication, Culture, and Community.* Oslo; 2002). Moreover, in the chapter on the history of music therapy, Joke Bradt traces the use of music in healing practices back to shamanism. She puts music into a broader context of healing rituals across the globe.[10] And Jrg Fachner, a Professor of Qualitative Research at Witten/Herdecke University, explains in his interview with Dr. Sundar: "…when we start to believe that music or art can be used in a standardized [sic] manner we start limiting the possibilities that art can open…The therapeutic process has nothing to do with applying for a passport at the appropriate desk or checking boxes on a questionnaire. There are rituals which are connected to music which seem to have the quality of a repeatable process, but the inner experiences and the focus of attention of those involved will always be different according to the uniqueness of the situation of the rituals happening".[11]

Example (sample: Bhajan de Kabir)
In Dinkar Kaikini performance of Kabir bhajan (a genre of Hindu devotional music), one can experience a steady predictable rhythm and a rather intricate, ornate melody that develops over the rhythm. The melody pattern is complex; it is the rhythmic pulsation of Satwa-tal, the 7-beat rhythm with the accent on the first one, which keeps everything together.

The piece starts with introduction of a rhythmic pattern, which contains syncopation. The offbeat is striking, and it offers an unpredictable development, especially when paired with the up and down scale development of the melody. This creates enough space for a patient to project her/his disturbing physical and/or emotional sensations and emotions. Both melodic and rhythmic intensity of the piece meet a patient's tension, and allow the reliving of strong emotions from the past, which may lead to culmination and, ultimately, catharsis. The voice of the singer, with all its imperfections, nuances, lyricism and expressionism, adds to the intensity of this bhajan. Now soft and pleading, now loud and demanding, it creates a range of emotions that can be experienced while listening to this composition.

Some of the same criteria utilized in the Helen Bonny Method of Guided Imagery in Music (GIM) to support the patient's deep relaxation are at work here:

- medium or slow tempo;
- steady predictable rhythm;
- simple structure with recognizable melodies or themes;
- simple, consonant harmony without sudden modulations.[12(p110)]

If one follows the scheme offered by Wigram, this piece cannot be used for deep relaxation with patients suffering from pain. However, it can be used for tension-release model, where the patient is met where he or she is at the moment.

From this perspective, it is interesting to note that T.V. Sairam considers bhajans, with their simple melodic structures, slow tempo, low-pitched notes repeated over and over, to be able to impart a relaxing and soothing feeling of spaciousness and reduce stress.[13]

Value of Rhythm and Drumming
Similarly to the melodic aspect of rāga music, the *tāla*, or beat, constitutes another crucial part of the performance and therapy. The healing aspect of drumming has been widely researched in the last decades. It is believed to induce changes in perception of the subjects, which involve changes in body-image, passing of time, and sometimes provoke intense imagery that leads to re-experiencing near-birth, or some traumatic events from the past.[14]

It is important to note the cyclical nature of rhythm in Indian music, especially Hindūstāni music. All the *tālas* (rhythmic cycles) are arranged in a rhythmic sequence followed by a return to beat 1, or *sam*. Within one rhythmic cycle, every beat has a different weight, and some are omitted altogether. The omission usually signals a return to the beginning. In other words, *sam* becomes an important reference point for both singer and instrumentalist, to come back to the original point. In between, the music can be freely improvised, but the return is important (*sample: Rāga Chayanat - Jor*).

This idea, offers rich potential for therapeutic entry points within a music therapy session. When working with narcissistically injured patients, for example, Diane Austin makes use of a number of techniques, "holding" being one of them. This particular technique creates "a containing environment by sustaining chords...", and thus provides a feeling of support that might have been absent in client's childhood years.[15]

Indian and Persion Music Traditions in Music Therapy

The use of drone as a holding technique for patients experiencing acute pain crises will be further discussed as well. In this sense, a feeling of going back, returning to the safety of one's self might be a powerful one. In terms of pain management, one could build a succession of tension and release patterns that would parallel the rhythmic sequence of leaving the predictable pattern, going into the world, and coming back to the beginning of the cycle.

History of Persian Classical Music

In this tradition, a mode is called *dastgāh*, as opposed to *rāga* in Indian music or *maqam* in Turkish and Arabic. Even though it is tempting to draw parallels with Indian music, the concept of dastgāh is different. According to Hormoz Farhat, dastgāh consists of a number of pieces that are grouped together, and most of them are composed in their individual modes.[16] The initial mode dominates, and the melody comes back to it frequently throughout the composition. However, from the initial mode the melody can shift with variation, unlike in Indian rāga, where the unity of one mode is preserved throughout the whole piece. In Persian Classical music, frequent modulations and sudden shifts of rhythmic patterns provide an interesting playground for a music therapist to explore therapeutic qualities of change (*sample 3*: *Seven-Beat Rhythm, Dastan Trio*).

Nevertheless, the structure of a traditional piece in Classical Persian music shares common features with Hindūstāni and Karnatik. Beginning with an instrumental introduction, it develops into a vocal improvisation, and builds to a climactic ending by way of a virtuoso solo. The structure of such a piece would appear as such:

- *Pish daramad*: a measured instrumental introduction to a performance;
- *chaharmezrab*: a virtuoso drum solo piece;
- *avaz*: a vocal non-metric improvisation set to a piece from classical poetry;
- *tasnif*: a vocal composed piece, usually folk, lyrical in nature;
- *reng*: fast tempo instrumental dance piece, also folk.

Call-Response, Question-Answer
Another powerful concept is a *question-answer* structure of instrumental performance in both Indian and Persian traditions (*samples: Prelude to Dastgah-e Mahur, Modulation - Dastan Trio)*. As the dialogue between string and percussion instruments continues, the mood of mutual understanding and encouragement is developed. The roles of percussion and strings alternate between supporting and leading, rendering both a feeling of

support and the possibility of a dialogue, instead of confrontation. This quality is clearly present at every moment. Again, this process can be compared to the technique of dialoguing, used by Diane Austin in her therapeutic work.[15(p295)] However, as the piece develops and modulates, the mood intensifies, and the dialogue becomes more "heated" or passionate. Thus, even though it might be an excellent piece to use for a client who needs stimulation, it might not be the best fit for someone in need of deep relaxation.

Discussion

According to contemporary ideas on music application in therapy, it is very difficult, if even possible, to distinguish between *aesthetic* (non-therapeutic) and *psychological* (psychotherapeutic) functions of music experience.[12] This brings us back to the attempts of Indian scholars to research the emotional impact of *rasa*. According to the rāga-based approach proposed by Sumathy Sundar, a therapist pays particular attention to swara patterns, embellishments and rhythm.[4] In a different study, rāga music was shown to improve the quality of sleep of patients with Major Depressive Disorder.[17] However, it has not been determined yet which particular elements of rāga are responsible for such a calming effect.

It seems that using rāga for therapeutic purposes can be a very subjective yet truly rewarding experience, since "music can be arousing, hypnotic, anxiety provoking, mind healing or shattering, a source of inspiration or spiritual vision – it is like a magic mirror enabling the listener...to find answers to deep existential questions".[12] A therapist has to be able to use his/her judgment, based on experience and intuition, as to which piece is appropriate for a particular condition.

Application of Hindūstāni Music Elements to Modern Music Therapy Practice

This section of the chapter will explore the clinical application of *Hindūstāni* music elements in (Western) music therapy practice to address pain management (see note 2). The following material was culled from my training and immersion in a clinical approach to the treatment of pain being studied at Beth Israel Medical Center, in New York. I will first describe my personal rationale for using such elements in music therapy, followed by a discussion of specific techniques I utilized with the patients enduring acute and chronic pain.

Indian and Persion Music Traditions in Music Therapy

Rationale
The rationale for incorporating Hindūstāni music elements into music therapy stems from its historical use in healing. I would like to discuss my own impetus for use of these elements as well, to give context for my approach to, and affinity for, this music.

It is an early Sunday evening and I am about four years old, sitting in the family room on a ledge jutting out from the fireplace. My father is in the corner of the room taking out a flat, square cardboard case. This is a weekly occurrence, one that I have come to love. I go over to him and he shares with me his small music ritual: taking out a reel tape and placing it on the reel to reel player. I can tell even as a young child how much the player means to him. It amazes me how sound comes out of it. I have no understanding yet of speakers, tape, and how audio recordings are made. To me it is as if the singers themselves are wound up into that brown tape, as if their bodies are magically transformed onto it. And as the tape moves from reel to reel through the machine, the voices of these people are pressed out of it, adding to their plaintive quality, especially in the slow songs sung by the longing voices of playback singers Lata Mangeshkar and Mukesh, Kishore Kumar, Mohammed Rafi, and Mahendra Kapoor and Asha Bhosle. As I do not know these names as a young child, I think of them solely as "he" and "she," as hero and heroine from the Indian (Bollywood) movies. I am familiar with the songs more than with the movies, and the hero and heroine are composites in my mind of all the images of the Indian actors and actresses that I have seen.

In the introduction of many of the slow songs, an instrument with a hauntingly beautiful sound is played before the vocals enter. This instrument's sound moves me incredibly and always seems to pull the most tender of emotions out of me. The instrument's wailing, nasal timbre and the way the melody moves cause me to imagine that its sound is floating out of the reel to reel player in wisps and streams of soft color, the way paint being introduced into a glass of water unfurls when the paintbrush is dipped into it. What constitutes the color flow as a wisp or a stream depends on the strength and loudness of the melody. This floating inkiness seems to dart and dance in the air around

> it, depending on the melodic movement of the song. Something about this sound soothes me, as if the melody is pouring into all the empty spaces in some musical porous landscape and filling its holes. I later will come to know this sound as the sarangi, a bowed lute from India. But I do not yet know this; it is still an amorphous liquid of sound floating in whirls and swaths of moving color in the air. My journey to know the names of the singers, the movies the songs come from, the way audio recordings are made, and the name of this instrument is still before me. As the music continues I take my place on the fireplace ledge – my "stage" – to act out the songs and sing with them. My musical play has begun.

Much later on my journey, a lecturer/performer of Hindūstāni music in an undergraduate course piqued my interest in this music tradition. Not having heard it in its pure form while growing up, I was instantly drawn into its sounds and felt a deep nostalgia upon hearing it. It reminded me of something I could not identify, which I later realized to be the Indian film music my father used to play long ago. (Indeed much of older film music derives from Indian classical music and *rāgas*).[18] I wondered where I could study this tradition.

This brought me to graduate study in ethnomusicology under Professor Stephen M. Slawek, a specialist in Hindūstāni music and senior sitār disciple of Pandit Ravi Shankar. While in school I had the opportunity to study sitār with Professor Slawek and voice with Anita Slawek, a reputable Hindūstāni singer and teacher. I chose this genre because my family is from North India (see note 3): My parents immigrated to the United States from there and took us to visit almost yearly when I was growing up. This helped foster a connection to the country and my family there.

Further along in my journey I took a sound healing class (see note 4) with Silvia Nakkach, a music therapist, sound healer, and Hindūstāni music vocalist who studied under the late Ustad Ali Akbar Khan. As I developed an interest in using music for healing purposes and in music therapy, the natural growth of this was to integrate what I had learned about Hindūstāni music, and then find a way to utilize the music in my sessions.

It is noteworthy for me to consider how my use of "adapted" Indian musical elements in some way reflects my own cultural identity. Ruud[19] and Swamy[20] discuss how music choices reflect one's identity. Neither completely Indian nor American, I have over time adapted my Indian background to fit my American one and vice versa. A product of the first generation, I continue to navigate/negotiate between these two parts of myself, taking from each what best suits me and shedding off what does not. Similarly, I take from Hindūstāni music what I feel best serves the patient and leave behind what I believe does not. I combine both Western and Indian musical elements to achieve patient goals. For example, I use guitar instead of the tānpura and sing with more of a Western timbre in my voice than an Indian one. Overall, these choices also reflect what I feel most comfortable doing musically.

To this end, I use elements influenced from and an adaptation of Hindūstāni music in clinical practice. I do not use the music in its pure form for several reasons. Firstly, I do not have the expertise and length of training required to improvise fully in various rāgas with patients. Secondly, the rules of each rāga are strict and even if I was proficient in playing them, I would want to adapt their form at times (e.g., note order) to fit the needs of the patient. (This is not to imply, however, that one cannot effectively use Hindūstāni or Karnatak music in its pure form in music therapy). Thus to maintain respect for the genre, I stress that I only employ musical devices that are influenced by the genre itself (see note 5).

Specific Techniques Used in Clinical Work

Musical Elements

How do Hindūstāni music elements figure into pain management in music therapy practice? Here my aim is not to present evidence for how these elements cause pain to go away; I do not purport to claim that music makes pain disappear. Rather my use of these elements is an attempt to refocus patients' attention and/or relax them in an effort to assist them in better managing their pain. Relaxation is a large part of the work I do in addressing pain management. Recent studies in pain medicine point to how relaxing during a pain episode can help one better cope with and manage pain.[21] This includes releasing muscle tension and reducing heart and respiration rates. Pain is not just a physical symptom but has physiological and psychological components as well.[22] As I observed in patients, pain and anticipation of it can cause stress and anxiety and, especially in the case of chronic pain, lead to depression and feelings of frustration. It can trigger irritability, disrupt sleep, and exacerbate feelings of loss of control.[21(p75)]

Below I will describe Hindūstāni music elements such as the drone and Hindūstāni-influenced vocalizations and how they are utilized in music therapy practice. I will then consider how breath focusing, use of imagery, mantra chanting, and singing sacred chakra vowels work in conjunction with these elements.

Music and Medicine: Integrative Models in the Treatment of Pain

Drone
A Hindūstāni music performance generally features three main components: the soloist (instrument or voice), the drone player (or electric drone), and the rhythm instrumentalist.[7(p23)] The soloist delivers an exposition of the rāga (improvisation and composition) and the drone player provides a continuous sequence of notes that stress the tonic of the piece. The rhythm instrumentalist maintains the beat and provides the rhythmic cycle on which the piece is based.

The drone is played on the *tānpura*, a lute with four or five strings. This instrument has a slight nasal and buzzing quality which is not always palatable to the Western ear. Thus in my music therapy interventions, I play drone on guitar. While the drone can consist of the fourth or seventh scale degree, it most commonly consists of the 5th scale degree, moving to the upper tonic, repeating the upper tonic, and then moving to the lower tonic. This pattern is repeated throughout a musical piece. As background to the changing melodic line of the soloist, the drone acts as a constant point of reference back to the tonic, creating a steadiness in the music. In this way it provides a stable tonal environment which, in a medical music therapy context, can help a patient feel held and safe.[23(pp55-56)]

The Musical Bubble
Carl Rogers contends that the therapist's way of interacting with a patient should produce a "climate of freedom and safety" in the therapeutic relationship.[24(p149)] I would like to extend from this idea and postulate that the music therapist's way of interacting (or making music) with a patient can create a sonic sanctuary through music. Making music can facilitate a sense of calm in the space for a patient in an ordinarily stressful or noisy environment.

One of the units in which I regularly conducted music therapy sessions housed individuals recovering from orthopedic surgery. Here I often encountered patients who were tired due to post-operative pain that kept them awake night and day. Contributing to their fatigue were the general noises and disruptions of a busy unit (monitors beeping, medical care team members performing necessary tests, foot-traffic in the halls, etc.). The hospital can be a tense environment with this cacophony of sounds, and I believe this tense quality can negatively impact the patients' personal environment and space, which may impede healing.

The aesthetics of the environment a patient is in can affect his or her well-being and healing. A music therapist can give meaning to this environment and offer the patient a "recluse" (John Mondanaro, personal communication, 2011) by the music he or she plays. The music therapy space, the room in which the patient and therapist create music can be thought of as sacred: It is a safe space allotted for healing. I often play a drone in music therapy sessions and sing Hindūstāni-influenced vocals over it. But before I start to sing, I play the drone by itself. The drone helps set up the room. Its vibrations create a mood in any room they permeate and seem to hold that space in suspended safety. Its notes are soothing to most patients and not too overwhelming. They are gentle and pervasive. Like the notes played on a tānpura, the notes I play consist of plucking and letting resonate (on the guitar) the fifth scale degree, to the tonic above it (which is then repeated), and then to the tonic below it. Inherent in the drone are thus the intervals of the octave, the perfect fifth, and the perfect fourth – all highly consonant intervals in Western music, to which most patients have exposure. These intervals create a pleasing sound, a non-dissonance. Playing them repeatedly perhaps adds to the holding quality of the music, and may contribute to creating a holding space (see note 6), adding to feelings of security when one experiences the disorienting sensation of pain.

When I play the drone for a patient and it enters the space, I like to think we are in a sort of musical bubble that absorbs and incorporates the already existing sounds that may be interfering with a patient's rest, making them more tolerable. By doing so it offers a recluse emotionally. Recently I asked a patient in pain how her experience with the drone and Indian vocalizations was after a session, and she replied that it took her to another place.

Musician, teacher, and sound healing practitioner Jonathan S. Goldman writes that "those using music as a therapeutic tool must first recognize the tremendous power of sonic vibrations to effect wholeness, health, and consciousness and then assume responsibility for working with the immense transformational energy inherent in music."[25(p29)] Pain and the tension resulting from it can be thought of as blocked or misdirected energy, blood flow, stress hormones, etc. The drone itself is made up of sound vibrations that can move energy along and release blockages or tension felt in parts of the body.

Clinical Work

Case Study 1: Abe
Sometimes the drone allows patients who feel too weak or uncomfortable to sing to speak their feelings over the music. Its unwavering and stable melodic construction provides an effective and holding foundation over which one can express one's feelings. It seems to invite a person into a meditative state with its relaxing qualities. I had one such an experience with Abe. In his early seventies, Abe had Chronic Obstructive Pulmonary Disease (COPD) and was HIV positive. The chaplain had referred him to

music therapy to provide an additional context for emotional support as well as a forum for his expression as she felt he seemed depressed. He was also experiencing shortness of breath due to his COPD.

In our session, he wanted to hear music but felt too tired and short of breath to sing or participate actively with instruments. Once I started to play the drone however, he began to speak about his feelings about his life and the many things he had done. Here speech became a musical statement over the drone. Moreover, listening to him speak about his life and his creative endeavors was bearing witness to who he was separate from his diagnosis. (John Mondanaro, personal communication, February 29, 2012).

Music therapy helped to remind him of his creative abilities, strength, and identity beyond that of a sick person. Acknowledging his need to express these aspects of himself through the music was a marked feature of our work together. The drone can act as a conduit to elevated mood and expression when a patient cannot participate in music making due to pain or discomfort, and the potential of such an intervention was exemplified in my work with Abe.

Patient Reactions to Drone
Often after I have stopped vocalizing for a patient, I keep playing the drone to maintain the sonic environment. Then I slowly and very gradually diminish the volume until it is almost inaudible. The effect is one of lingering tones in the air after the music has ended, which can sustain the holding environment even after the therapist leaves the room. Patients have often commented to me that they could still hear the drone after the music had ended and that it made them feel "at peace," and was "soothing." The drone supported them to still hear the Indian vocalizations I had just sung. The results of this intervention ranged from patients actively integrating the music to achieve deepened states of rest and meditation to those who were in need of sleep.

Hindūstāni-Influenced Vocals
Hindūstāni music is based on melody, on the intricacies of the unfolding of one melody at a time.[7(p24)] Its melodic vehicle is known as rāga.

As previously mentioned, each rāga has its own rules regarding note order, e.g., ascent and descent up the rāga's scale. Each one has its own characteristic melodic phrases (or stock phrases). In addition to this, most rāgas have chief notes and secondary chief notes that figure prominently in the melodic exposition. Some rāgas have stricter rules than others.

In clinical work I pattern the melodies I sing over the drone after the rules that govern rāgas. The notes used in an improvisation and the order in which they are sung can affect the outcome of the overall sound and the mood produced. Each note can be thought of as a person or personality. The arrangement of notes is akin to the collection of personalities or people in a group in a contained space. If one person is missing, it can change the dynamics of the group entirely. The same is with notes. If a group of people is standing in a line, the energy that will be evoked from the group depends on who is standing next to whom. Is the troublemaker next to the timid person? Is the sweet person next to the happy one? All this can affect the overall dynamics of a space. The same goes for the notes of a melody and the order in which they are sung.

I also pay attention to intervals according to the mood I wish to create. I avoid singing large intervals if I want the mood to be more relaxing. In this case, I tend to use slides between the notes, especially in descent from one note to another. The upper note is held steadily, almost elongating the tone, and then slides down to rest on the note a step below. This resting note is not sustained as long. I jump between larger intervals when I want the music to stimulate a patient. The timbre I use is shakier and I quicken the pace of the drone to match the energy of the melody.

The way the melody and notes are sung affects the patient. Long tones are sung in the lower register to relax. Short tones are sung in the higher register to stimulate. The choice of what syllable to sing is important as well. Vowel choice can affect pitch contour. The sounds "a" and "ah" lead to more stable intonations (low standard deviations from the mean pitch), than "ee," "oo," and even more so than "r," and "ra."[6] Though this may be only slightly discernible to a patient, I believe everything can contribute to something sounding more stable. And the more stable the less tension may be evoked in the patient, even if this occurs below their conscious understanding.

Below I will discuss more in depth how I use melody with patients vis-à-vis the intervention of tension release.

Tension-Release Intervention

Pain can generate tension, whether this includes contracting one's muscles or experiencing anxiety. The goal is to meet a patient where he or she is presently (emotionally and physically), and then shift their current state to one more conducive to healing, such as relaxation. With this in mind, music is first played to the patient that evokes the tension they feel. The therapist follows the breath of the patient and adjusts her music/rhythm to the patient's respiration rate, until patient's breath and therapist's music entrain to each other in rhythmic synchrony. As the music continues, the therapist alternatively creates passages of tension and relaxation with gradual emphasis given to those of relaxation. Through the principle of entrainment the patient's breath slows to a more relaxed pace, leading to a natural state of tension release and a more optimal state for healing.

Tension can be created in music through various mechanisms: harmonically by delaying the V-I chord cadence, dynamically through crescendo, or rhythmically through acceleration of tempo. Through the influence of Hindūstāni music elements, I like to create tension and release through melodic movement.

In Western voice leading, the leading tone wants to resolve to the tonic, the fourth scale degree often wants to move to the third, and the second to the tonic. Similar rules of melodic movement in Hindūstāni music can aid in the creation of melodic tension when a note is not resolved melodically to where the listener anticipates it to go. By delaying melodic movement to the tonic, be it the higher or lower one, the therapist can build tension.

Most Hindūstāni rāgas are associated with stock phrases that characterize it. In adaptation of this musical device, the therapist sings a stock melodic phrase repeatedly over the course of an improvisation, so the ear gets accustomed to it. Then to build tension, the therapist sings the stock phrase and intentionally leaves out the last note, and then repeats this phrase with the omission. The ear anticipates the last note, but it does not arrive.

Case Study 2: Jean and Melodic Elaboration known as Vistār.
One way to create melodic tension is by exploring melody through the Hindūstāni music concept of *vistār* (expansion). Vistār is a type of melodic elaboration used in improvisation (Anita Slawek, personal communication, 1997). One of its objectives is to gradually introduce the listener to each note of a rāga, so that he or she becomes accustomed to its sound. Below is an excerpt of a session with a patient Jean to further illustrate vistār and melodic tension release. Jean is an 87-year old French man with leukemia, who was hospitalized for a staphylococcus infection and weakness following chemotherapy. The Clinical Nurse Specialist reported that he had been quite demanding of hospital staff during a previous admission. Recalling his fondness for music during that admission, she now referred him for music therapy to help him better manage and cope with his present hospitalization. With this patient I patterned the melodic elaboration of my vocal improvisation on the concept of *vistār alāp*. Although the way I explore notes may not exactly resemble this concept, my improvisation is influenced by it.

I began playing the drone on a guitar to clear a sonic space in Jean's hospital room. Singing very softly on the tonic (the beginning of vistār type improvisation), I produced notes that were primarily the neighboring tones of the tonic. Eventually I extended the range of notes to the lower register below the tonic in stepwise motion (down to the fifth scale degree). Subsequently I moved back to the tonic and then begin to explore the middle register using a specific paradigm of melodic elaboration. In this paradigm, I tend to improvise upward to a note, and then move stepwise back to the tonic and rest on it. Then I sing up the scale again, but sing one note higher than the one I ascended to previously, followed by a stepwise return to the tonic. In this way, I elaborate melodically into the middle and upper part of the scale until I reach the high tonic.

While exploring the middle register, the melodic motion is not always strictly stepwise, as I pattern my ascending and descending vocal lines on the rules of melodic motion in rāga Yaman Kalyan. Rāga Yaman Kalyan uses a major scale, modified to include a sharp on the fourth scale degree. This note collection is similar to that of the Lydian mode, however the pattern of notes and the sequence in which they are sung moves beyond the Lydian scale. At times I used vocal slides and/or grace notes in the movement from one note to another. I execute these ornamentations in a manner consistent with the prescribed stock phrases of this rāga.

The goal of a vistār alāp is to reach the high tonic, and I focus on this same goal in my vocal improvisation for Jean. However, movement up to the high tonic is delayed in ways to produce tension, e.g., singing the leading tone and then moving down to the 6th scale degree. Singing the upper tonic is a culminating moment when it occurs, as the tension is resolved. After this goal has been achieved, I then vocalize a quick descent back to the lower tonic. This acts as a melodic denouement. The improvisation section of the rāga has finished, and the next section occurs (end of vistār type improvisation). I then begin to sing a small composition I learned in rāga Yaman Kalyan. I sing it very slowly, and extend the pacing of the melody in order to sustain the patient's relaxed state. I also refrain from the words of the composition, and instead focus my singing on the use of "ah" and "mm" so that Jean's experience is not disrupted. I am mindful of this because I have found that associations to the meaning of words inevitably occur when words are introduced, and in this work, such mechanisms of the intellect have the potential to distract a patient away from achieving a purely meditative state.

While doing all this, I watch the movement of Jean's chest in effort to entrain my drone rhythm to the pace of his breath. This presents a challenge so instead I try to align parts of the rhythm of the melody I sing to his breath (entrainment), starting a melodic phrase on an inhale and ending it on one of his exhales. His face looks relaxed: He seems content by his facial expressions. His eyes are closed and it looks like he has been in a relaxed state for some time.

Music and Medicine: Integrative Models in the Treatment of Pain

Breath Focusing, Imagery, Mantra, and Sacred Vowels
Breath work and imagery use with patients can further enhance relaxation. Before starting the drone, I ask the patient to think about a place that he likes (real or imagined), somewhere that gives him ease of mind. I ask him to describe this place to me. After the drone has begun, I ask the patient to focus on the natural pace of his breath, the rise and fall and physical sensations of inhalation and exhalation. I have him imagine he is in the place he likes and suggest physical sensations relating to it (e.g., if the ocean, I say "you can feel the warm sand under your feet"). Evoking imagery of a familiar place hopefully puts patients at ease and creates continuity between the hospital and their life outside of it, helping to establish normalcy. Deep breathing can help one relax, and relaxation in turn effects physiological changes such as decreased heart and respiration rates and blood pressure.[21] One can inform patients to use these techniques in future instances of pain: To focus on their breath and visualize their imagined place.

To induce relaxation, Schaffer and Yuchi, according to Benson, support using a "mental device" or a "constant stimulus on which the patient focuses, such as . . . a repeated word or phrase."[21(p78)] I use chant or mantra with patients to engage coping mechanisms for when the therapist is not there, as in the case of Alicia.

Case Study 3: Alicia
Alicia was a Latina woman in her late forties, who was admitted to Beth Israel Medical Center for severe back pain. Her hospitalization was anxiety provoking for her due to this pain for which she was undergoing diagnostic testing. The testing had yet to divulge the genesis of her discomfort and subsequently the medical team was challenged in the task of creating an effective treatment plan. She was understandably frustrated, worried, and unable to sleep. She was referred for music therapy services to help her manage her pain and anxiety. At the onset of our session her pain level was controlled with medication, and she reported her pain to be at a level of 2 out of 10 on a Visual Analog Pain Scale (VAS). She confided however that she was very worried the pain meant something was horribly wrong with her, something that would necessitate a drastic lifestyle change or be life-threatening. She asked to play something together that would help her release the anxiety she felt surrounding her pain and condition. She asked if I knew any mantras she could use in moments of stress, to help her when music therapy was not available. Feeling at a loss to deliver a mantra in that moment, I suggested that we create one that expressed what she felt while making use of her inner resources.

We talked about times in her life when she had felt hardship and how she had coped with these situations. She recounted that in these instances, she had consistently showed resilience and perseverance. Her mantra thus became: "I have the strength to get through this." We repeated this several times while focusing on her breath. I then asked her to repeat it in her mind while synchronizing her words to the rhythm of her inhales and exhales. The rationale behind this was that the mantra would give her strength as well as a sense of agency that when coupled with breath work, would help her focus and move through any tension and pain she was feeling. The pace of her breath, in the absence of music, would also act as a "rhythm track" to which she could organize the mantra's words. With the mantra, Alicia was able to create something that spoke personally about who she truly is, something that was uniquely hers. She crafted something that she could use in the future when she felt she needed it; something helpful to implement that transcended the time boundaries of a music therapy session and could have a lasting effect.

Giving patients a resource that can be called upon when needed can reinforce existing coping skills and provide incentive to reach therapeutic goals. Such intervention also empowers the patient during treatment by encouraging an active role in the care being received. Here the therapist honors the patient's wishes and facilitates the patient in actively designing his or her therapy, which reflects a Rogerian approach.[24(p149)]

Alicia was a major agent in the mantra creation process. Granting her control and restoring parts of her autonomy were in some way central to her process and showed her the inner power she possessed. This was an important factor to Alicia as with many patients experiencing a loss of control in so many arenas of their lives. The mantra here acted to reduce anxiety felt surrounding her pain.

Case Study 4: Marie
A patient in her mid-fifties named Marie had received spinal fusion. Marie was in pain but had refused pain medication, because it made her feel too drowsy and confused. Music therapy was referred for her to provide a forum for tension release and engage coping skills for pain management, especially as a non-pharmalogic method. She reported her pain was at a level of 4 of 10 on the pain scale when she did not move. However when movement was necessary, she was quite uncomfortable. I tried several musical styles in the service of a tension-release intervention including the use of the drone and Hindūstāni-influenced singing, but she was unable to refocus or relax. I eventually offered Hindūstāni-influenced music as well, but she was too uncomfortable and kindly requested we end the session.

Marie's pain was too great to allow her the clarity or ability to integrate the music therapy session, and this scenario rears the question as to whether proper pain intervention had been assessed and rendered pharmacologically.

Discussion

Some of the patients I discussed were able to relax or drift into sleep during the music therapy intervention, but it is not clear as to how pain medication may have been a factor. My music therapy interventions with Indian musical elements are mostly receptive in that patients choose to listen, however an active component exists as well. A therapeutic forum is provided, which patients are invited to speak about their lives over the drone. In other instances where the patient chooses not to verbalize their process, or is unable to physically participate in music due to pain, engagement through active listening can become the most viable option for receiving treatment.

In working with pain management, I occasionally provide music therapy as a co-treatment for a patient receiving Reiki. As the Reiki therapist works on the patient I play the drone and sing Hindūstāni-influenced vocalizations that align with the physical movement of the Reiki therapist's hands. I improvise on notes above the tonic while her hands hover above a part of the body. When she takes her hands away from the patient's body to dispel energy, I sing a downward melodic slide, coming to rest on the tonic once she brings her hands back to the patient.

During these sessions, I may also integrate Yogic philosophy, where there are chakras (energy or life force centers) in the human body that are associated with a sacred vowel sound.[26] I sometimes sing on the appropriate vowel that corresponds to the chakra on which the Reiki therapist is working. Thus if she is concentrating on the head, I sing the vowel "eeh" which corresponds to the crown chakra. While there is no concrete evidence for what this practice might do, it is my goal that singing these sacred vowels help activate the related chakra and move the energy within it, thus affecting how the patient feels the flow of energy in relation to the specific pain in the body.

Certainly the range and variation of outcomes warrants important questions about treatment efficacy. How does using Hindūstāni music elements to assist with pain management integrate with other therapies including pharmacologic treatment? How might the therapeutic impact of treatment integration be evaluated? The indication for research on the effects of music therapy in conjunction with other types of intervention, both non-pharmacologic and pharmacologic in the treatment of pain is great. With the latter, dosage and frequency of medication administering in conjunction with the timing of the music therapy intervention is an important factor for consideration. The effectiveness of co-treatment with other non-pharmacologic therapies may also be worthy of research, when determining efficacy of treatment practice.

Conclusion

In this chapter we have discussed some of the therapeutic possibilities of connecting elements of Indian and Persian music traditions with contemporary music therapy practice, specifically to address pain management. As these traditions in their vastness and complexity require many years to understand and master, we view this chapter as a contribution to an ongoing dialogue about how to implement these traditions in clinical practice. We hope that our work will inspire an exchange with others across diverse fields to further explore the therapeutic potential that is possible in this area, not only here in the United States but in the practice of music therapy in India, Iran, and other countries (see note 7).

References

1. Nettl B. An ethnomusicological perspective. *International Journal of Music Education.* 2005;23(2):131-133. doi: 10.1177/0255761405052407
2. Bruscia K. *Defining Music Therapy. 2nd ed.* Gilsum, NH: Barcelona Publishers; 1998.
3. Shiloah A. *Music in the World of Islam: A Socio-Cultural Study.* Detroit, MI: Wayne State University Press; 1995.
4. Sundar S. Traditional Healing Systems and Modern Music Therapy in India. *Music Therapy Today* (Online). 2007; VIII (3): 397-407. http://musictherapyworld.net
5. Hamel PM. *Through Music to the Self: How to Appreciate and Experience Music Anew.* Element Books; 1984.
6. Rao S. *Acoustical Perspective on Raga-Rasa Theory.* New Delhi: Munshiram Manoharlal Publishers; 2000.
7. Wade B. *Music in India: The Classical Traditions.* New Delhi: Manohar; 1991.
8. Ruckert G, Widdess R. Hindustani raga. In: Arnold A, ed. *Garland Encyclopedia of World Music.* Vol.5: South Asia: The Indian Subcontinent. Routledge; 1999: 64-88
9. Shanker R. *Music Therapy: Indian Classical Music Perspective.* http://www.rajamsmusictherapy.com/music-therapy--indian-classical-music-perspective.html

10. Bradt J. The History of Music Therapy. In: Brooks S, ed. *Creative Arts Therapy Manual*. Springfield, IL: Charles C Thomas; 2006: 168-174.
11. Sundar S. Addressing Diversities in Music Therapy Theory, Practice and Research: Major Challenges. Jörg Fachner interviewed by Sumathy Sundar. *Voices: A World Forum for Music Therapy*. 2007; 7 (1).
https://normt.uib.no/index.php/voices/article/view/468/377
12. Wigram T, Pedersen I, Bonde L. *A Comprehensive Guide to Music Therapy: Theory, Clinical Practice, Research and Training*. London: Jessica Kingsley Publishers; 2004.
13. Sairam TV. *Raga Therapy*. Chennai: Nada Centre for Music Therapy; 2004.
14. Szabó C. The Effects of Listening to Monotonous Drumming on Subjective Experiences. In: Aldridge D, Fachner J., eds. *Music and Altered States*. London: Jessica Kingsley Publishers; 2006: 51-59.
15. Austin D. The Musical Mirror: Music Therapy for the Narcissistically Injured. In: Bruscia K, ed. *Case Studies in Music Therapy*. Barcelona Publishers; 1991: 291-307.
16. Farhat H. *The Dastgāh Concept in Persian Music*. Cambridge University Press; 1990.
17. Desmukh A, Sarvaiya A, Seethalakshmi R, Nayak A. Effect of Indian Classical Music on Quality of Sleep in Depressed Patients: a Randomized Controlled Trial. *Nordic Journal of Music Therapy*. 2009; 18 (1): 70-78.
18. Morcom A. *Hindi Film Songs and the Cinema*. Hampshire, UK: Ashgate; 2007.
19. Ruud E. *Music Therapy: Improvisation, Communication, and Culture*. Gilsum, NH: Barcelona; 1998.
20. Swamy S. "No, she doesn't seem to know anything about cultural differences!": Culturally centered music therapy supervision. *Music Ther Perspect*. 2011;29(2):133-137.
21. Schaffer SD, Yucha CB. Relaxation & pain management: The relaxation response can play a role in managing chronic and acute pain. *Am J Nurs*. August 2004;104:75-82.
22. Davis BD. *Caring for People in Pain*. London: Routledge; 2000.
23. Down K. Sound Synergy: The Significance and Use of the Musical Drone in Music Therapy [master's thesis]. New York: New York University; 2009.
24. Raskin NJ, Rogers CR, Witty MC. Client-centered therapy. In: Corsini RJ, Wedding D, eds. *Current Psychotherapies*. 9th ed. Belmont, CA: Brooks/Cole; 2011:148-195.

25. Goldman JS. Toward a new consciousness of the sonic healing arts: The therapeutic use of sound and music for personal and planetary health and transformation. *Music Ther.* 1988;7(1):28-33.
26. Judith A. *Eastern Body, Western Mind: Psychology and the Chakra System as a Path to the Self.* New York, NY: Celestial Arts; 2004.

Music and Medicine: Integrative Models in the Treatment of Pain

APPENDIX A

CDs:

1. Rāga Chayanat by Sanjukta Biswas: private copy (permission of the author granted).

2. Dastan Trio: Journey to Persian. Arc Music, 2003.

3. Ramnad Krishnan: Vidwan. Music of South India. Elektra Nonesuch, 1988.

4. Indie du Nord: Dinkar Kaikini. Ocora France, 1997.

Note about Diacritical Marks and Pronunciation

An 'a' without a symbol represents the sound 'uh', as in "must".

An 'ā' represents the sound 'ah', as in "father". Another transliteration of this sound is "aa".

An 'ī' represents the sound 'ee', as in "meet".

An 'ū' represents the sound 'oo', as in "food".

APPENDIX B

Notes

1. All music samples in this part of the paper are available through Dropbox. Interested readers should contact Oksana Rosenblum at oksana.rosenblum@gmail.com with the request to send them the shared link.
2. The musical elements used and described below come from Hindūstāni (North Indian classical) music. While some of these elements may hold for both North and South Indian classical music, in an effort to simplify, I concentrate on the former, as this is the tradition in which I have trained.
3. While Hindūstāni music is the classical music genre from the part of India my family hails, it is not the principle music of my Punjabi, Sikh cultural heritage.
4. Sound, Voice, and Music Healing is a 9-month certificate program offered at the California Institute of Integral Studies in San Francisco. For more information, see http://www.ciis.edu/About_ CIISPublic_Programs/Certificate_Programs/Sound_Certificate.html
5. The concept of showing respect to the genre and lineage of Indian classical music, North or South, runs deep among its practitioners and includes, but is not limited to, respect for one's guru as well as respect for the instruments and performers (i.e., removing one's shoes when playing, not stepping directly over an instrument, and audience members not sitting at a level above the performer). This reflects how the concept of respect pervades Indian culture and extends to its artforms.
6. It must be noted that there are contraindications of using the drone as well.[23(p21-22)]
7. While there are other scholars and clinicians looking at implementing these music traditions in music therapy practice, due to various constraints, it is unfortunately not possible to discuss their work in the present chapter. Some of these clinicians include but are not limited to: Eric Fraser, DeBorah Green, M. Hai Haran, Ranjana Kirthi, Veena Kumar, Monique McGrath, Silvia Nakkach and Aaron Shragge. There are also those with whom the authors are as yet unacquainted, who we graciously look forward to meeting.

Music and Medicine: Integrative Models in the Treatment of Pain

CONTRIBUTORS

Melanie May Po Acosta MA, LCAT, MT-BC, NRMT holds an MA in Music Therapy from NYU and a BA in Communication Studies from Vanderbilt University. She also holds a Post-Master's Level I Advanced Training Certificate from the Nordoff Robbins Center for Music Therapy. Melanie is the Asthma Initiative Program (AIP) music therapist researching the effects of music therapy through the use of wind instruments in children and adolescents with Asthma. Melanie has also provided music therapy services for children, adolescents and adults diagnosed with a variety of developmental disabilities, including autism spectrum disorders, mental retardation, and cerebral palsy. Melanie comes to the music therapy field with 15 years experience as a professional singer, bringing with her a deeply rooted philosophy and belief in the power of music as a form of communication and as a tool to form healthy physical, emotional, and spiritual connections. Melanie is a member of the American Music Therapy Association, Certification Board of Music Therapists, Actor's Equity Association, Screen Actor's Guild and the American Federation of Television and Radio Artists.

Erik Baumann Cornejo MMT is an International Research Scholar at the Louis Armstrong Center for Music and Medicine. He was born in Lima, Peru, where he earned a bachelor's degree in clinical psychology. There he worked as a psychotherapist, and was involved in several community development projects with at-risk populations. He subsequently earned his Music Therapy Masters degree from the Universitat de Barcelona, Spain, where he focused his music therapy training on the child-parent bond. Erik speaks six languages and is a traveler of the world. He is a published writer and has presented his work in Spain, Sweden, and most recently at the Gestalt Center in his native Peru.

Thomas J. Biglin, Jr. MA, MT-BC received his master's degree in Music Therapy from New York University and his bachelor's from the University of Pennsylvania. Working with such organizations as the Roosevelt Children's Center, the JCC of Manhattan, and the Institute for Music and Neurologic Function in the Bronx, Tom applies his integrative, multi-instrumental, music therapy approach to a varied population including medically fragile children, adolescents with developmental delays, as well as adults recovering from stroke and those with various forms of dementia.

Frank Bosco MA, MT-BC, LMT, RPP, SEP, LCAT is the founder/director of Sound Health Studio, a center specializing in body/mind wellness and therapy. He has been in private practice for over 30 years integrating a wide range of somatic/psychotherapy practices. He specializes in body-oriented psychotherapy (primarily Gestalt Therapy) processing with the use of music and sound. As one of the first few New York professionals to be trained in Somatic-Experiencing® (an approach for "renegotiating" trauma), he has specialized in incorporating music and sound therapy for pain reduction and trauma resolution. Frank has been an adjunct faculty member in the graduate music therapy program at New York University for over 20 years facilitating group process classes and conducting workshops in the application gestalt theory to music therapy. He has been an active member of the New York Institute for Gestalt Therapy, and is currently serving a term as Vice President.

Jenny Branson BA, MT-BC is the Clinical Coordinator and Supervisor of Norton Healthcare, Louisville, KY. She provides clinical coordination and supervision for medical music services throughout Norton Healthcare in Louisville, Kentucky. As a medical music therapist, she works with adults in an acute care medical hospital, in both inpatient and outpatient settings. Jenny's program provides music therapy intervention, a music listening library, a visiting artist program, education, and outreach services to the Norton Healthcare System. She has presented her work in intensive care medical music therapy, music therapy co-treatment, and percussion in therapy locally and regionally. A classically trained percussionist, Jenny is active in the local music community, performing with a variety of groups on a regular basis.

Soniya K. Brar MA, MM, MT-BC is a music therapist who holds a Master's in Ethnomusicology. Her clinical training is in medical adult and pediatric settings as well as in work with the neurologically-impaired. Her interests include using elements of North Indian classical music in music therapy practice to address pain management and anxiety and utilizing a holistic approach to patient treatment. In addition to this is how the culture of therapist and client can affect and inform music therapy practice. Ms. Brar is a former music educator at the community-college level and has published on Sikh religious music in the 2001 2nd edition of the New Grove Dictionary for Music and Musicians (London: Macmillan).

Bernardo Canga MMT holds a Superior Degree in Music from Conservatorio de Oviedo (Spain), specialized in Violin and Viola. His commitment to underserved populations led him to participate in international programs that combine Global Health and At-Risk Youth. He earned a Masters in Music Therapy from the Pontifical University of Salamanca. His Master Thesis on

Contributors

Non-verbal Processes of Communication in Intellectual Disabilities was presented at the VIII European Music Therapy Congress. He completed a clinical fellowship at Beth Israel Medical Center prior to joining the music therapy staff of the Louis Armstrong Center for Music and Medicine. He is currently participating in research studies of Music Therapy and Oncology, Heart Disease, Chronic Obstructive Pulmonary Disease, and Environmental Music Therapy, and has been central to program development as the primary music therapist in the inpatient oncology unit at Roosevelt Hospital in New York, NY.

Maya Charlton MA, MT-BC is a music Therapist at Children's Hospital & Research Center Oakland, Oakland, CA. She graduated from New York University in 1998 with a Master's in Music Therapy. She has established and directed music therapy programs throughout the Bay Area serving children and adolescents in medical and mental health settings. Since 2008 Maya has directed the Jared Kurtin Music Therapy Program at Children's Hospital & Research Center Oakland where she specializes in trauma, hematology, oncology and palliative care.

Cheryl Dileo PhD, MT-BC is the Carnell Professor of Music Therapy, Director of the PhD Program and Director of the Arts and Quality of Life Research Center at Temple University. She is a founding member of the International Association for Music and Medicine and is a Past-President of the World Federation of Music Therapy and National Association for Music Therapy. She was the former McAndless Distinguished Professor at Eastern Michigan University and is currently an Honorary Associate Professor at the University of Melbourne (Australia) and a member of the PhD Advisory Board at Aalborg University, Denmark. She is the recipient of the Lifetime Achievement Award, Research/Publications Award and Award of Merit from the American Music Therapy Association, and the Faculty Research Award from Temple University. She has published extensively and is a co-author of 6 Cochrane reviews and author/editor of 13 books and more than 100 chapters and articles. She lectures internationally on a regular basis.

Natalia Garrido MMT was born in Madrid, Spain, where she earned her Masters degree in Music Therapy from the Universidad Autonoma of Madrid. Her post-graduate work in Madrid was focused extensively on children living with physical and neurologic impairment, and emotional disturbance, as well as with pediatric patients admitted to cardiac unit of the Gregorio Marañon Hospital. Continuing this work internationally, Natalia provided music therapy to physically and emotionally challenged children from underprivileged areas and low resources in Mexico and India. Subsequently, Natalia accepted the position as the 2010/11 Research Fellow for the Louis Armstrong Center for Music and Medicine in New York, NY. She is currently building a music therapy program in the oncology unit of the Hospital de Jaen, Spain where her work focuses on developing environmental music therapy, conducting research within the chemotherapy infusion suite, and providing individual music psychotherapy. Natalia has presented her work internationally, and most recently participated in the 2012 World Music Therapy Congress in Bangkok, Thailand.

Suzanne Hanser EdD, MT-BC is founding chair of the Music Therapy Department at Berklee College of Music in Boston, MA. She is Past President of both the World Federation of Music Therapy and the National Association for Music Therapy, and is founding member of the International Association for Music and Medicine. Dr. Hanser has served as Music Therapist at Dana-Farber Cancer Institute and Research Scholar at the Women's Studies Research Center at Brandeis University. She received a National Research Service Award from the NIA and was a Senior Postdoctoral Fellow at Stanford University School of Medicine. She is the author of "Manage Your Stress and Pain through Music" (with S Mandel). In 2006 she was named by the Boston Globe as one of eleven Bostonians Changing the World. In 2009 she was awarded the Sage Publications Prize for her article, "From ancient to integrative medicine: Models for music therapy." She received the Lifetime Achievement Award from the American Music Therapy Association in 2011.

Annie Heiderscheit PhD, MT-BC, LMFT is a board certified music therapist and licensed marriage and family therapist. She is an assistant professor in the Center for Spirituality at the University of Minnesota and adjunct faculty in the music therapy program at Augsburg College. She is the Director of the Arts and Healing Initiative at the Center and the 2010-2012. A Marilyn Sime Research Fellow, Dr. Heiderscheit is also a clinical music therapist at The Emily Program and at the University of Minnesota Amplatz Children's Hospital. She is the secretary/treasurer of the World Federation of Music Therapy. She actively conducts research based on her clinical practice. She has authored several book chapters and articles based on her clinical work and research. Dr. Heiderscheit frequently presents her research and clinical work nationally and internationally. Her areas of expertise are in working with clients with eating disorders at various levels of care, adults and children medical settings.

Jillian Hicks MA, MT-BC works as a Board Certified Music Therapist at Willamette Valley Hospice in Salem, OR providing psychological, physiological, and emotional support to people during the end of life process. Jillian attended Lewis & Clark College, Marylhurst University, and received her Masters in Music Therapy at New York University. She was the 2011-12 Music Therapy Fellow at the Louis Armstrong Center for Music and Medicine at Beth Israel Medical Center where she specialized in the application of music therapy in medical settings. Jillian was a presenter at the 2012 International Association for Music & Medicine Conference in Bangkok, Thailand.

Nancy A. Jackson PhD, MT-BC is a board certified music therapist with more than 19 years of clinical experience in areas including music psychotherapy and medical music therapy in both group and individual formats. She is the Director of Music Therapy at Indiana University, Purdue University Fort Wayne, IN. She received both her Master's in Music Therapy, and Doctor of Philosophy in Music Therapy degrees from Temple University. Her research interests include the understanding of anger and other emotions within the music psychotherapy process, music therapy for chronic pain and chronic illness; experiential learning in music therapy education, collaboration in the music therapy profession, and professional supervision. Dr. Jackson frequently presents at regional, national, and international conferences and professional meetings. She is Director of Music Therapy at Indiana University – Purdue University Fort Wayne.

Robert E. Krout EdD MT-BC is Professor and Director of the Music Therapy Program in the Meadows School of the Arts at Southern Methodist University (SMU) in Dallas, Texas, where he was named the Outstanding Teaching Professor for 2010-2011. Prior to joining SMU, Robert was Director of Music Therapy at Massey University in Wellington, New Zealand. He was previously Music Therapy Manager and Internship Director at Hospice of Palm Beach County, Florida, and Associate Professor at the State University of New York at New Paltz from 1982-1997. In 2005 he received the Research and Publication Award of the American Music Therapy Association.

Yi-Ying Lin MA, MT-BC was born in Taipei, Taiwan, and has lived there for 26 years. She studied counseling and elementary education at the Bachelor's level and is currently completing her Master's Degree in Music Therapy in Montclair State University. She completed a clinical internship within the Louis & Lucille Armstrong Music Therapy Program at Beth Israel Medical Center from 2011 to 2012, with concentration in the areas of environmental music therapy, radiation oncology, NICU, COPD, and The Music and Health Clinic. She is completing her thesis research study on understanding Asian international music therapy students' peer group experiences.

Joanne V. Loewy DA, LCAT, MT-BC is the Director of the Louis Armstrong Center for Music and Medicine, which among many populations is serving musicians and their unique ailments including chronic fatigue, chemical dependency, performance anxiety and overuse. She oversees the Department of Music Therapy which she started at Beth Israel in 1994. She has conducted research in sedation, assessment, pain, asthma and NICU music therapy. Her areas of specialty are assessment, hermeneutic research, trauma and supervision. Dr. Loewy is the co-Editor in Chief of the international, peer reviewed journal 'Music and Medicine' and serves on several editorial boards including the Cochrane Palliative Care Review and the Journal for Complementary and Alternative Medicine. She received her doctorate from NYU and has edited several books including Music Therapy in Pediatric Pain, Music Therapy in the NICU, and she co-edited Music Therapy at End of Life and Caring for the Caregiver: Music Therapy in Grief and Trauma and Advances in Integrative Medicine: Music, the Breath and Health. She is a founding member of the International Association for Music and Medicine and guest lectures at the Albert Einstein College of Medicine and teaches at Hahnemann Creative Arts Therapy graduate music therapy program at Drexel University in Philadelphia, Molloy College and Temple University.

Susan E. Mandel PhD, MT-BC is a music therapy consultant to Lake Health in northeast Ohio, where she manages the music therapy program and is the principal investigator of music therapy research studies in cardiac rehabilitation, diabetes education, and integrative medicine. Dr. Mandel is a faculty member of the School of Advanced Studies of the University of Phoenix.

John F. Mondanaro MA, LCAT, MT-BC, CCLS is the Clinical Director of the Louis & Lucille Armstrong Program at Beth Israel Medical Center in New York, NY where he oversees inpatient services, the Clinical Internship Program, the Visiting Artist Series, the Observation & Orientation Program, and the International Scholar Program. Earning a MA in Music Therapy from New York University, and BA in Art from St. Ambrose University, John is licensed by the New York State Education Department as a mental health practitioner in Creative Arts Therapy. He maintains board certification by the Certification Board of Music Therapy, and certification in Child Life Practice by the Child Life Council. Working from an integrative philosophy, John has published numerous articles on the arts in healthcare and has additionally composed and produced two full-length recordings of original music. He teaches Medical Music Psychotherapy at the New School and is a member of the International Association of Music and Medicine, American Music Therapy Association, the Certification Board of Music Therapists, and the American Society of Composers, Artists, & Publishers.

Paul Nolan MCAT, LPC, MT-BC is the Director of Hahnemann's Music Therapy Programs in the Department of Creative Arts Therapy at Drexel University in Philadelphia, PA. He has clinical experience in adult inpatient and outpatient psychiatry, gerontology, child and adult medical settings. Paul has numerous publications; has been invited to present both the nationally and internationally. He has juried numerous presentations, and has served on many editorial boards related to the arts and health.

Stephan J. Quentzel MD, JD, MA is the Medical Director for both the Louis Armstrong Center for Music and the Psychiatry Institute for Urban Family Health at Beth Israel Medical Center, New York, NY. Triple boarded in psychiatry, family medicine and holistic/integrative medicine, Dr. Quentzel practices clinically with a comprehensive view of the patient. As Medical Director of the Louis Armstrong Center for Music and Medicine he provides clinical management of a unified bio-psycho-musical service geared to the health needs of musicians and performing artists, and as a private practitioner he employs an "all things are connected" framework. His approach integrates brain sciences and psychiatry with general medicine, psychology, philosophy, preventative, herbal medicine and nutrition in pursuit of comprehensive and optimal health and wellness. He is a founding member of the International Association for Music and Medicine and an editorial reviewer for the 'Music and Medicine' journal. He is an assistant professor at the Albert Einstein College of Medicine.

Trisha Ready PhD holds a PhD in Clinical Psychology from Pacifica Graduate Institute and practices clinical psychology at Fairfax Hospital in Seattle, WA. Her dissertation and research were based on using self-selected music as a means of emotional containment and expression for people experiencing early stages of psychosis. She has articles published or forthcoming in the American Journal of Hospice and Palliative Medicine, Music and Medicine, and Psychoanalysis, Culture, and Society. She currently uses music as an adjunct to group and individual therapy with patients at an acute psychiatric hospital in the Seattle area.

Music and Medicine: Integrative Models in the Treatment of Pain

Oksana Rosenblum MA graduated from JTS with the Master's in Jewish Art and Visual Culture in 2005. She gained her Bachelor's and Master's degrees in Cultural Anthropology from Ukraine in 2001. Since 2005, Oksana has been free-lancing as a visual researcher in the field of Jewish art and history, contributing her talents to the newly created museums of Jewish History in Warsaw and Moscow. After finishing the Certificate Program in Creative Arts Therapy at The New School in 2011, Oksana volunteered as a research assistant at Beth Israel Hospital in NYC, helping with the research study on music therapy and its effect on cancer patients. Oksana studies Persian and Indian music in her free time, and occasionally performs with ethnic group ensembles. She lives in Brooklyn, NY and can be contacted at oksana.rosenblum@gmail.com

Andrew Rossetti MMT, MT-BC coordinates the Radiation-Oncology Programs located in Phillips Ambulatory Care Center and BI West through the Louis Armstrong Center for Music and Medicine of Beth Israel Medical Center in New York, NY. He has developed several music therapy programs in hospitals both in the United States and in Spain including a comprehensive NICU music therapy program at Advocate Lutheran General Hospital in Chicago as well as programs in acute and out-patient psychiatric units at the Hospital del Mar, and the Centre Forum Psychiatric Facility in Spain where he was a professor in the music therapy masters program at Pompeu Fabra University in Barcelona. In private practice in Spain, Andrew developed a multi-modal model along with Psychiatrist Dr. Javier Rubio for their co-treatment of psychiatric patients. Andrew received his Masters in Music Therapy from the Facultad de Psicologia Blanquerna at Ramon Llull University in Barcelona Spain. He studied at the Julliard School and holds a Bachelor's in classical guitar performance from the Westchester Conservatory of Music. Andrew's extensive experience as a professional musician has allowed him to tap into the emotional and metaphoric power of music, employing it in a variety of arenas in clinical practice.

Gabriel A. Sara MD is the Medical Director of The Roosevelt Hospital Chemotherapy Infusion Suite. He is a Senior Attending Physician in the Division Of Hematology/Oncology at St. Luke's and Roosevelt hospitals (SLR) as well as the Executive Director of the Patient Services Initiative at The Continuum Cancer Center Of New York (CCCNY), a unique philanthropy program he has developed since 2005. In his various titles, he oversees operations in the chemotherapy Infusion Suite, takes on clinical care, research and teaching responsibilities in the division of hematology/oncology at SLR and continues to enhance the vast philanthropy program that has dramatically impacted the patients' care at CCCNY. Dr. Sara has

Contributors

served in several hospital committees. After receiving his medical degree from the Faculté Française de Médecine in Beirut, Lebanon in 1980, Dr. Sara completed his residency training at the State University of New York (SUNY)-Downstate Medical Center in Brooklyn. He then completed a medical oncology and hematology fellowships at SLR and at New York Presbyterian Hospital/Columbia University Medical Center. Dr. Sara is board certified in internal medicine, hematology and medical oncology. His areas of expertise include breast cancer, lung cancer, lymphoma, gastrointestinal cancers and solid tumors as well as hematologic malignancies. He is a member of the American Society of Internal Medicine, the American Society of Clinical Oncology, the New York Metropolitan Breast Cancer Group and the New York Cancer Society. He received the St. Luke's-Roosevelt Hospital Center's 2004 "Wholeness of Life" award and since 1997 has been yearly cited in the Hematology/Oncology section of "Top Doctors: New York Metro Area" by Castle Connolly. Since 2008, he has been yearly cited in the "Super Doctors" edition of the New York Times Magazine (http://www.superdoctors.com/) and was among New York Magazine's "Best Doctors" for 2008, as listed in the June 16, 2008 edition of the magazine. The New York Magazine list is excerpted from Castle Connolly's annual guidebook, "Top Doctors: New York Metro Area." In 2005, Dr. Sara established the Helen Sawaya Fund, in memory of his patient and friend Helen Sawaya, a philanthropy program which mission is to enhance the experience of cancer patients through art, music, reflexology, a travel program and more. Dr. Sara grew up surrounded by music at home and plays several instruments. He also sings regularly in a choir. His love for music made him a strong advocate in implementing music therapy at CCCNY where it is now an integral part of the routine treatment of patients.

Benedikte B. Scheiby MA, MMEd, DPMT, CMT, AMT, LCAT is the Director of Music Therapy Training and Supervision, and Senior Clinician Music Psychotherapist at the Institute for Music and Neurologic Function in the Bronx, NY. She is the Director of the Postgraduate Institute for Analytical Music Therapy in New York, where she holds a private practice working with clients interested in personal growth, wellness, psychological and physical challenges like anxiety, depression, addiction, attachment challenges, social skills, eating disorders, emotional, medical or spiritual challenges. She is a licensed clinical music psychotherapist, Analytical Music Therapist (Priestley method) and certified body psychotherapist in the United States who has been an adjunct professor at the Masters Music Therapy Program at New York University for 20 years. She provides individual and group music therapy supervision, and has been a music psychotherapist for 30 years, working with populations including adults, children, couples, the elderly

Music and Medicine: Integrative Models in the Treatment of Pain

both in the context of wellness, psychiatry and in a medical paradigm.

Brian H. Schreck MA, MT-BC is a Music Therapist/Coordinator at Cincinnati Children's Hospital Medical Center in Cincinnati, OH, where he has recently developed the Children's Pediatric Hospice Program. His training in music therapy includes a Bachelor's Degree from Berklee College of Music in Boston and a Master of Arts Degree from New York University. Prior to his current position, Brian introduced and established music therapy in palliative care to Saint Vincent Catholic Medical Center in New York. He enjoys exploring new instruments, playing and performing in acoustic and electric bands, and painting.

Fred Schwartz MD is an anesthesiologist in practice at Piedmont Hospital in Atlanta, Georgia. He has utilized music in numerous patient populations, and has studied and written about the use of music in the NICU, operating room, and cardiac care. He founded Transitions Music in the late 1980's and developed music for babies incorporating womb sounds as well as music and guided visualization for adult sleep, relaxation, and surgery. Dr. Schwartz is treasurer and a founding member of the IAMM (International Association for Music in Medicine). He is an active member of SAMA (Sound and Music Healers Association), American Music Therapy Association (AMTA), MHTP (The Music for Healing and Transition Program), and ISMM (International Society of Music Medicine). His interests include finding bridges between various professional groups who use music for healing. He has used music with hospital patient for over 30 years. Interests include music and NICU, operating room, Labor & Delivery, and the cardiac patient. He has produced the *Transitions* womb sound music series and was the medical spokesman for Governor Zell Miller in bringing music to babies in Georgia.

Ralph Spingte MD is currently Director of the Dept of Algesiology & Interdisciplinary Painmedicine, Regional Pain Centre DGS at Sportklinik Hellersen; Luedenscheid Germany.He is a Board Certified Anesthesiologist, Board Certified for Pain Medicine, and for Occupational Health. Lifetime Professor of MusicMedicine at University of Music and Drama, Hamburg; former Adjunct Professor at the Institute for Music Research, University of Texas at San Antonio, former Associate Editor International Journal of Arts Medicine MMB Saint Louis, Co-Editor-in-Chief of the Journal Music and Medicine SAGE Los Angeles, Co-Editor Journal for Music and Health/Musik und Gesundheit, Bremen. He got his German Approbation and Dr.med. from the Medical Faculty at the Rheinisch-Westfaelische Friedrich Wilhelms University Bonn in 1981.His doctoral dissertation deals with music as psychophysiological therapeutic against perioperative anxiety and stress. He has 30 years experience in clinical medicine (Anaesthesia, Intensive Care, Internal Medicine, Pain Medicine and Occupational Health Care). Spintge conducted a series of psychophysiological studies about the anxioalgolytic effects of music in Surgery, Anaesthesia, Pain Medicine, Obstetrics, and Dentistry during several stays abroad and in cooperation with scientists, medical doctors, music therapists and psychologists from the University of Hirosaki, Japan, the University of Vienna/Austria, the Erasmus University Rotterdam/The Netherlands, the University of Marburg/Germany, the Free University of Berlin/Germany, the University of Osnabrueck/Germany, the New South Wales State Conservatorium of Music Sydney/Australia, the University of Bonn/Germany. He was co-investigator within a 10-years collaborative research program about "Rhythmicity, HRV and The Neurovegetative Status in Man" with the German Max-Planck-Society, The Institute for Physiology at Free University of Berlin, The Institute for Synergetic Mathematics at University of Stuttgart and the National Research Centre Juelich, based on a grant from Sporthilfe e.V.. Spintge inaugurated the term MusicMedicine describing scientifically based clinical use of musical stimuli. His current area of research is focused upon the impact of musical stimuli on Heart Rate Variability in chronic pain, burn-out & fatigue, sleep disorders and sports, as well as the importance of music in human evolution including epigenetics. Spintge´s publications comprise numerous articles and 22 books about innovations in anesthesia, pain medicine and applications of medicofunctional music / MusicMedicine. He is founding member (1982) and President of the International Society for Music in Medicine ISMM Inc., member of the International.Association.for the Study of Pain IASP, German Association for Pain Medicine DGS, German Society for Medical Psychology, Honorary Member of the Music Therapy Association of Catalonia/Spain. He is lecturing within the Music Therapy Master course at the Institute for Music Therapy at University for Music and Drama Hamburg.

Angela Thompson MA, MT-BC is a music therapist specializing in the Neonatal Intensive Care Unit of The Louis Armstrong Center for Music and Medicine at Beth Israel Medical Center and St. Luke's Roosevelt Hospital, New York, NY. She is a graduate of Montclair State University where she received the David Ott Scholarship award for outstanding music therapist and holds a BA in vocal performance from West Virginia University. Angela was team member of the Heather on Earth multi-site NICU research study at Beth Israel since in its inception. Additionally, Angela piloted and instituted a music therapy program for homeless infants in Jersey City where she continues to practice today.

Iris Valentin BM, Music/Socialtherapist is a Music/Socialtherapist currently practicing Germany. Born in New York City, Iris moved to Berlin, Germany in 1967 where studying music and clarinet she received a degree in Music Education and Classical Clarinet Performance. After 25 years of teaching and concert engagements, she pursued postgraduate coursework in music and social therapy. Her subsequent work in a rehabilitation clinic in Saarland, Germany led to the opening of an out-patient medical office specializing in the treatment of tinnitus, oncology and psychosomatic patients. It was here that she developed her model of Audio Communication Therapy. Iris is a published writer and lecturer with several articles in music therapy journals. She has offered workshops and seminars in her model of Audio-Communication Therapy, and is a member of the German Musictherapst 'Association (DMtG) and International Society of Music and Medicine (ISMM).

Christine Vaskas MS, MT-BC received a M.S. in Music Therapy from Molloy College and a B.S. in Music from Long Island University. As both the 2012/13 Music Therapy Research Fellow for the Louis Armstrong Center for Music and Medicine at Beth Israel Medical Center and St. Luke's Roosevelt Hospital, and member of the Louis & Lucille Armstrong Music Therapy Team, she has contributed to research focusing on the effect of music therapy on the resiliency in adults undergoing infusion therapy, and in the study of Environmental Music Therapy in the Surgical Intensive Care Unit. Christine has clinical experience in pediatrics, oncology, the NICU, the BIMC HIV/AIDS clinic, and palliative care. At this writing, Christine is also completing training as a Child Life Specialist.

INDEX

A

Abandonment, 376, 412
Abdominal pain, 374
Abuse, 116
Acquired Immunodeficiency Syndrome (AIDS), 134, 373, 409
Acupuncture, 191
Acute Myeloid Leukemia (AML), 135
Acute pain, 29, 136, 182, 215, 260, 302, 335
Adrenaline, 22, 255
Advanced disease process, 405
Adverse psychological implications, 422
Aesthetic awareness, 291
Aesthetic creation, 384
Aesthetic experience(s), 85, 91, 284
Aesthetic sensibility, 390
Aesthetic(s), 287, 397, 455, 486
Affected voice, 219
Affective analgesia, 84
Agitation, 414, 437
Allodynic pain, 97
Alopecia, 422
Altruism, 377, 384
Amygdala, 84
Analgesics, 52, 85
Analgetics, 30
Analytical Music Therapy (AMT), 153, 158, 177
Ancient healing tradition(s), 473
Anesthesia, *Anesthesia*, 29, 115
Anesthetics, 30
Anger, 357, 368, 383, 422
Anorexia Nervosa (AN), 349, 360
Antidepressant(s), 98, 183, 184, 187, 303
Anxiety, 16, 44, 67, 79, 80, 97, 100, 134, 142, 181, 216, 217, 256, 266, 275, 277, 281, 283, 286, 299, 303, 312, 321, 378, 380, 386, 404, 407, 423, 433, 436, 437, 485, 492
Anxioalgolytic Music (AAM), 30
Anxiolytic(s), 183, 187, 303
Apnea, 405
Arthritic pain, 98
Asian culture(s), 465
Asian scale(s), 456
Assessment, 96, 99, 135, 146, 220, 312
Association(s), 196, 324
Attachment, 320
Attia Behavioral Pain Scale, 313
Attunement, 193, 194, 199, 200, 205
Audiating, 82
Audio-Communication, 254, 255, 258
Auditory focal point, 48
Autonomic balance, 305
Autonomic Nervous System (ANS), 255, 259, 284, 297
Autonomy, 51, 134, 137, 501
Awareness, 222, 261, 265, 389

B

Basal stress level, 297
Beauty, 80, 85, 238, 384, 394, 397
Behavioral pain reaction, 311
Beneficence, 51, 52
Beta blocker drug(s), 298
Betrayal, 376
Biocultural Model of Pain, 53
Biopsychosocial-spiritual aspect(s), 136
Blood draws, 310
Body aches, 386
Body awareness, 254, 275
Body dissatisfaction, 353
Body-image, 480
Body-mind resonance, 100
Bonding, 319
Bonny Method of Guided Imagery and Music (BMGIM), 53, 184, 348, 352, 480
Borderline personality, 360
Bossa nova, 436
Brain Derived Neurotrophic Factor (BDNF), 14
Brain tumor, 407
Breast cancer, 271, 425, 428, 429, 433, 437
Breath, 145, 215, 222, 223, 323
Breath work, 137, 139, 394, 396, 492
Breathing, 226, 386
Brief Pain Inventory, 15
Bulimia Nervosa (BN), 349, 364

C

Call-response, 481
Cancer, 44, 80, 87, 134, 136, 138, 144, 196, 266, 403, 422, 479
Cardiac illness, 47
Cardiac Surgical Intensive Care Unit (CSICU), 278
Caregiver(s), 287, 422, 433

Cathartic release, 435
Central hypersensitivity syndrome, 13
Central Nervous System (CNS), 312, 406
Certification Board of Music Therapists (CBMT), 61
Chant(s), 475, 492
Chemotherapy, 267, 277
Childbirth, 47
Chinese culture, 464
Chronic illness, 59, 134, 238
Chronic Obstructive Pulmonary Disease (COPD), 487
Chronic pain, 11, 12, 19, 29, 55, 80, 105, 151, 181, 182, 183, 185, 189, 261, 298, 302, 305, 312, 340, 421
Chronic stress, 299
Classical Indian music, 474, 484
Classical Persian music, 474
Clinical intuition, 278, 462
Clinical voice, 219
Cognitive realm, 82
Collaborative music-making, 161
Color Analysis Scale (CAS), 280, 433
Communication skill(s), 264
Communicative musicality, 196, 197, 205
Community, 381
Complex grief, 195
Complimentary treatment, 183
Compulsive behavior(s), 349
Confidentiality, 377
Conflict resolving strategies, 264
Confusion, 422
Congested breathing, 405
Control, 267
Coping skill(s), 378
Cortisol, 22, 196, 301, 351
Countertransference, 54, 161, 166, 198, 199, 205
Creative expression, 394
Creativity, 80
CRIES Neonatal Pain Scale, 314
Crisis stabilization, 194
Cultural factor(s), 55, 424
Cultural identity, 423, 425
Cultural universality, 218
Culturally informed music therapy, 427
Culturally sensitive, 337
Culturally sensitive approach, 335
Culturally specific music therapy, 479

D

Deep breathing, 338, 492
Dementia, 413
Depression, 16, 136, 141, 181, 183, 300, 303, 320, 378, 386, 422, 423, 425, 454
Developmental approach, 316
Disclosure, 385
Disorganization, 195
Dissonance, 240
Distorted body image, 349
Distress, 254, 406, 410, 412
Drone, 481, 486, 487, 489, 493, 494
Drum & Bass, 142
Drumming, 137, 141, 338, 384, 387, 388, 393, 480
Dysfunctional thought(s), 349
Dysphagia, 395
Dyspnea, 134, 422

E

Eating Disorder Not Otherwise Specified (ED-NOS), 348, 349
Échelle Douleur Inconfort Nouveau-Né, Neonatal Pain and Discomfort Scale (EDIN), 314
Electronic grooves, 397
Electronic music, 142
Embodiment, 199, 339
Emotion avoidance, 350
Emotion(s), 195, 275, 285, 362, 384, 479
Emotional awareness, 254
Emotional connection, 456
Emotional content, 299
Emotional Detonisation Training (EDT), 32
Emotional discomfort, 350
Emotional distress, 194, 277, 357
Emotional dysregulation, 195, 350
Emotional pain, 145, 165, 194, 242, 378, 407, 410, 411, 413
Emotional realm, 83
Emotional regulation, 194, 200
Emotional release, 388
Emotional response(s), 98, 217, 285
Emotional state, 217, 238
Emotional stressor(s), 336
Emotional support, 30, 378, 488
Emotional trauma, 317
Emotional vitality, 258
Empathy, 86, 309, 464
Empowerment, 344, 394

Index

End of life, 48, 403, 422
Endocrine system, 406
Endogenous system of pain modulation, 315
Endorphin(s), 30, 255, 282, 315
Endotracheal tube suctioning, 310
Entrainment, 31, 48, 93, 96, 182, 217, 219, 299, 322, 326, 406, 413, 489
Environmental Music Therapy (EMT), 99, 105, 275, 279, 286, 291, 319, 451, 461
Ethical principles, 51
Eutectic Mixture of Lidocaine and Prilocaine (EMLA), 315
Existential crisis, 422
Expression of feelings, 407

F

Family dynamics, 394, 424
Family Systems Psychology, 136
Family-centered care, 133, 136, 315, 318, 337, 342
Fatigue, 181, 266, 386, 387, 422, 425, 454
Fear, 312
Fetal heart rhythms, 299
Fibromyalgia, 13
Fifth vital sign, 312
Fight or flight, 14, 265, 285, 320
Fixed gestalt, 124
Fragile environment(s), 291
Fragile population(s), 277, 325
Frustration, 386
Functional pain, 97

G

Gaiting, 85
Gastro-intestinal bowel irritation, 389
Gastrointestinal cancer, 430
Gate control theory, 137, 277, 281, 291, 406
General anesthesia, 301
Generalized anxiety disorder, 360, 364
Gestalt therapy, 116, 121, 122
Gestational age, 313
Grief, 367, 368
Group cohesion, 377, 384
Group dynamic(s), 254, 263
Group singing, 80
Guided imagery, 49, 198
Guided music meditation, 384, 387
Guilt, 376

H

Harmonics, 137
Harmonization, 259
Harmony, 384, 406
Headaches, 374
Healing vibration, 478
Health related quality of life (HRQOL), 336
Heart rate, 216, 286
Heart rhythm, 299
Heart variability (HRV), 297
Hepatitis, 374
High-risk behavior(s), 378
Holding environment, 487, 488
Holistic effect of music therapy, 272
Holistic pain management, 44
Hospice, 239, 398, 407
Human Immunodeficiency Virus (HIV), 134, 373, 409
Humanistic philosophy, 279
Humming, 145
Hyperalgesia, 302
Hyperalgesic pain, 97
Hypothalamus, 22

I

Identity, 195, 424
Imagery, 182, 185, 187, 189, 228, 324, 343, 355, 358, 368, 397, 406, 492
Improvisation, 80, 85, 142, 184, 338, 383, 387, 390, 406, 434, 476, 491
Improvisational music therapy, 149, 226, 380
Improvisational singing, 215, 218, 220, 222, 224, 228
Independence, 339
Individualized care, 421
Inflammation, 404
Inflammatory pain, 12, 98
Informed consent, 51
Instinctive sound(s), 218
Integrated music therapy approach, 405
Integrated treatment team, 403
Integration, 96
Integrative music therapy, 403
Intensive care unit (ICU), 277
Interdisciplinary, 63, 135
Interpersonal realm, 83
Interval(s), 489
Intervention(s), 337
Iso principle, 60, 217, 219, 223, 413
Isolation, 350, 376, 378, 381, 410, 422

J

Joy, 256

L

Legacy, 238
Leukemia, 490
Life review, 405
Listening, 49, 254, 405, 406, 464, 494
Live music, 241, 387, 399, 434
Live music making, 101
Loss, 362, 367, 374, 376, 436
Loss of control, 197, 501
Lower back pain, 98
Lullaby, 324, 379
Lyric analysis, 386, 407
Lyric discussion, 406
Lyric substitution, 384, 388

M

Major Depressive Disorder, 14, 360, 364, 482
Maladaptive pain, 97
Mantra, 432, 435, 485, 492, 493
Mastery, 379
Maternal heartbeat, 299
Maternal-fetal dialog, 299
Meaningful connection, 197
Medical fragility, 309, 311
Medical Intensive Care Unit (MICU), 277, 398
Medical music psychotherapy, 99, 156
Medical music psychotherapy assessment, 101
Medical music therapy, 62, 157, 237, 486
Medical rehabilitation, 149
Medical trauma, 149, 162, 177
Medical-psychosocial integration, 96
Medicofunctional music, 30, 33
Meditation, 479
Meditative state, 487, 491
Melody, 406, 475, 479
Memories, 362, 405, 432
Metabolic abnormalities, 351
Methadone, 382, 385
Migraine headaches, 98
Milieu therapy, 194
Mind-body, 17, 367, 453
Mindfulness, 127, 338
Mini Mental Status Exam, 85
Mis-attunement, 198
Mood, 136, 194, 217, 286, 406, 422
Mortality, 311

Mother's voice, 299
Multicultural approach(es), 473
Multicultural perspective(s), 439
Multidisciplinary, 239, 353
Multi-individual process, 287
Multi-modal therapy, 253, 254
Muscle relaxant(s), 183
Muscle tenseness, 258
Music as medicine, 21, 22, 215, 219
Music as therapy/in therapy, 474
Music child, 216
Music elicited fantasy, 406
Music engagement, 85
Music improvisation(s), 82, 159, 432
Music listening, 89, 182
Music medicine, 245, 260, 272
Music psychotherapy, 20, 21, 100, 151, 152, 232, 278, 279, 367, 436, 464
Music sedation, 102, 103, 109
Music therapy, 21, 52, 59, 87, 96, 137, 140, 144, 155, 216, 254, 260, 261, 262, 287, 299, 315, 327, 344, 375, 389, 404, 423, 427, 473, 478, 494
Music therapy assessment, 133, 429, 434
Music therapy entrainment, 53, 55
Music therapy improvisation, 79, 80, 85
Music therapy pain assessment, 96
Musical idioms, 324
Musical visualization, 96
Musicality, 216
Music-assisted imagery, 45
Music-assisted relaxation, 60, 184, 186, 338
Music-centered work, 215
Music-induced positive emotion, 88
Myelopathy, 374
Myofascial pain, 116

N

Natural singing voice, 220
Nausea, 266, 422
Negative emotion(s), 196
Neonatal Intensive Care Unit (NICU), 277, 299, 309
Neonatal morbidity, 311
Neural sensitization, 404
Neuroendocrine, 30
Neurohormonal mechanism(s), 299
Neuroimmune receptors, 30
Neurologic music therapy, 60
Neurological gaiting, 79, 93
Neurological pain, 216

Index

Neurological stimulation(s), 217
Neurology, 30
Neuromatrix theory, 277, 282, 291
Neuromodulators, 22
Neuropathic nerve disruption, 385
Neuropathic pain, 12, 13, 97, 98, 275, 374
Neurophysiological mechanism(s), 53
Neuroplasticity, 14, 152, 154, 155, 312
Neurotransmitter dysregulation, 14
Neurotransmitter(s), 13, 22, 404
Newborn Individualized Developmental Care and Assessment Program (NIDCAP), 317
Nociception, 120, 283
Nociceptive, 275
Nociceptive pain, 12, 97
Non-compliance, 338
Non-inflammatory/non-neuropathic pain, 13, 97, 98
Nonmaleficence, 51, 52
Non-malignant chronic pain, 182
Non-medical intervention(s), 403
Non-nutritive suck, 326
Non-pharmacologic therapies, 375
Non-Small Cell Lung Cancer (NSCLC), 393
Non-steroidal anti-inflammatory drug(s), 336
Nordoff-Robbins, 215, 216
Norepinephrine, 13, 22, 196

O
Obsessive thought(s), 349
Obsessive-compulsive disorder, 360
Oligoanalgesia, 53
Oncology, 254, 277
Opiate(s), 19
Opioid tolerance, 55
Opioid(s), 85, 299, 336
Opportunistic bacterial infection(s), 375
Orthopedic surgery, 134
Ovarian cancer, 412
Oxytocin, 196

P
Pain, 80, 303, 310, 423, 433
Pain assessment, 99, 312
Pain control, 404, 406, 411
Pain episode(s), 336
Pain intensity, 302

Pain management, 74, 219, 275, 378, 403, 415, 473, 474, 478, 482, 485, 494
Pain medicine, 29, 30, 33
Pain memory, 256, 261
Pain pattern, 115
Pain perception, 53, 183, 189, 217, 222, 253, 256, 261, 275, 276, 406
Pain response, 310, 404
Pain scale, 313
Pain score(s), 66
Pain signaling, 14
Pain stimulus, 310
Pain threshold, 30
Pain tolerance, 30
Painful procedure(s), 311
Pain-relieving experience(s), 256
Palliative, 30, 33, 136, 245, 260, 398
Pancreatitis, 374
Panic, 422
Parasympathetic Nervous System(s) (PNS), 297, 406
Pathophysiology, 97, 298
Patient outcomes, 63
Patient satisfaction score(s), 67, 74
Pediatric Intensive Care Unit (PICU), 277
Peer support, 377
Pentatonic, 455, 456
Perception of noise, 280
Perfectionism, 353, 355
Performance, 339
Perinatal stress, 298
Peripheral Nervous System (PNS), 406
Peripheral neuropathy, 422
Persistent pain, 84
Personality disorders, 194
Physical complication(s), 351
Physical pain, 150, 165, 182, 191, 239, 384, 393, 410, 412
Physical trauma, 149
Physiologic Consequences of Perioperative Stress, 300
Physiologic pathology, 297
Physiologic trauma, 318
Physiological distress, 351
Physiological pain, 226
Physiological realm, 83
Physiological response(s), 133
Pleuritus, 374
Pneumonia, 374
Polyvagal theory, 284, 291, 320

517

Poor body image, 349
Positive physician-patient relationship, 266
Positive thinking, 338
Post Traumatic Stress Disorder (PTSD), 360, 390
Postpartum depression, 299
Post-surgical pain, 228
Post-surgical stress, 136
Preferred music, 194, 195, 200, 338
Premature Infant Pain Profile (PIPP), 313
Preoperative music, 301
Pre-term infants, 310
Preventive Approach to Traumatic Experience by Resourcing the Nervous System (PATTERNS), 316
Preverbal trauma, 199
Procedural support, 108, 379, 437
Progressive muscle relaxation, 260
Progressive relaxation, 223, 224, 232
Projective identifications, 198
Psoriatic arthritis, 374
Psychoacoustic variable(s), 286
Psychoactive treatment(s), 20
Psychodrama, 254
Psychoeducation, 137, 377
Psychoemotional aspect(s), 133
Psychoemotional goal(s), 398
Psychogenic pain, 150, 151
Psychological distress, 350, 351
Psychological pain, 116, 150, 155
Psychological stress, 160, 351, 422
Psychoneuroimmunology, 254, 259
Psychopathology, 20, 84, 200
Psychopharmacology, 20
Psychosis, 195
Psychosocial assessment, 17, 18, 20, 138, 411
Psychosocial stress, 181, 341, 406
Psychosocial support, 376
Psychosocio-cultural components, 259
Psychotherapeutic support, 374
Psychotherapy, 20, 118, 133

Q
Quality of life, 80, 336, 398, 403, 424

R
Racial stereotyping, 336
Radiation oncology, 452
Radiation therapy, 277, 289, 407
Rāga music, 480
Randomized controlled trial(s), 31, 47, 82

Receptive music therapy, 228, 261, 262
Receptive-regulative music therapy, 253
Reconciliation, 197
Reconstitution, 108, 316, 322, 323
Recorded music, 67, 96
Recording, 239, 244, 251, 339, 340
Referred pain, 119
Reflection, 80, 86, 88
Refocusing, 53
Regional anesthesia, 299
Regulative music therapy, 261, 262
Rehabilitation, 265
Reiter's syndrome, 374
Relaxation, 47, 215, 220, 224, 226, 231, 253, 254, 256, 261, 267, 270, 287, 319, 383, 384, 389, 404, 406, 432, 436, 437, 438, 439, 475, 492
Release, 96, 133, 404
Religion, 424
Reminiscence, 405
Remo ocean drum, 323, 396, 428, 431, 434, 438
Repressed grief, 256
Repression, 268
Repressive behavior, 261
Resilience, 137, 141, 339, 341, 344, 398
Resonance, 205, 219, 222, 223
Respiratory distress, 395, 397
Respiratory rate, 216
Rhythmic pattern, 479
Rhythm(s), 137, 205, 217, 218, 258, 384, 406, 475, 479
Rorschach, 194, 204

S
Sacred chakra vowel(s), 485
Sadness, 357, 368
Saudade, 436, 437
Schizophrenia, 194, 196, 201, 203, 364, 385
Secondary gains, 337
Sedation, 97, 102, 226, 323
Self-acceptance, 271
Self-advocacy, 397
Self-affirmation, 271
Self-awareness, 254, 268, 291
Self-depreciation, 350
Self-determination, 266, 269
Self-directed neuroplasticity, 154, 155
Self-esteem, 144, 261, 265, 271, 349, 379, 384, 397
Self-expression, 339, 383, 384

Index

Self-perception, 263
Self-reflection, 254, 266
Self-regulation, 265, 312, 322, 323, 327
Self-selected music, 199
Self-understanding, 270
Sense of control, 134, 339, 380, 407
Sense of self, 195
Sensory experience, 312
Serotonin, 13
Shame, 348, 349, 351, 357, 368
Sharing music, 196
Sickle cell anemia, 90, 91, 98
Sickle Cell Disease (SCD), 335
Singing, 49, 105, 182, 216, 323, 327, 390, 392, 405, 414, 429, 474, 485, 491
Sleep disturbances, 422
Social engagement, 327
Social therapy, 254
Social withdrawal, 350
Socioeconomic status, 336
Somatic complaint(s), 182
Somatic pain, 374
Somatic responses, 217
Song choice, 390
Song of kin, 103, 241, 324, 325, 326, 379
Song sensitation, 195, 383, 386
Songwriting, 80, 105, 184, 338, 340, 381, 384, 390, 406
Sound environment, 465
Sound healing, 484
Sound vibration(s), 487
Soundbath, 398
Soundscape, 452
Speech prosody, 224
Spinal fusion surgery, 227
Spine surgery, 45
Spiritual distress, 407, 409, 410, 412
Spiritual needs, 427
Spiritual pain, 150, 151, 408
Spiritual realm, 83
Spirituality, 55, 424, 425, 430
Spontaneous expressions of emotions, 218
State, 275
State anxiety, 29, 280, 284, 289, 479
State of trauma, 320
State-Trait Anxiety Inventory Scale, 45
Static emotions, 476
Stigmatization, 376
Story song, 437, 438
Strength, 399
Stress, 44, 134, 142, 196, 217, 261, 297, 302, 310, 321, 327, 336, 349, 404, 406, 423, 485
Stress hormone(s), 258, 311
Stress management, 59
Stress regulation, 24
Stress response, 22, 60, 300, 301, 305, 312, 323
Stress-Relaxation, 32
Substance abuse, 378, 385
Substance related issues, 194
Surgical Intensive Care Unit (SICU), 277
Sympathetic Nervous System (SNS), 115, 297, 298
Symptom management, 398
Synerdisciplinary team approach, 404

T

Tachycardia, 312
Tactile perception, 260
Tape removal, 310
Tempo, 137, 217, 218, 258, 406
Tension, 137, 422
Tension release, 137, 139, 145, 288, 396, 436, 490, 493
Therapeutic alliance, 137, 143, 145, 394
Therapeutic change, 219
Therapeutic communication, 220
Therapeutic goal, 53
Therapeutic presence, 390
Therapeutic process, 199, 200, 356, 406
Therapeutic rapport, 195, 343
Therapeutic refocusing, 22
Therapeutic relationship, 21, 190, 219, 270, 323, 391, 392, 397, 399, 411, 424, 432, 486
Therapeutic soundscape, 466
Therapeutic voice work, 338
Timbre, 220, 221, 222, 489
Tinnitus, 253
Tinnitus retraining therapy, 264
Tonal intervallic synthesis, 96, 143
Toning, 96, 182, 221, 223, 323, 327, 341
Trance, 142
Transcendence, 80
Transference, 198, 261
Transformation, 190
Transition, 436, 438
Transitional object(s), 324, 343
Transitional support, 319
Trauma, 116, 155, 316, 321, 353, 358, 378, 423, 438

Trauma-informed approach, 317
Traumatic crisis, 196
Traumatic event(s), 480
Traumatic experience(s), 363
Traumatic mechanism(s), 134
Traumatic response(s), 135, 144
Treatment efficacy, 95
Treatment plan, 136
Trigger points, 116
Trust, 377

U

Uncertainty, 380
Unity of mood, 475
Universality, 377
Unresolved emotions, 190

V

Vagus nerve, 298
Vaso-occlusive crises (VOC's), 336
Venipuncture, 310
Verbal reflection, 79
Vibration(s), 141, 217, 218, 219, 223, 341

Vibratory resonance, 221
Victimization, 116
Viral infection(s), 374
Visceral pain, 374
Visual Analog Scale (VAS), 15, 280, 431, 492
Visualization, 120, 137, 228, 263, 384, 394, 396, 430
Vitality, 399
Vocal improvisation, 217, 220, 481
Vocal intonation, 284
Vocal melodic phrase(s), 437
Vocal music therapy, 215, 219, 225
Vocal prosody, 145
Voice disorder(s), 221
Volume, 137

W

Wholistic healing, 182
Wong-Baker Faces Scale, 430, 433
World music traditions, 474

Y

Yin and Yang, 297